CHILD AND ADOLESCENT PSYCHIATRY FOR THE SPECIALTY BOARD REVIEW

This new, thoroughly revised fifth edition of *Child and Adolescent Psychiatry for the Specialty Board Review* offers a comprehensive study guide of child psychiatry.

New authors incorporate the latest evidence-based content while still offering the questions and detailed answers format of previous editions. Part I includes chapters covering normal development, diagnostic categories, treatments, and special issues, whilst Part II includes new case problems that test knowledge of assessment and treatment planning. This book includes hundreds of multiple-choice questions, modelled on board examination questions, and includes references from leading textbooks, providing a comprehensive review of the field.

Both general and child/adolescent psychiatrists will find this fifth edition essential, not only as a guide for preparing for their first successful board examination but also as a review in preparing for important recertification exams.

Caitlin R. Costello, MD, is an Associate Clinical Professor in the Department of Psychiatry and Behavioral Sciences, Division of Child and Adolescent Psychiatry, at the University of California, San Francisco, USA. She is the training director of the child and adolescent psychiatry fellowship program and the medical director of child and adolescent outpatient services at Langley Porter Psychiatric Hospital and Clinics. Her interests include medical education, curriculum development, obsessive-compulsive and tic disorders, the interface between psychiatry and the legal system, and juvenile justice.

Lauren T. Schumacher, MD, is an Assistant Clinical Professor in the Department of Psychiatry and Behavioral Sciences, Division of Child and Adolescent Psychiatry, at the University of California, San Francisco, USA. She specializes in child and adolescent psychiatry with a particular interest in attention-deficit/hyperactivity disorder (ADHD) and anxiety disorders. She has presented at national conferences and is the author of multiple book chapters on pharmacological treatment of ADHD. She is also active in child and adolescent psychiatry fellowship training and medical student education.

CHILD AND ADOLESCENT PSYCHIATRY FOR THE SPECIALTY BOARD REVIEW

Fifth Edition

Caitlin R. Costello and
Lauren T. Schumacher

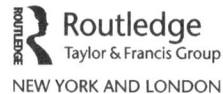

Routledge
Taylor & Francis Group

NEW YORK AND LONDON

Designed cover image: Nayanba Jadeja © Getty Images

Fifth edition published 2024
by Routledge
605 Third Avenue, New York, NY 10158

and by Routledge
4 Park Square, Milton Park, Abingdon, Oxon, OX14 4RN

Routledge is an imprint of the Taylor & Francis Group, an informa business

Fourth edition published by Routledge 2015

Library of Congress Cataloging-in-Publication Data
Names: Costello, Caitlin R., author. | Schumacher, Lauren T., author.
Title: Child and adolescent psychiatry for the specialty board review / Caitlin R. Costello and Lauren T. Schumacher.
Description: Fifth edition. | New York, NY : Routledge, 2024. | Revised edition: by Hong Shen and Robert L. Hendren. Fourth edition. 2015. | Includes bibliographical references.
Identifiers: LCCN 2023027361 (print) | LCCN 2023027362 (ebook) | ISBN 9781032307831 (paperback) | ISBN 9781032312576 (hardback) | ISBN 9781003308805 (ebook)

ISBN: 978-1-032-31257-6 (hbk)
ISBN: 978-1-032-30783-1 (pbk)
ISBN: 978-1-003-30880-5 (ebk)

DOI: 10.4324/9781003308805

Typeset in Times
by Apex CoVantage, LLC

CONTENTS

Part I: Multiple-Choice Questions

Part II: Clinical Cases

ACKNOWLEDGMENTS

We would like to thank Robert Hendren, DO, and Hong Shen, MD, for all their hard work in writing the prior editions of *Child and Adolescent Psychiatry for the Specialty Board Review* upon which this book was built.

INTRODUCTION

Child and Adolescent Psychiatry for the Specialty Board Review is a study guide for the child and adolescent specialty board review and has been highly regarded and popular since the first edition was published more than 25 years ago. Eight years have passed since the fourth edition was published by Robert Hendren, DO, and Hong Shen, MD. Tremendous advances and changes in the field of child and adolescent psychiatry have occurred in the past few years. The principal textbooks referenced in the fourth edition have new editions. This fifth edition, written by new authors Caitlin Costello, MD, and Lauren Schumacher, MD, is carefully revised, offering updated information, along with the most recent references and knowledge reflected in those changes.

Not only will general and child/adolescent psychiatrists, residents, medical students, and other professionals find this new edition invaluable as a study guide in preparing for board examinations, recertification examinations, PRITE exams, and the medical students' clerkship shelf exams, but it will also serve as an excellent review of the latest knowledge in the field for those wishing for an up-to-date review. This revision updates references and many of the questions are brand-new, which will help readers review and learn new information and be better prepared for their examinations and their practice. This edition features problem-based clinical cases similar to the board examinations' linked-item set questions which highlight the material's relevance to clinical treatment.

REFERENCES

Note: With dramatic advances continually being made in the clinical sciences, it is a challenge for physicians to keep abreast both of the modifications in treatment that such advances require and of the new drugs being introduced each year. The authors and publisher of this volume have taken care to make certain that the doses of drugs and schedules of treatment are correct and compatible with standards generally accepted at the time of publication. However, it is essential for the reader to become fully cognizant of the information on the instruction inserts provided with each drug or therapeutic agent prior to administration or prescription.

Further, as some of the topics are by nature ambiguous, it is suggested that the reader consult the indicated reference sources for clarification should there be a discrepancy between the answer selected and that which appears in the book.

Each question, answer, and explanation can be found in one or more of the basic books on child and adolescent psychiatry, reference books, and published journal articles listed here or in the answers to the questions. The references are cited by number and the appropriate section following each answer in the text.

1 Dulcan, M. K., & American Psychiatric Association (Eds.). (2022). *Dulcan's textbook of child and adolescent psychiatry* (3rd edition). American Psychiatric Association Publishing.
2 Dulcan, M. K., Ballard, R. R., Jha, P., & Sadhu, J. M. (2018). *Concise guide to child and adolescent psychiatry* (5th edition). American Psychiatric Association Publishing.
3 Martin, A., Volkmar, F. R., & Bloch, M. (Eds.). (2018). *Lewis's child and adolescent psychiatry: A comprehensive textbook* (Fifth edition). Wolters Kluwer.
4 American Psychiatric Association (Eds.). (2013). *Diagnostic and statistical manual of mental disorders: DSM-5* (5th edition). American Psychiatric Association.

5 Sadock, B. J., Sadock, V. A., & Ruiz, P. (Eds.). (2017). *Kaplan & Sadock's comprehensive textbook of psychiatry* (10th edition). Wolters Kluwer.

6 Boland, R. J., Verduin, M. L., Ruiz, P., Shah, A., & Sadock, B. J. (Eds.). (2022). *Kaplan & Sadock's synopsis of psychiatry* (12th edition). Wolters Kluwer.

PART I
MULTIPLE-CHOICE QUESTIONS

1

NORMAL GROWTH AND DEVELOPMENT

DOI: 10.4324/9781003308805-2

QUESTIONS

Directions: Select the best response for each of the questions 1–70.

1 What percentage of genes in humans is responsible for regulating the growth and development of the central nervous system (CNS)?

 a About 5%

 b About 10%

 c At least one-third

 d At least 50%

 e At least 75%

2 All of the following statements regarding migration of neurons are correct *except*:

 a During corticogenesis the newly formed glutamatergic projection neurons migrate along with radial glial cells guides.

 b Migration of neurons starts during late-stage embryonic development of the nervous system.

 c Some cytoskeletal proteins, molecular motor, and adhesion molecules are needed for the process.

 d Decreased expression of certain microtubule-binding protein can interfere with the migration process.

 e Abnormal distribution of GABAergic neurons could be underlying the pathogenesis of certain psychiatric conditions.

3 Which of the following neurotransmitters can impact coordinating the modulation of the entire neocortex and regulate theta rhythms on EEG?

 a Dopamine

 b Serotonin

 c Norepinephrine and epinephrine

 d Histamine

 e Acetylcholine

4 Which of the following neurotransmitters inhibits prolactin release?

 a Dopamine

 b Serotonin

 c Norepinephrine and epinephrine

 d Histamine

 e Acetylcholine

5 Which of the following neurotransmitters is responsible for the regulation of arousal state, vigilance, and stress response?

 a Dopamine

 b Serotonin

 c Norepinephrine and epinephrine

 d Histamine

 e Acetylcholine

6 Which of the following neurotransmitters is responsible for the regulation of autonomic and neuroendocrine processes?

 a Dopamine

 b Serotonin

 c Norepinephrine and epinephrine

 d Histamine

 e Acetylcholine

7 Which of the following neurotransmitters may be implicated in Alzheimer's disease and rapid eye movement (REM) sleep?

 a Dopamine

 b Serotonin

 c Norepinephrine and epinephrine

 d Histamine

 e Acetylcholine

8 By the age of 3 years, most children can perform all of the following tasks *except*:

 a Riding a tricycle

 b Copying a square

 c Copying a circle and a cross

 d Building a tower of 9 to 10 cubes

 e Feeding self well and putting on shoes

9 Piaget postulated four stages of cognitive development. Which one of the following sequences of development describes the stages given by Piaget?

 a Concrete operational → sensorimotor → preoperational → formal operational

 b Preoperational → sensorimotor → concrete operational → formal operational

 c Sensorimotor → preoperational → formal operational → concrete operational

 d Sensorimotor → preoperational → concrete operational → formal operational

 e Sensorimotor → concrete operational → preoperational → formal operational

10 Lawrence Kohlberg described three major levels of moral development: (I) preconventional morality, (II) morality of conventional role conformity, and (III) morality of self-accepted moral principles. He proposed two types/stages in each level, going from type 1/stage 1 as the lowest to type 6/stage 6 as the highest. His theory integrated the concepts of development of which of the following theorists?

 a Jean Piaget

 b Carol Gilligan

 c Harry Harlow

d John Bowlby

e Mary Ainsworth

11 Margaret Mahler described an attachment theory based on psychoanalytic theory including a complex sequence that infants gradually develop step by step. Which one of the following sequences describes the corresponding stages of "separation-individuation" proposed by Mahler?

a Symbiosis → normal autism → differentiation → practicing → reapproachment → object constancy (individuation)

b Differentiation → reapproachment → symbiosis → practicing → normal autism → object constancy (individuation)

c Practicing → differentiation → symbiosis → normal autism → reapproachment → object constancy (individuation)

d Normal autism → differentiation → reapproachment → symbiosis → practicing → object constancy (individuation)

e Normal autism → symbiosis → differentiation → practicing → reapproachment → object constancy (individuation)

12 Fetus brains and brains of toddlers have a larger number of neurons and synaptic connections than brains of adults. What term is used to describe the process by which the overproduction of synapses is reduced?

a Extermination

b Pruning

c Excitotoxicity

d Enucleation

e Trimming

13 Based on the "temperament theory" developed by Stella Chess and Alexander Thomas, all of the following are behavioral dimensions of young children *except*:

a Activity level

b Adaptability

c Intensity

d Mood lability

e Rhythmicity

14 Based on neuroanatomical distribution, all of the following neurotransmitter systems originated from small groups of densely packed neurons that project to their target areas using long-ranged projection fibers *except*:

a Glutamatergic system

b Serotonergic system

c Dopaminergic system

d Noradrenergic system

e Cholinergic system

15 Which of the following serotonin receptors is coupled to an ion channel?

a 5-HT_1

b 5-HT_2

c 5-HT_3

d 5-HT_4

e 5-HT_5

16 Operant conditioning is *best* described by which one of the following phrases?

a Behaviors that are strengthened or weakened as a function of the events that follow them

b Presentation or removal of an event after a response that increases the frequency of the response

c Removing the presence of a reinforcing event after a response that decreases the frequency of the previously reinforced response

d Certain stimuli coming to elicit reflex response

e Reinforcement of the gradual approximation of a desired behavior

17 All of the following are true regarding Baumrind's parenting styles *except*:

a Children with authoritative parents tend to do well academically and socially.

b Authoritarian parents have high expectations and high responsivity.

c Parents with low responsivity and low demandingness are categorized as neglectful.

d Authoritarian style may be associated with a positive outcome in some minority families.

e Parents with a permissive style are highly responsive to their children's needs and have few expectations.

18 Based on cognitive behavioral theory, Spivak and Shure proposed five problem-solving steps that children can be taught. All of the following are those steps *except*:

a Problem identification, definition, and formulation

b Negative thought elimination

c Choosing a new strategy

d Implementing the new strategy

e Evaluating the new strategy

19 At which of the following age ranges do children start to show an understanding of object permanence?

a Age of 0–2 months

b Age of 2–7 months

c Age of 7–18 months

d Age of 18–36 months

e Age of 36–48 months

20 There are many forces that may interfere with normal developments of infants and toddlers, such as regulatory disturbances. The followings are all such regulatory disturbances *except*:

a Sleep disturbances

b Excessive crying or irritability

c Eating difficulties

d Low frustration tolerance

e Prolonged separation from caregivers

21 Mary Ainsworth developed a research instrument known as the Strange Situation procedure to assess the security of attachment in infancy. All of the following statements are accurate *except*:

a Attachment can be defined as secure and insecure.

b Within insecure attachment, there are three types: avoidant/dismissive, resistant/anxious-ambivalent, and disorganized/disorientated.

c Securely attached infants tend to be more resilient, self-reliant, emphatic, and confident in developing adult relationships.

d Resistant or anxious-ambivalent infants tend to develop an adult pattern of aloofness and detachment.

e Disorganized-disorientated infants may be associated with an unresolved and disorganized pattern in adults.

22 What is the correct order of Erikson's eight stages of the life cycle?

a Trust vs. mistrust, autonomy vs. shame and doubt, initiative vs. guilt, industry vs. inferiority, identity vs. role confusion, intimacy vs. isolation, integrity vs. despair, generativity vs. stagnation

b Trust vs. mistrust, autonomy vs. shame and doubt, industry vs. inferiority, initiative vs. guilt, identity vs. role confusion, intimacy vs. isolation, generativity vs. stagnation, integrity vs. despair

c Trust vs. mistrust, autonomy vs. shame and doubt, initiative vs. guilt, industry vs. inferiority, identity vs. role confusion, intimacy vs. isolation, generativity vs. stagnation, integrity vs. despair

d Trust vs. mistrust, initiative vs. guilt, autonomy vs. shame and doubt, industry vs. inferiority, identity vs. role confusion, intimacy vs. isolation, generativity vs. stagnation, integrity vs. despair

e Trust vs. mistrust, autonomy vs. shame and doubt, initiative vs. guilt, industry vs. inferiority, intimacy vs. isolation, identity vs. role confusion, generativity vs. stagnation, integrity vs. despair

23 Which one of the following enzymes is the rate-limiting enzyme responsible for the synthesis of serotonin?

a Tyrosine hydroxylase

b Tryptophan hydroxylase

c Monoamine oxidase (MAO)

d Catecholamine-O-methyltransferase (COMT)

e Dopamine hydroxylase

24 Which of the following is the metabolite of serotonin?

a Vanillylmandelic acid (VMA)

b Homovanillic acid (HVA)

c 3-methoxy-4-hydroxyphenylglycol (MHPG)

d 5-hydroxindoleacetic acid (HIAA)

e 3,4-dihydrophenylacetic acid (DOPAC)

25 Which of the following neurotransmission systems is crucial for inhibiting excitatory neurons?

a Cholinergic neurotransmission

b GABAergic neurotransmission

c Noradrenergic neurotransmission

d Cholinergic neurotransmission

e Glutamatergic neurotransmission

26 Which of the following neurotransmission systems is crucial for forming of memory?

a Cholinergic neurotransmission

b GABAergic neurotransmission

c Noradrenergic neurotransmission

d Dopaminergic neurotransmission

e Glutamatergic neurotransmission

27 Which of the following ages represents the time when children first begin to be involved with pretend play?

a 2 years

b 4 years

c 6 years

d 8 years

e 10 years

28 By which of the following ages do *most* children develop a stable gender identity?

a 12–18 months

b 3 years

c 5 years

d 7 years

e 9 years

29 Which of the following neuroimaging methods requires the administration of radioactive tracers?

a Magnetic resonance imaging (MRI)

b Magnetic resonance spectroscopy (MRS)

c Computer tomography (CT)

d Single photon emission computed tomography (SPECT)

e Magnetoencephalography

30 Diffusion tensor imagining (DTI) utilizes which of the following neuroimaging methods?

a Magnetic resonance imaging (MRI)

b Magnetic resonance spectroscopy (MRS)

c Computer tomography (CT)

d Single photon emission computed tomography (SPECT)

e Magnetoencephalography (MEG)

31 All of the following statements about magnetic resonance spectroscopy (MRS) are correct *except*:

a In contrast to MRI, MRS provides biochemical information of the subject in the form of a spectrum.

b ^{31}P MRS is the most sensitive technique.

c Using spatial encoding and localization, MRS is able to acquire not only a spectrum of a single voxel but also spectra of 2-D matrix and 3-D multiple voxels.

d MRS can measure the concentrations and distributions of metabolites within the brain, such as N-acetyl aspartate (NAA), total creatine (tCr), and total choline (tCh).

e Reduction of NAA and tCh are found in adolescents with bipolar disorder.

32 All of the following statements regarding electroencephalography (EEG) and magnetoencephalography (MEG) are correct *except*:

a EEG has superior ability to measure brain electrical activity more directly than those of PET and SPECT.

b EEG has poorer spatial resolution than PET, SPECT, and MEG.

c EEG is relatively inexpensive and becomes a more expansive procedure when combined with MRI.

d MEG has poorer temporal resolution than PET and SPECT.

e Neither EEG nor MEG can measure activity in subcortical structures.

33 All of the following are the stages of children's understanding of the concepts of death *except*:

a Irreversibility

b Finality (nonfunctionality)

c Causality

d Inevitability (universality)

e Acceptability

34 At what age do children acquire the concepts of irreversibility, nonfunctionality, and universality related to death?

a Years 2–3

b Years 3–5

c Years 5–7

d Years 7–9

e Years 9–11

35 During which of the following age ranges do children acquire the ability to understand conservation?

a The first year of life

b Years 1–2

c Years 2–7

d Years 7–11

e Years 11–end of adolescence

36 During which of the following age ranges do children develop the ability for symbolic thought?

a Birth to 5 months

b 5–9 months

c 9 months–1 year

d 1 year–18 months

e 18 months–2 years

37 During which of the following age ranges do children begin using hypotheticodeductive thinking?

a The first year of life

b Years 1–2

c Years 2–7

d Years 7–11

e Years 11–end of adolescence

38 All of the following statements regarding neurobiological changes in adolescence are correct *except*:

a Recent studies show dramatic neurobiological changes in the adolescent brain especially in regions of the forebrain and mesocortical and limbic systems.

b Massive pruning leads to the loss of about 50% of the cortical synaptic connections prior to puberty.

c Loss of inhibitory GABAergic inputs in the prefrontal cortex is prominent.

d A longitudinal MRI study of youth aged 7–19 years showed that intelligence was associated with the trajectory of cortical development.

e Executive functioning continues to improve throughout adolescence.

39 Which of the following developmental sequences correctly describes the process of puberty in girls?

a Menarche → pubic hair → breast development → height spurt

b Breast development → pubic hair → height spurt → menarche

c Breast development → height spurt → menarche → pubic hair

d Height spurt → breast development → pubic hair → menarche

e Menarche → height spurt → breast development → pubic hair

40 In general, studies of the effects of the timing of maturation suggest that early maturation is more advantageous in terms of popularity, self-esteem, and intellectual ability for:

a Boys

b Girls

c Both boys and girls

d Neither boys nor girls

e Unknown because no clear pattern has been identified

41 Which of the following descriptions correctly defines the concept of polymorphisms:

a One of the variant types of a gene at a particular locus on a particular chromosome

b A suspected gene that might be involved in a disease

c The location of a specific gene that is located on a chromosome

d A variable segment of DNA with known physical location, and its inheritance can be followed

e A common variation of DNA in the sequence that occurs ≥1% among individuals

42 All of the following statements of linkage analysis are correct *except*:

  a Linkage studies analyze the probability of a given phenotype being transmitted together from one generation to another.

  b Parametric and nonparametric linkage analyses are two basic approaches.

  c Linkage analysis is good for detecting common susceptibility variants of relatively small effect.

  d LOD score of 3 and above indicates a linkage to a marker (1000:1 odds in favor).

  e Parametric approach is powerful in investigating Mendelian disorders, while nonparametric approach is more robust in investigating disorders with no known clear mode of inheritance.

43 Fluorescence in situ hybridization (FISH) is primarily used in which type of the following genetic studies?

  a Study of patterns of inheritance and transmission

  b Linkage analysis

  c Genetic association

  d Molecular cytogenetics

  e Sequencing of human genome

44 All of the following statements regarding genomic microarray technology are accurate *except*:

  a Genetic polymorphisms can be arrayed on glass or nylon substrates/slides.

  b Numerous sequential reactions are needed to identify many genetic markers.

  c In genome-wide studies, it increases the efficiency and lowers the cost.

  d It can conduct genome-wide gene expression profiling.

  e Large sample sizes are required to obtain the needed level of significance.

45 Based on contemporary theories and studies, all of the following statements regarding the cultural impact on developmental stages are accurate *except*:

  a "Precocity baby phenomenon" occurs more commonly in Europeans and Americans.

  b Japanese and Chinese American infants are less excitable using rhythmicity and activity as measurements of their temperament.

  c While Japanese parents believe their children's academic achievement depends on effort, American parents believe in their children's innate ability.

  d To avoid cultural bias, *cultural-free tests* and *culture-fair tests* have been developed to evaluate children's IQ across cultures.

  e Girls in industrial countries have a tendency of reaching menarche earlier than girls in developing countries.

46 All of the following statements regarding the evaluation/assessment of development of infants and toddlers are correct *except*:

  a There is a characteristic developmental pattern for children with *failure to thrive*.

  b Social environmental disturbance can interfere with language and communication development.

  c Qualitative observation of children's interactions is important in evaluating children with seemingly appropriate developmental profiles.

  d Qualitative observation is also important in children with *scattered* developmental profiles across different domains.

  e Assessment of the development of young children should serve a role in facilitating referrals to appropriate educational or rehabilitative services and collaborations among providers.

47 From approximately which of the following ages have children achieved the development of a theory of mind?

  a Years 3–4

  b Years 4–5

  c Years 5–7

  d Years 7–9

  e Years 9–11

48 All of the following statements regarding children's play are correct *except*:

  a Pretend play requires children's ability to symbolize.

  b Children under age 3 are more likely to choose to play by themselves or be involved in parallel play.

  c Children 3 to 4 years old start engaging more with other children.

  d During therapeutic play with children, the therapist may join in with children's play, which can be more productive than interpreting the play.

  e It is easy to distinguish whether preschool children play with a normative imaginary friend by asking them if the friend is real or not.

49 All of the following statements regarding separation are accurate *except*:

  a With limited coping capacity, preschoolers face more difficulties in dealing with separation than older children.

  b Emerging symbolic capacity and capacity of object constancy help young children to cope with separation.

  c Continued contacts with a previous teacher or nanny make it harder for children to become familiar with a new teacher or nanny, and thus a clean break would be a better approach.

  d Separation is more difficult for children with parents who are separated or divorced.

  e Consistency, structure, and predictability are critical for visitations of young children with their parents who are divorced.

50 All of the following statements regarding aggression in children are correct *except*:

a As one of the most common reasons for child psychiatric consultation, aggression may reflect a balance between the child's reaction to frustration versus assertiveness and individuation.

b Aggression in children always expresses some of their needs and feelings.

c Younger children with few words may exhibit more physical aggression than their counterparts who are more verbal.

d By age 5 or 6, aggression tends to diminish.

e Preschoolers' aggression usually leads to aggression in grade school children.

51 Which of the following concepts did Piaget use to describe the preoperational child?

a Mastering the concept of conservation

b Abstract thinking

c Egocentrism

d Circular reactions

e Seriation and classification

52 Clinically, attachment theory is useful in all of the following circumstances *except*:

a Predicting the inevitable consequences/outcomes of early insecure attachment

b Understanding the nature of development of child psychopathology

c Understanding child abuse/neglect

d Understanding delinquency

e Treatment of mental illnesses in childhood

53 Temperament is viewed as individual differences in the reactivity and behavioral style that individuals utilize in different situations. Which of the following statements about temperament is *not entirely accurate*?

a Temperament is determined by three primary dimensions: activity level, adaptability, and sense of humor.

b Temperament can be categorized into three constellations: easy, difficult, and slow to warm up.

c *Goodness of fit* is used to describe the compatibility of traits between children and their parents.

d Genetic factors, as well as environmental factors, contribute to temperament.

e Certain alleles of a dopamine receptor gene DRD4 are associated with novelty-seeking temperamental traits.

54 All of the following statements regarding early adolescent development are correct *except*:

a Early adolescence starts around the ages of 12–14 years.

b Growth spurt occurs 1–2 years earlier in girls than in boys.

c Youngsters in this stage tend to show more interest in spending time with peers and to be more aware of appearance and style.

d At this stage, some youngsters experiment with tobacco, alcohol, and marijuana.

e Epidemiologic studies show that at this stage adolescents are characterized by overwhelmed alienation, profound angst, and significant disruptive family relationships.

55 All of the following statements regarding middle adolescent development are correct *except*:

a Middle adolescence roughly covers the ages of 14 to 16 years.

b A lot of adolescents in this stage have clear goals of being independent.

c Solid identity formation occurs.

d Boys are more prevalent in using cocaine than girls based on the Youth Risk Behavior Surveillance System (YRBSS-2005).

e Their drive for autonomy may create conflicts between them and their parents.

56 All of the following statements regarding late adolescence development are correct *except*:

a Late adolescence generally covers the ages of 17 to 19 years.

b Identity formation is gradually solidified with openness for refinement during young adulthood.

c Completion of high school and transition into college or job training often occurs.

d The use of tobacco, alcohol, and marijuana is lower than middle adolescence.

e Neuroimaging studies showed continued prefrontal cortex neural network development during this stage.

57 All of the following statements regarding adolescent pubertal development are correct *except*:

a A surge of gonadotropin-releasing hormone (GRH) from the hypothalamus starts puberty development.

b GRH stimulates pituitary glands to release gonadotropinluteinizing hormone (GLH) and follicle-stimulating hormone (FSH).

c GLH and FSH stimulate the secretions of a variety of androgens, testosterone, estradiol, and other peptides.

d Two additional hormones (thyroxin and prolactin) play pivotal roles in regulating growth hormone.

e The increase of both weight and height is a sign of puberty, which is often called growth spurt.

58 All of the following statements regarding adolescent sexual development are correct *except*:

a In boys, secondary sexual characteristics (increased length and width of penis) occur after a surge of androgens from enlarged testes.

b Tanner staging rates sexual maturity into five stages (1–5).

c Tanner staging uses genital maturity to rate boys and uses breast development to rate girls.

d   The primary sex characteristic in females is ovulation, or the release of eggs from ovaries.

e   The primary sex characteristic in males is development of facial hair.

59   At which of the Tanner stages does menarche usually occur?

a   Tanner stages 1–2

b   Tanner stages 2–3

c   Tanner stages 3–4

d   Tanner stages 4–5

e   After stage 5

60   According to Lawrence Kohlberg, morality can be divided into three levels: preconventional, conventional, and postconventional. Each level can be further divided into two stages (up to a total of six stages—also called types). If an adolescent has an ability to interpret moral dilemmas—that is, the concept of *extenuating circumstances* is understood—which level and stage of moral development has the adolescent reached?

a   Preconventional Level, stage 1

b   Preconventional Level, stage 2

c   Conventional Level, stage 3

d   Conventional Level, stage 4

e   Postconventional Level, stage 5

61   All of the following statements regarding adolescents' self-esteem are correct *except*:

a   The primary features of good adolescent self-esteem are related to their perceptions of positive physical appearance and high value to peers and family.

b   The secondary features of adolescent self-esteem are related to their academic achievement, athleticism, and other special talents.

c   Adolescents' self-esteem is mediated by external factors, such as feedback from peers and family.

d   A recent report indicated that younger adolescents (ages 13 to 17) have higher self-esteem than older adolescents (ages 18 to 22).

e   During adolescence, boys have a more significant drop in their self-esteem than do girls.

62   All of the following statements regarding adolescent brain development are correct *except*:

a   Abstract reasoning, planning, and affect modulations are the most dramatic changes of cognition in adolescents.

b   In the frontal cortex, increased myelinization of axons occurs during puberty, which increases transmission speed.

c   There is a linear increase in white matter in the frontal and parietal cortexes and a nonlinear decrease in gray matter density (synaptic pruning) in the frontal lobes.

d   Being responsible for mediating executive function, the prefrontal cortex matures more slowly than the other areas of the brain.

e   Functional MRI shows that boys have diminished activities in the amygdala when presented with fearful faces.

63   The dysfunction of the hypothalamic-pituitary-adrenal axis (HPA) neuroendocrine pathway may be related to the following psychiatric disorders/conditions *except*:

a   Major depressive disorder (MDD)

b   Posttraumatic stress disorder (PTSD)

c   Schizophrenia

d   Psychosocial short stature

e   Substance-related and additive disorders

64   Initiation of neurotransmission is accomplished by all of the following actions *except*:

a   Release of presynaptic neurotransmitter

b   Binding of the neurotransmitter to the presynaptic receptor

c   Binding of the neurotransmitter to the postsynaptic receptor

d   Activation of the postsynaptic receptor

e   Regulation of the second messengers

65   All of the following statements regarding the basal ganglia are correct *except*:

a   They modulate motor and some cognitive functions.

b   The basal ganglia include the caudate nucleus, putamen, globus pallidus, subthalamic nucleus, and substantia nigra.

c   Portions of the basal ganglia may be involved in the etiology of obsessive-compulsive disorder (OCD).

d   They may be involved in the etiology of attention-deficit/hyperactivity disorder (ADHD).

e   They can initiate particular movements.

66   All of the following statements regarding memory in children are correct *except*:

a   Children's lack of conscious memory of the first three years of their life is referred to as infantile amnesia.

b   Nondeclarative memory is not fully developed until age 3.

c   Infantile amnesia seems to be related to failure to adequately store memories.

d   Gradual development and differentiation of the neocortex limits the appearance of declarative memory during infancy.

e   Memory capacity increases with increased language ability.

67   All of the following statements regarding masturbation, genital self-stimulation, and sex play are correct *except*:

a   Genital self-stimulation is normal in babies and increases between the ages of 15 and 19 months.

b   Younger children may acquire playmates and show curiosity about their own and others' genitalia.

c   It is unusual for couples with steady relationships to masturbate.

d   Masturbation becomes pathological when it becomes a compulsion.

e   In early adolescence, teenagers may engage in sex play with partners both of the same sex and of the opposite sex.

68 Which of the following is *not* a phase of normal physiological responses to sexual stimulation?

a Desire

b Excitement

c Orgasm

d Resolution

e Desire aversion

69 All of the following statements regarding adolescent homosexuality are accurate based on the current state of our knowledge *except*:

a Homosexual play and contacts are most frequent in early adolescence, which does not necessarily lead to a homosexual orientation in adulthood.

b Following APA's suit, WHO finally removed homosexuality as a disease from ICD-10 in 1992.

c There are both genetic and environmental influences in homosexuality.

d Research data shows strong correlations between different levels of sex hormones among heterosexual and homosexual individuals.

e Homosexuality may be strongly influenced by the amount and time of certain prenatal hormonal exposure.

70 Which of the following statements regarding resilience is *incorrect*?

a There are two fundamental components of resilience: significant risk (or adversity) and positive adaptation.

b The authoritative parenting style is considered less optimal in fostering children's resilience.

c There is an important genetic influence on resilience.

d Community factors such as mentors and informal support groups, religious affiliations, and strong teacher–child relationship can positively influence resilience.

e Internal locus of control, feeling of self-efficacy, and high emotional intelligence are protective factors.

Matching

71–75 Match the following descriptions or examples to the corresponding frequently used terminology in the preschool period:

a Animism

b Attachment

c Egocentrism

d Parallel play

e Symbolic play

71 Children use play objects in representational ways, such as using a doll as a baby.

72 A child plays with a truck while another child is stacking up blocks, and they are both aware of each other.

73 The capacity of a child having an internal representation of the availability of their caregivers.

74 A child tells his mother that a rock needs to drink water just like his dog.

75 Lack of understanding of others' perspectives.

76–79 Match each term used by Freud to describe a developmental stage with one of the following corresponding descriptive terms used by Erikson:

a Identity

b Autonomy

c Basic trust

d Initiative

76 Oral

77 Anal

78 Phallic

79 Adolescence

80–86 Match each of the following hormones to one of the following corresponding regulating hormones:

a Corticotropin-releasing hormone

b Thyrotropin-releasing hormone

c Luteinizing-hormone-releasing hormone

d Gonadotropin-releasing hormone

e Somatostatin

f Growth-hormone-releasing hormone

g Progesterone, oxytocin

80 Adrenocorticotropic hormone

81 Prolactin

82 Growth hormone (stimulated)

83 Growth hormone (inhibited)

84 Follicle-stimulating hormone

85 Luteinizing hormone

86 Thyroid-stimulating hormone

87–92 For each of the named major figures in developmental psychiatry, choose from the following terms or descriptions the one that is *most* associated with his or her theory:

a Transitional object

b Attachment theory

c Assimilation, accommodation

d Developmental lines

e Reparation

f Goodness of fit

87 Bowlby

88 Piaget

89 Winnicott

90 Melanie Klein

91 Chess and Thomas

92 Anna Freud

93–108 Match each defense mechanism listed with the one of the following examples that *best* describes it:

a An adolescent "forgets" to tell her parents about a failing grade in school.

b   An adolescent who is angry with a teacher berates a sibling for no apparent reason.

c   An adolescent denies any feeling of abandonment or rejection by the noncustodial parent after a divorce.

d   An adolescent returns to childish and dependent behavior following a family move to a new city.

e   An adolescent mother resents the demands that caring for her child makes on her. However, she repeatedly tells herself and others how wonderful motherhood is. At times, she worries unnecessarily that some harm will come to her child.

f   An adolescent experiencing repeated trouble with the law claims that all of the problems are the fault of law enforcement officers, who have it in for him.

g   An adolescent with a terminal illness volunteers to work as a hospital aide.

h   When asked about the automobile accident in which his father was killed, an adolescent begins discussing the mechanics of trauma, velocity of impact, safety rules, and changing trends in life expectancy.

i   An adolescent, in a cool and unemotional manner, describes the circumstances of a serious automobile accident in which he received multiple injuries.

j   A hospitalized adolescent views each member of the medical staff as being all "good" or all "bad."

k   An adolescent repeatedly engages in risk-taking behavior.

l   An adolescent laughs about an embarrassing encounter with a teacher.

m   An adolescent explains her drug abuse by saying that "everybody" does it.

n   An adolescent girl who is angry at her family after being grounded runs away from home without verbally expressing her anger.

o   An adolescent identifies with a rock star or an athletic coach whom he admires.

p   An adolescent whose father recently died of a myocardial infraction begins a vigorous exercise program.

93   Denial

94   Projection

95   Splitting

96   Acting out

97   Regression

98   Counterphobia

99   Identification

100   Reaction formation

101   Repression

102   Displacement

103   Isolation of affect

104   Rationalization

105   Intellectualization

106   Sublimation

107   Humor

108   Altruism

109–112 For each of the brain regions listed, select from the following the neurotransmitter that is *most* associated with it:

a   Dopamine

b   Serotonin

c   Norepinephrine

d   Acetylcholine

109   Locus ceruleus

110   Substantia nigra

111   Raphe nuclei

112   Nucleus basalis of Meynert

ANSWERS AND EXPLANATIONS

1 **(c)** Even though the exact number of genes expressed within CNS is unknown, it is estimated that at least one-third of the human genes is involved in regulating the growth and development of the CNS. *(Ref. 3, Ch. 3.3.1, Genes and the Building of the Brain section)*

2 **(b)** The migration of neurons starts in the early embryonic development. It has been established that the newly formed glutamatergic projection neurons migrate along with radial glial cells providing guidance during corticogenesis. Double-cortin is a microtubule-binding protein, which is a necessary component in the neuron's migration process. Replicated data show that abnormal GABAergic cells in prefrontal regions of the cortex could be underlying the pathogenesis of certain psychiatric conditions, such as schizophrenia. *(Ref. 3, Ch. 3.3.1, Migration of Neurons section)*

3 **(b)** Only a limited number of neurons produce serotonin, but these neurons innervate different target fields and have enormous influence in all aspects of CNS function. Serotonergic neurons have different cellular morphologies; some of them have fine fibers, while others have beaded varicosities. Innervated by both fiber types, each cortical neuron is modulated by at least 200 serotonergic varicosities, and each serotonin neuron may affect up to half a million target neurons. Serotonin has an impact on the coordinated modulation of the entire neocortex and regulates theta rhythms. *(Questions 3–7: Ref. 5, pp. 61–75)*

4 **(a)** Dopamine neurons are located in the midbrain substantia nigra and ventral tegmental area (VTA) along with some other areas, and their mesoaccumbens pathway is responsible for reward. Their degeneration is responsible for Parkinson's disease; blockage of their receptors by antipsychotics may induce extrapyramidal effects. Blocking dopamine release may also disinhibit prolactin release causing hyperprolactinemia, sometimes found in patients taking certain antipsychotics.

5 **(c)** Norepinephrine is produced by neurons in the locus ceruleus (LC) and the lateral tegmental noradrenergic nuclei. These neurons provide projections to the neocortex, hippocampus, thalamus, and midbrain tectum, where they play a role in the regulation of arousal state, vigilance, and stress responses.

6 **(d)** Known for its involvement with allergies, histamine is produced in the tuberomammillary nucleus, and histaminergic fibers project diffusely to many different areas of the brain and spinal cord, but the hypothalamus receives the densest innervation, where histamine plays a role in the regulation of autonomic and neuroendocrine processes.

7 **(e)** Projecting to either distant brain regions (projection neurons) or contacting local cells (interneurons), cholinergic neurons are found in both the forebrain complex and the mesopontine complex. Degeneration of nucleus basalis of Meynert is found in patients with Alzheimer's disease, and the degree of neuronal loss correlates with the severity of dementia, which indicates that a cholinergic deficit may be underlying pathology of the disease, which is also supported by the fact that

drugs that promote acetylcholine signaling are beneficial to the disorder. Cholinergic neurons in the mesopontine complex continue to fire in REM sleep and may have a role in inducing REM sleep. Cholinergic neurons have local contact projections to the striatum (interneurons), and modulation of their cholinergic transmission may play a role in the anti-Parkinsonian effects of anticholinergic agents.

8 **(b)** By the age of 3 years, children can ride a tricycle, jump from the bottom steps, and alternate feet going up steps. A child at 2 can imitate vertical and circular strokes; by age 3, a child can copy a cross, and by age 5, a square. At age 3, children can build towers of 9–10 cubes, and also can put on their shoes, unbutton buttons, and feed themselves. *(Ref. 6, Table 32-3)*

9 **(d)** Four major stages of cognitive development are described by Piaget. They are (1) a sensorimotor stage (0 through 18–24 months), (2) a preoperational stage (2 through 5–7 years), (3) a stage of concrete operations (6–7 through 11 years), and a stage of formal operations (11 years to adulthood). *(Ref. 6, Table 32-5)*

10 **(a)** Piaget believed moral development parallels the four major stages of cognitive development that he described. Having integrated Piaget's concepts of cognitive development, Lawrence Kohlberg proposed three levels of morality. The levels are as follows:

Level I. Preconventional morality

Type 1/Stage 1. Punishment and obedience orientation

Type 2/Stage 2. Agreement to obey in return for reward

Level II. Morality of conventional role conformity

Type 3/Stage 3. Good-boy morality

Type 4/Stage 4. Authority-maintaining morality

Level III. Morality of self-accepted moral principles

Type 5/Stage 5. Morality of democratically accepted law

Type 6/Stage 6. Morality of individual principles of conscience. *(Ref. 5, p. 710)*

11 **(e)** Margaret Mahler described an attachment theory based on psychoanalytic theory including a complex sequence that infants gradually develop step by step as *Stages of Separation-Individuation* including: normal autism (ages 0 to 2 months), symbiosis (ages 2 to 5 months), differentiation (ages 5 to 10 months), practicing (ages 10 to 18 months), reapproachment (ages 18 to 24 months), and object constancy (individuation) (ages 2 to 5 years). *(Ref. 6, Table 32-9)*

12 **(b)** Studies of a variety of mammalian species support the hypothesis that competitive interactions between two or more populations of neurons early in development play a significant role in the elimination of the initial population of axons and in the later segregation of their synapses. This competitive elimination process is referred to as *pruning*. Some of the cells that have served their function during brain development by producing neurotropic or growth factors are programmed to die and are eliminated, which is a process named *apoptosis*. *(Ref. 6, Ch. 32.1, Pruning section)*

13 **(d)** Having observed the inborn differences and variety of autonomic reactivity and temperament among infants and toddlers, Chess and Thomas proposed nine reliable behavioral dimensions: activity level, distractibility, adaptability, attention span, intensity, threshold of responsiveness, quality of mood, rhythmicity, and approach/withdrawal. Mood lability is not one of them. *(Ref. 6, Table 32-7)*

14 **(a)** Neurotransmitter systems can be divided into two groups based on anatomic distributions. The first group originates from small, densely packed neurons in certain areas of the forebrain or brain stem, projecting to the target areas with long-ranged projection fibers, which includes serotonergic, dopaminergic, cholinergic, and noradrenergic systems. The second group includes glutamatergic and GABAergic systems that are more widely distributed throughout the brain. *(Ref. 3, Ch. 6.1.1, Neurotransmitter Systems section)*

15 **(c)** All serotonin receptors are coupled either to phospholipase C or to G-protein but 5-HT$_3$ receptors are coupled to an ion channel. *(Ref. 3, Ch. 6.1.1, Serotonergic System section)*

16 **(a)** Answer (a) is a definition of operant conditioning. Operant has some influence (operate) on the environment; answer (b) is a definition of reinforcement; answer (c) is a definition of extinction; answer (d) is a definition of classical conditioning that is concerned with stimuli (such as noise, light, taste) that evoke involuntary or automatic responses; and answer (e) is a definition of shaping. *(Ref. 3, Ch. 6.2.2, Cognitive-Behavioral Model section)*

17 **(b)** The authoritative style is characterized by high responsivity and high demandingness and is associated with the best outcomes for children overall. The authoritarian style is characterized by low responsivity and high demandingness; it is associated with good outcomes in some minority families. Permissive style consists of high responsivity and low demandingness. Neglectful/uninvolved style consists of low responsivity and low demandingness. *(Ref. 3, Ch. 2.1.3, Home and Family section)*

18 **(b)** Negative thought elimination is not a step that was proposed by Spivak and Shure. Problem identification, definition and formulation, generation of alternative solutions, choosing a new strategy, implementing the new strategy, and evaluating the new strategy are the five steps that are often the foundation of behavioral skills training strategies in group and individual therapies of children. *(Ref. 3, Ch. 6.2.2, Anxiety Disorders section)*

19 **(b)** At the age of 2–7 months, infants start to show understanding of object permanence when they gradually achieve cognitive ability to create mental representations of objects and people that can exist even when they are no longer within their sight. This allows infants to play peek-a-boo with their caregivers, and it is a prerequisite skill for imaging and visual differentiation between caregivers and strangers. By age 18 months, they solidly grasp the concept. *(Ref. 3, Ch. 2.1.1, Five Qualitative Stage of Infancy)*

20 **(e)** Many forces may interfere with the normal development of infants and toddlers, such as regulatory disturbances, social/ environmental disturbances, psychophysiological disturbances, developmental delays, genetic and metabolic disorders, exposure to toxins, CNS damage, and prematurity. A prolonged separation from caregivers is a social/environmental disturbance but is not necessarily a regulatory disturbance. Sleep disturbances (frequent waking), excessive crying or irritability, eating difficulties (finicky eating or food refusal), low frustration tolerance, and self-stimulatory/unusual movements (rocking, head banging, excessive finger sucking) are considered regulatory disturbances. *(Ref. 3, Table 2.1.1.1)*

21 **(d)** Attachment can be defined as secure and insecure. Within insecure attachment, there are three types: *avoidant/dismissive*, *resistant/anxious-ambivalent*, and *disorganized/disorientated*. Securely attached infants tend to be more resilient, self-reliant, emphatic, and confident in developing adult relationships. *Avoidant or dismissing* infants tend to develop a pattern of aloofness and detachment to defend against loss and separation, and may be more vulnerable to adult disorders such as borderline, histrionic, and dependent personality disorders. *Resistant/anxious-ambivalent* infants tend to experience their past attachments through confusion, anger, and fear of abandonment, and develop excessive dependency and fear in their adult life. *Disorganized-disorientated* infants may be associated with unresolved and disorganized patterns in adults, which can lead to more disturbed self-object relations. *(Ref. 5, p. 886)*

22 **(c)** Erickson conceptualized psychosocial development as occurring in predetermined phases across the lifespan. Each phase is dependent on proper development of the prior phases. *(Ref. 5, pp. 900–901)*

23 **(b)** Serotonin is produced from hydroxylation and decarboxylation of the amino acid tryptophan. The rate-limiting step is the hydroxylation of tryptophan to form 5-hydroxytryptophan, catalyzed by the enzyme tryptophan hydroxylase. Tyrosine hydroxylase, on the other hand, is the rate-limiting enzyme for the synthesis of dopamine and norepinephrine. *(Ref. 3, Figure 6.1.1.4, Figure 6.1.1.5)*

24 **(d)** The serotonin metabolite on the list is 5-HIAA. Metabolites of neurotransmitters can be found in cerebrospinal fluid, blood, and urine. Studies measuring metabolites of neurotransmitter ontogeny have helped us understand neurochemistry of normal development. Monoamine oxidase (MAO) and catechol-amine-O-methyltransferase (COMT) are two main enzymes responsible for the metabolism of many neurotransmitters. The metabolites of norepinephrine are MHPG and VMA. HVA is the principal metabolite of dopamine. *(Ref. 3, Figure 6.1.1.4)*

25 **(b)** GABAergic interneurons (short-ranging neurons) can be found in the cortex, thalamus, striatum, cerebellum, and spinal cord; long-ranging neurons can be found in the basal ganglia, septum, and substantia nigra. GABAergic neurons in the cortex and thalamus are crucial for inhibiting the excitatory neurons. This inhibition is believed to benefit the treatment of anxiety disorders, insomnia, and agitation. *(Ref. 3, Ch. 6.1.1, GABAergic System section)*

26 **(e)** Glutamatergic neurons can be located in different areas throughout the brain, affecting brain functions in many ways by binding to NMDA, AMPA, and kainate receptors. Binding of glutamate to glutamatergic neurons and NMDA receptors in the hippocampus is crucial in the formation of memory

resulting from the creation of long-term potentiation. *(Ref. 3, Ch. 6.1.1, Glutamatergic System section)*

27 **(a)** Children begin pretend play around age 2 when they have the capacity to allow a real object to stand for another or for something imaginary, such as brushing the hair of a doll (real object), to represent a real action (something imaginary). *(Ref. 3, Ch. 2.1.2, Play section)*

28 **(b)** A child's basic sense of self as male or female is defined as gender identity regardless of chromosomal constitution, gonadal/hormonal secretions, or genitalia. With both biological and environmental psychosocial influences, most children develop a stable gender identity by age 3. *(Ref. 3, Ch. 2.1.3, Major Lines of Development section)*

29 **(d)** Both single photon emission computed tomography (SPECT) and positron emission tomography (PET) require the administration of radioactive tracers. Even with limited exposure to radiation (less than the dose of a chest x-ray), they are much less acceptable in research than other neuroimaging methods, such as magnetic resonance imaging (MRI), magnetic resonance spectroscopy (MRS), functional MRI, and EEG/magnetoencephalography. CT uses conversational x-ray (not radioactive tracers). New technology combines PET and CT to image blood flow and neurotransmitter systems. *(Ref. 6, Ch. 1.1, Neuroimaging section)*

30 **(a)** As a modality of MRI, DTI uses mathematically described directional diffusion of water in brain tissues in vivo, and it can provide information on the direction and integrity of neural fiber tracks. Thus, it is useful in studying the connectivity of white matter and its color-coded maps can help parcellate some tissues that are difficult to segment with conventional methods. *(Ref. 5, pp. 270–271)*

31 **(b)** ^{1}H (not ^{31}P) MRS is the most widely used technique because of its greatest sensitivity in detecting signals compared to other nuclei used in vivo, such as phosphorus (^{31}P) and carbon 13 (^{13}C). Studies show alteration of NAA, rCh, glutamate, glutamine, and GABA in patients with certain mental illnesses, such as major depression, bipolar disorder, panic disorder, and attention hyperactive/impulsive disorder. *(Ref. 6, Table 1-24)*

32 **(d)** EEG and MEG measure electrical activity of the brain with a temporal resolution on the order of milliseconds. MEG also has better spatial resolution than conventional EEG, and it is less prone to motion artifact because it does not require scalp electrodes. But the hardware of MEG is much more expensive than that of EEG and a magnetically shielded room is required. *(Ref. 5, p. 4010)*

33 **(e)** Acceptability is not a stage in children's understanding of the concepts of death. But irreversibility, finality (nonfunctionality), causality, and inevitability (universality) are the four stages that have been consistently noted in the studies. *(Ref. 3, Ch. 7.2.5, Children's Concepts of Death section)*

34 **(c)** A review by Speece and Brent indicated that children between ages of 5 and 7 can acquire the concepts of irreversibility, nonfunctionality, and universality, and found that the earlier studies that cited older age of acquisition had significant methodological flaws. *(Ref. 3, Ch. 7.2.5, Children's Concepts of Death section)*

35 **(d)** Children acquire the concept of conservation between the ages of 7 and 11, which is equivalent to the concrete operational stage of cognitive development proposed by Jean Piaget. With the understanding of conservation, children can recognize that objects are still the same (characteristics of the objects are conserved) even if their shape has changed. Around the same time, children usually achieve an understanding of the concept of reversibility, where they recognize that one thing can turn into another and back again (i.e. water and ice). *(Ref. 6, Ch. 34.1, Stage of Concrete Operations section)*

36 **(e)** During the last part of the sensorimotor stage proposed by Jean Piaget, between the ages of 18 months and 2 years, children develop symbolic thought while they use symbolic representation of event and objects, and attain object permanence. *(Ref. 6, Table 34-2)*

37 **(e)** Hypotheticodeductive thinking is the highest organization of cognition, and occurs after children reach formal operational stage (age 11 through the end of adolescence) based on the cognitive development theory of Piaget. At this stage some children can use deductive and inductive reasoning, and can make hypotheses and test them. However, some children may regress to an earlier stage of thought process, and some adolescents or adults may never reach this stage. *(Ref. 6, Table 34-1)*

38 **(c)** Loss of excitatory glutamatergic inputs especially predominant in the prefrontal cortex is one of the results of synaptic remodeling. Neuropsychological tasks of executive functioning as well as inhibition that are associated with prefrontal cortical functioning continue to improve in adolescence. Developmental changes in GABAergic neurons and their synapses may play a role in fine-tuning of inhibitory control. Disruption of such developmental changes may be linked to people with schizophrenia. *(Ref. 3, Ch. 2.1.4, Physical Changes section)*

39 **(b)** In girls, puberty begins with breast development followed by the growth of pubic hair, height spurt, and finally the onset of menstruation. The timing of each physical characteristic relative to the others can vary from individual to individual. For girls, puberty begins at an average of 9 to 11 years of age, approximately 2 years earlier than in boys. Boys follow the developmental sequence of pubic hair, penile and testicle growth, and height spurt. *(Ref. 3, Ch. 2.1.4, Physical Changes section)*

40 **(a)** Studies show that early maturation is more socially advantageous for boys especially in terms of their popularity, self-esteem, and intellectual ability. However, it is also associated with increased risk for delinquent behaviors. Early maturation in girls is associated with lower self-esteem, increased risk for developing depression and anxiety, and risk-taking behaviors, although the impact also depends on social and environmental factors. *(Ref. 3, Ch. 2.1.4, Physical Changes section)*

41 **(e)** A polymorphism is a common variation in the sequence of DNA that occurs in ≥1% of the population. Single nucleotide polymorphisms (SNPs) are variations at a single nucleotide that occur in approximately 1/1000 bases in human DNA. These variations are commonly used to track inheritance in families and have been widely used in linkage studies. They are considered as common SNPs if the frequency is greater than 1% in a population. Answer (a) is the definition of allele. Answer (b) is the definition of candidate gene. Answer (c) is the definition of locus. And answer (d) is the definition of marker. *(Ref. 3, Table 3.3.2.1)*

42 (c) Linkage analysis uses LOD scores to describe the level of linkage, 2.2–3.6 being considered suggestive linkage, 3.6–5.4 statistically significant, > 5.4 highly significant. Association analysis examines gene frequencies within populations; its ability to look at large sample sizes makes it more powerful for detecting common susceptibility variants of relatively small effect compared to linkage analysis which needs larger genetic effects due to the limits on sample size inherent in studying families. While a parametric approach is more useful in studying Mendelian disorders, a nonparametric approach has greater advantage in studying disorders without any known clear mode of inheritance. *(Ref. 3, Ch. 3.3.2, Approaches to Gene Discovery section)*

43 (d) Fluorescence in situ hybridization (FISH) is one of the most popular and useful techniques in molecular cytogenetic studies. The technique uses molecular probes to detect susceptible genes by identifying individuals with particular chromosomal abnormalities, such as translocations, deletions, and duplications. *(Ref. 3, Table 3.3.2.1)*

44 (b) Arrays of SNPs can be fabricated on glass or nylon slides, which allows researchers to investigate hundreds of thousands of genetic markers simultaneously in a single reaction. This provides a way to screen and survey polymorphisms across the entire genome. This technology has transformed molecular biology into a new era, and significantly improved efficiency and decreased cost in genome studies. *(Ref. 3, Ch. 3.3.2 Genome-Wide Association section; Ref. 5, Ch. 37, Genome-Wide Association section)*

45 (a) Precocity of babies occurs in traditional and nonindustrialized societies; that is, African babies raised in traditional fashions reach more advanced levels of motoric functioning during infancy than do their European and American counterparts. This was believed to be due to the deliberate teaching of infants by caregivers in African countries regarding how to walk and sit and the encouragement of practice. *(Ref. 3, Ch. 2.2.1, Cultural Impact on Developmental Stages section)*

46 (a) Children with failure to thrive may present with developmental difficulties in many areas, but do not have a characteristic diagnostic developmental pattern. Language/communication development is linked with social/environmental factors and influences. Qualitative observation of children's interactions with others in different settings, such as their motivations, problem-solving processes, and affective states, is an important part of assessing children even if they have average developmental profiles. It is also important in evaluating children with discrepancies across different developmental domains. *(Ref. 3, Ch. 2.1.1, Forces that May Compromise Normative section)*

47 (b) Development of a theory of mind is a developmental achievement that allows children to see the world in both physical and nonphysical ways through the lens of mental states. Their understanding of themselves and others is greatly expanded. During an early stage, the capacity can fluctuate, especially in stressful situations. The development of this capacity can be delayed in disadvantaged children, such as children with severe traumas and/or neglect. *(Ref. 3, Ch. 2.1.2, Emerging Minds section)*

48 (e) Preschool kids may play with imaginary friends when there are no real friends nearby. Some surveys show that they often insist on their reality and their boundary between reality and fantasy is often blurred. Creating imaginary friends may reflect their concerns and anxiety. It is often *not* easy to distinguish whether their use of imaginary companionship is normal or not, especially in younger children, which may require evaluating them in multiple settings over time. *(Ref. 3, Ch. 2.1.2, Play section)*

49 (c) Preschoolers need reassurance that indicates their teachers or nannies did not leave because of them, and visiting with their previous teachers and nannies may be helpful, as well as pictures, letters, and phone calls. "Clean breaks" rarely help with their separations. *(Ref. 3, Ch. 2.1.2, Separation section)*

50 (e) Even though certain significant behavioral problems in early childhood are predictive of later behavioral difficulties, aggression in preschoolers does not necessarily predict aggression in school-aged children. Actually, by ages 3 and 4, children's physical aggression is transformed into more verbal aggression, such as shouting, yelling, and name calling because of their improved language skills. By ages 5 and 6, overall aggression diminishes and tends to focus more on their social situations and needs, compared to younger children, whose aggression focuses on their physical needs and desires. *(Ref. 3, Ch. 2.1.2, Aggression section)*

51 (c) The preoperational child is extremely egocentric. Piaget used the concept of circular reactions in describing the sensorimotor stage. Children are not capable of mastering the concepts of conservation, classification, and seriation until the concrete operational stage. The ability to think abstractly does not fully appear until the stage of formal operations. *(Ref. 6, Table 32-5)*

52 (a) Clinical studies of attachment are helpful in understanding most of the situations listed. Insecure attachment can potentially foreshadow later development problems; however, the outcomes may be influenced by many factors and may not be necessarily fixed or inevitable. *(Ref. 3, Ch. 5.15.3, Interactions of Attachment section)*

53 (a) Measures of temperament developed by Chess and Thomas include nine dimensions: activity level, rhythmicity, approach-withdrawal, adaptability, responsiveness, intensity of reactions, quality of mood, distractibility, and attention span. Three constellations of temperament were proposed: easy temperament, difficult temperament, and slow-to-warm-up temperament. Recent studies showed that certain alleles of a dopamine receptor gene DRD4 are associated with novelty-seeking temperamental traits, which highlighted the genetic influences on temperament. However, studies also showed significant environmental influences. *(Ref. 5, Table 39-1, Table 39-4)*

54 (e) Epidemiologic studies did not provide any evidence to show that at this stage adolescents are characterized by overwhelmed alienation, profound angst, and significant disruptive family relationships, even though most striking changes can be seen in terms of their physical, emotional, and behavioral presentations. *(Ref. 5, p. 3366)*

55 (c) Adolescents in late adolescence may gradually move to solid identity formation when they continue to actively explore their academic pursuits, musical and artistic talents, athletic participations, and social bonds. The other statements in the questions correctly describe the characteristics of middle adolescence. *(Ref. 5, p. 3367)*

56 **(d)** The 2005 YRBSS study showed the use of tobacco, alcohol, and marijuana in late adolescence is higher than in middle adolescence, and also showed that about 14% of 12th graders drove after consuming alcohol and 27% of 12th graders also took rides with drivers who had been drinking. *(Ref. 5, p. 3367)*

57 **(d)** Two additional hypothalamic peptides (growth-hormone-releasing hormone and somatostatin) play a role in puberty development by promoting growth hormone from the pituitary gland. *(Ref. 5, p. 3368)*

58 **(e)** The primary sex characteristic in males is development of sperm by the testes and ejaculation. Thickening of the skin, broadening of shoulders, and the development of facial hair are all secondary sexual characteristics in males. *(Ref. 5, pp. 3368–3369)*

59 **(c)** Adolescent girls' ovarian follicles produce sufficient estrogen in Tanner stages 3–4 when menarche occurs. During these stages ovulation occurs every 28 days until menopause. *(Ref. 5, p. 3368)*

60 **(e)** Lawrence Kohlberg proposed three levels of morality, which are further divided into six types/stages. In the postconventional level and in stage 5, adolescents are more flexible in their thinking of "right" or "wrong" and they have achieved abilities to interpret complex moral dilemmas, and the concept of "extenuating circumstances" is understood. Here are the stages:

Level I. Preconventional morality

Type 1/Stage 1. Punishment and obedience orientation

Type 2/Stage 2. Agreement to obey in return for reward

Level II. Morality of conventional role conformity

Type 3/Stage 3. Good-boy morality

Type 4/Stage 4. Authority-maintaining morality

Level III. Morality of self-accepted moral principles

Type 5/Stage 5. Morality of democratically accepted law

Type 6/Stage 6. Morality of individual principles of conscience. *(Ref. 5, p. 710)*

61 **(e)** During adolescence, girls have a more significant drop in their self-esteem than boys according to a recent study on global measures of self-esteem in adolescence and young adulthood. The data might reflect the "inflated" self-esteem of school-aged children, which was realized by late adolescents when they became more aware of their shortcomings and had more realistic views of themselves. *(Ref. 5, p. 3370)*

62 **(e)** Based on recent functional MRI studies of social cognition, girls (not boys) demonstrate diminished activities in the left amygdala when presented with fearful faces, and also show higher activities in the dorsolateral prefrontal cortex, which may reflect increased maturity in the regulation of emotions compared to their male counterparts. *(Ref. 5, p. 3371)*

63 **(d)** Neuroendocrine influence in the early stage of development can be long-lasting and permanent. The HPA axis is one of the neuroendocrine pathways (among others, such as the somatotropic axis, hypothalamic-pituitary-thyroid axis, and hypothalamic-pituitary-gonadal axis) that may play important roles in regulating brain development. All the listed conditions can be related to the dysfunction of the HPA axis *except* for the psychosocial short stature that is believed to be associated with the hyposecretion of growth hormone (a dysfunction of the somatotropic axis). *(Ref. 3, Figure 6.1.1.7)*

64 **(b)** The initiation of transmission is accompanied by (1) the release of the presynaptic neurotransmitter, (2) the binding of the neurotransmitter to postsynaptic receptors, (3) the activation of receptors, and/or (4) the regulation of secondary messengers. The termination of the transmission is the result of (1) the ending of the excitation of the presynaptic terminal, (2) the depletion of the neurotransmitter, (3) the binding of the neurotransmitter to the presynaptic receptors, which turns off the release of the neurotransmitter, (4) the reuptake of the neurotransmitter by the presynaptic terminal, and/or (5) metabolism of extracellular enzymes, which depletes the neurotransmitter available in the synaptic cleft. *(Ref. 3, Figure 6.1.1.2)*

65 **(e)** The basal ganglia, consisting of five subcortical interconnected parts (caudate nucleus, putamen, globus pallidus, subthalamic nucleus, and substantia nigra), plays an important role in maintaining and regulating motor and some autonomic functions through its connections/circuits to the cortex. It is also believed that dysfunction of the basal ganglia or/and the associated circuits is involved in some neuropsychiatric conditions (especially the conditions related to motor and attention dysfunctions) such as Parkinson's disease, OCD, and ADHD. The basal ganglia appear to participate in enabling particular movements and controlling their sequencing, rather than directly initiating their occurrence. *(Ref. 6, Ch. 33, Basal Ganglia section)*

66 **(b)** The capacity for declarative memory is not fully developed during the first three years of a child's life. Nondeclarative memory develops early in infancy. Instead of having difficulty in retrieving early memories, children do not store their conscious declarative memories in organized ways. The early memories are formed in very fragmented ways, which are tied to the specific context of an infant's understanding of the world, and not imbued with meaning or a complex understanding of the events. *(Ref. 5, p. 743)*

67 **(c)** Even though condemned by many cultures for a long time, masturbation is very prevalent throughout people's lifetime. Studies showed couples in a steady relationship continue to masturbate. When masturbation becomes a compulsion and out of the person's willful control, it is considered pathological. It is also considered to be abnormal if it is the only sexual activity of the person who has an available intimate partner. *(Ref. 5, 1961)*

68 **(e)** Desire aversion or sexual aversion is not a phase of normal physiological responses to sexual stimulation. The normal phases include *desire*, *excitement*, *orgasm*, and *resolution*. Under DSM-5, major sexual dysfunctions include delayed ejaculation, erectile disorder, female orgasmic disorder, female sexual interest/arousal disorder, genito-pelvic pain/penetration disorder, male hypoactive sexual desire disorder, premature (early) ejaculation, and substance/medication-induced sexual dysfunction. *(Ref. 4, pp. 423–450; Ref. 5, p. 1959)*

69 **(d)** The overwhelming majority of research examining the endocrine system failed to show significant correlations between atypical levels of sex hormones and homosexuality. However, recent studies showed possible correlations between the timing and amount of prenatal exposure to certain hormones (such as androgen) and subsequent sexual orientation. Homosexual contacts are more frequent in early adolescence, some of which are transient and do not necessarily predict sexual orientation. Strong evidence exists to support both genetic and environmental influences in the establishment of homosexuality based on twin studies. *(Ref. 5, pp. 1991–1995)*

70 **(b)** The authoritative parenting style is considered generally optimal in fostering children's resilience, which is characterized by the appropriate balance of parental warmth and firm, consistent, and reasonable supervision and control. Warmth and control are two essential elements of "good parenting." High warmth plus lax discipline and control or low warmth plus strict discipline/control are both less optimal approaches. *(Ref. 3, Ch. 2.3, Familial Factors in Resilience section)*

Matching

71 **(e); 72. (d); 73. (b); 74. (a); 75 (c)** Symbolic play emerges in infancy when children begin to combine words and gestures in order to label objects in relationship to their needs, and to use the objects in representational ways. In younger children, parallel play is more dominant than reciprocal play that involves interactive reciprocal exchanges among the children. Secure attachment depends on the children's capacity of having a stable internal representation of the availability of their caregivers. The tendency of children's attribution of living qualities to a nonliving object is called animism. Egocentrism refers to the lack of ability of young children to see others' perspectives, being self-centered. *(Ref. 3, Ch. 2.1.2)*

76 **(c); 77. (b); 78. (d); 79. (a)** In addition to the foregoing relationships, Piaget's sensorimotor stage correlates with Freud's oral stage, his preoperational stage correlates with Freud's anal and phallic stages, his concrete operational stage correlates with Freud's latency stage, and his formal operational stage correlates with Freud's adolescence stage. *(Ref. 6, Table 34-10, Table 32-5)*

80 **(a); 81. (g); 82. (f); 83. (e); 84. (d); 85. (c); 86. (b)** Hormonal production and secretion are regulated by neuronal secretory products from the hypothalamus. Such products are considered as regulating hormones that are responsible for acting on the pituitary to regulate the release of target hormones that in turn directly act on other peripheral endocrine organs. *(Ref. 5, p. 166, Table 1.12-3)*

87 **(b)** John Bowlby utilized developmental psychology and evolutionary biology to propose that infant–mother attachment not only is a result of the mother's association with the gratification of urges, but also is due to species-typical behaviors that evolved to promote infant survival. *(Questions 87–92: Ref. 5, pp. 3359–3361; Ref. 6, Ch. 34.4)*

88 **(c)** "Assimilation" and "accommodation" were terms Piaget used to describe the way the organism creates and adapts to new knowledge.

89 **(a)** Winnicott used the term "transitional object" to describe the first "not-me" object such as a soft blanket or a cuddly toy used for comfort when the mother is unavailable to provide comforting.

90 **(e)** Klein postulated a rich inner life of the infant with many sexual and aggressive fantasies. "Reparation" was a term she used to refer to the return to the mother after she became the object of the infant's fantasized attacks for withholding gratification.

91 **(f)** In their New York Longitudinal Study, Chess and Thomas utilized the terms "goodness of fit" and "poorness of fit" to describe the match of the infant's temperament with the environment/caregivers.

92 **(d)** Anna Freud strove to create a developmental theory based on the unfolding of sexual and aggressive urges in relationship to the child's parents and environment.

93 **(c)** Denial is an unconscious mechanism that allows the adolescent to avoid awareness of thoughts, feelings, wishes, needs, or external reality factors that are consciously intolerable. *(Questions 93–108: Ref. 5, Table 6.1-2; Ref. 6, Table 34-12)*

94 **(f)** Projection (projection of guilt) is the unconscious mechanism whereby an unacceptable impulse, feeling, or idea is attributed to the external world.

95 **(j)** Splitting occurs when the adolescent unconsciously views people or events as being at one extreme or the other.

96 **(n)** Acting out takes place when unconscious emotional conflicts or feelings are expressed in an arena that is different from the one in which they arose. Generally, acting out is a feeling expressed in actions rather than in words.

97 **(d)** Regression is a partial or symbolic return to more infantile patterns of reacting or thinking.

98 **(k)** Counterphobia is seeking out experiences that are consciously or unconsciously feared.

99 **(o)** Identification occurs when a person unconsciously patterns himself or herself after some other person (role modeling or imitation is similar to identification but is a conscious process).

100 **(e)** Reaction formation unconsciously transforms unacceptable feelings, ideas, or impulses into their opposites.

101 **(a)** Repression (unconscious) and suppression (conscious) occur when unacceptable thoughts, wishes, or impulses that would produce anxiety are pushed out of awareness.

102 **(b)** Displacement takes place when emotions, ideas, or wishes are transferred from their original source or target to a more acceptable substitute.

103 **(i)** Isolation of affect is the separation of ideas or events from the feelings associated with them.

104 **(m)** Rationalization uses reasoning and "rational" explanations, which may or may not be valid, to explain away unconscious conflicts and motivations.

105 **(h)** Intellectualization controls affect and impulse by analyzing through excessive thought without experiencing the feeling.

106 **(p)** Sublimation unconsciously replaces an unacceptable feeling with a course of action that is personally and socially acceptable.

107 **(l)** Humor is used defensively to relieve anxiety caused by the discrepancies between what one wishes for himself or herself and what actually happens.

108 **(g)** Altruism is a seemingly unselfish interest in the welfare of others.

109 **(c)** Most noradrenergic neurons in the brain arise from the locus ceruleus and are thought to play a role in anxiety and panic disorders. *(Questions 109–112: Ref. 6, Ch. 33, Neurophysiology and Neurochemistry section)*

110 **(a)** Dopamine is the major neurotransmitter in the pigmented substantia nigra that degenerates in Parkinson's disease.

111 **(b)** The midline raphe nuclei contain serotonin, which is important in sleep and some types of depression.

112 **(d)** Cholinergic neurons have both long-ranged projections and short-ranged projections, and locate in the basal forebrain (septum, diagonal band, and nucleus basalis of Meynert).

2

NEURODEVELOPMENTAL DISORDERS

DOI: 10.4324/9781003308805-3

QUESTIONS

Directions: Select the best response for each of the questions 1–78.

1 Which of the following is *not* a diagnosis listed in the Neurodevelopmental Disorders chapter of DSM-5?

  a Global developmental delay

  b Childhood-onset fluency disorder

  c Attention-deficit/hyperactivity disorder

  d Reactive attachment disorder

  e Tourette's disorder

2 Significant changes have been made in DSM-5 regarding diagnosing autism spectrum disorders. All of the following descriptions reflect such changes *except*:

  a DSM-5 uses the term "autism spectrum disorder" to replace the pervasive developmental disorders in DSM-IV.

  b Autism spectrum disorder and ADHD are no longer mutually exclusive.

  c Asperger's disorder was singled out and was categorized somewhere else.

  d DSM-5 uses three levels to specify the severity.

  e DSM-5 also includes specifiers to describe patients' additional deficits in different areas.

3 Based on DSM-5, clinicians may use all of the following guidelines to evaluate children with possible intellectual disabilities *except*:

  a Children have to meet three criteria to be diagnosed with an intellectual disability.

  b The three criteria include Criterion A: deficits in intellectual functions, Criterion B: deficits in adaptive functioning, and Criterion C: onset of the deficits during the developmental period.

  c Criterion A calls for an IQ score below 70 to meet the threshold for a diagnosis of intellectual disability.

  d Clinicians should use specifiers to identify the severity of the intellectual disability.

  e There are four levels of severity: mild, moderate, severe, and profound.

4 All of the following statements regarding the diagnostic Criterion A (deficits in intellectual functions) of intellectual disability are correct *except*:

  a Intellectual functions are measured by tests of intelligence that give IQ scores.

  b Individuals with intellectual disability must have approximate scores of less than two standard deviations from population mean.

  c "Flynn effect" may lower the test scores.

  d Invalid scores can be due to the use of brief intelligence screening tests, and the overall IQ score becomes invalid if there are significant discrepancies across subtest scores.

  e Factors that can influence IQ scores include co-occurring disorders, the individual's social cultural background, and the individual's native language.

5 All of the following statements regarding the diagnostic Criterion B (deficits in adaptive functioning) of intellectual disability are correct *except*:

  a Adaptive functioning involves adaptive reasoning in three domains: conceptual (academic) domain, social domain, and practical domain.

  b Both clinical evaluation and psychometric measures are used to assess adaptive functioning.

  c Unspecified intellectual disability is considered when standardized testing is difficult or impossible to administer.

  d Impairments in at least two of the three domains are needed to qualify for Criterion B.

  e The impairments in Criterion B must be directly related to the intellectual deficits in Criterion A.

6 While overall general population prevalence of intellectual disability is approximately 1%, what is the approximate prevalence of severe intellectual disability?

  a 0.05%

  b 0.1%

  c 0.3%

  d 0.6%

  e 0.9%

7 Which of the following disorders or syndromes is *most* likely to have a course including periods of worsening intellectual functioning, followed by stabilization?

  a Global developmental delay

  b Unspecified intellectual disability

  c Sanfilippo syndrome

  d Rett syndrome

  e Cerebral palsy

8 All of the following are genetic or physiological risks and poor prognostic factors associated with intellectual disability *except*:

  a Certain chromosomal disorders

  b Inborn errors of metabolism

  c Neonatal encephalopathy related to delivery

  d Hypoxic ischemic injury

  e Female gender compared to male gender

9   All of the following statements regarding the differential diagnosis of intellectual disability are accurate *except*:

a   A diagnosis of intellectual disability can be assumed with the existence of a medical or genetic condition that commonly causes intellectual disability.

b   Intellectual disability falls under the category of neurodevelopmental disorder, which is distinct from the neurocognitive disorders.

c   Both intellectual disability diagnosis and specific learning disorder diagnosis should be made if full criteria for both conditions are met.

d   Intellectual disability is not unusual among children with autism spectrum disorder.

e   IQ scores of children with autism spectrum disorder can be unstable. Reassessment across developmental stages is important.

10   Which of the following conditions is the *least* common comorbidity with intellectual disability?

a   ADHD

b   Anorexia nervosa

c   Depressive and bipolar disorders

d   Anxiety disorders

e   Stereotypic movement disorder

11   Which of the following conditions is *only* diagnosed at the age of 5 years and older?

a   Autism spectrum disorder

b   Global developmental delay

c   Unspecified intellectual disability

d   Down syndrome

e   Fragile X syndrome

12   In DSM-5, the communication disorders include all of the following conditions *except*:

a   Language disorder

b   Phonological disorder

c   Speech sound disorder

d   Childhood-onset fluency disorder

e   Social (pragmatic) communication disorder

13   Difficulty with discourse is often shown in individuals with language disorder and is also an important diagnostic criterion for language disorder. Which of the following situations accurately describes the meaning of "impairment in discourse"?

a   A child of age 8 only speaks about 20 single words.

b   A child of age 8 talks about past events using present tenses.

c   A child of age 8 speaks sentences with incorrect sequences of words.

d   A child of age 8 can understand better than he can talk.

e   A child of age 8 cannot summarize an event using a narrative.

14   By which of the following ages are individual differences in language ability *first* felt to be stable and the diagnosis of language disorder more reliable over time into adulthood?

a   At the age of 2

b   At the age of 4

c   At the age of 6

d   At the age of 8

e   At the age of 10

15   Which of the following genetic syndromes or conditions has the *least* impairing effects on language and speech?

a   Williams syndrome

b   Fragile X syndrome

c   Down syndrome

d   Landau-Kleffner syndrome

e   Autism spectrum disorder

16   All of the following descriptions are important aspects of the difficulties found in children with social communication disorder *except*:

a   Children cannot greet people or share information either verbally or nonverbally in social contexts.

b   Children always speak in the same fashion and are unable to adjust their communication to fit into different settings or contexts.

c   Children often use monosyllabic whole-word repetitions.

d   Children cannot take turns while conversing with their peers and often miss verbal or nonverbal cues to regulate interaction.

e   Children have difficulty understanding inexplicit or ambiguous meanings of language (e.g., humor, metaphors, idioms, and making inferences).

17   Many studies have been conducted to investigate and explore the etiology of autism spectrum disorder. All of the following are neurobiological findings found in autism *except*:

a   Decreased peripheral serotonin levels more likely than increased

b   Increased head size (macrocephaly)

c   Failure to activate fusiform face region

d   Persistent "primitive" reflexes

e   High rates of EEG abnormality/seizure disorder

18   The performance deficits in face and facial expression recognition in people with autism spectrum disorder have been documented in many research studies that attempted to examine responsivity to the human face. Compared to typically developing individuals, a child with autism spectrum disorder is *more* likely to focus on which area of a frightening person's face?

a   Hair

b   Forehead

c   Upper half of the face (including eyes)

d   Ears

e   Mouth area

19 Which one of the following factors is the *most* consistently related to the outcome of autism spectrum disorder?

  a Amount of time spent in school

  b Rating of social behavior

  c Comorbid neuropsychiatric disorders

  d Communicative skills

  e Rating of social maturity

20 Which of the following is *least* likely to have co-occurring autism spectrum disorder?

  a Down syndrome

  b Angelman syndrome

  c Tuberous sclerosis

  d Fragile X syndrome

  e Phenylketonuria (PKU)

21 Which of the following genetic variations is *strongly* associated with Rett syndrome?

  a Mutations of MECP2 gene

  b Mutations of FMR1 gene

  c Deletion of an elastin gene

  d Deletion of chromosome 15p11q13

  e Trisomy 21

22 Treatment of autism spectrum disorder can often be challenging. All of the following statements regarding interventions used in treating autism spectrum disorder are accurate *except*:

  a Controlled clinical trials on secretin showed significant improvements compared to placebo.

  b Appropriate educational interventions foster the acquisition of basic social, communicative, and cognitive skills.

  c Behavioral modification procedures can help to promote appropriate behaviors and decrease inappropriate behaviors.

  d Psychotherapy is not usually indicated for children with autism spectrum disorder.

  e No pharmacologic agents used in the treatment of autism spectrum disorder are curative.

23 All of the following statements regarding DSM-5 diagnostic criteria for autism spectrum disorder are correct *except*:

  a Criteria A and B cover the areas of (1) impairments in social communication and social interaction and (2) restricted and repetitive patterns of behavior, interests, and activities, respectively.

  b All three core deficits from Criterion A and all four core deficits from Criterion B must be present.

  c Comorbid diagnosis of intellectual disability should only be made when the intellectual functioning is below that expected for the general developmental level.

  d Individuals with impairments in social communication but whose symptoms do not meet the criteria for autism spectrum disorder should be evaluated for social (pragmatic) communication disorder.

  e Specifiers should be used to identify children with autism spectrum disorder associated with a medical or genetic disorder, e.g. Rett syndrome, Fragile X syndrome.

24 Which of the following numbers reflects an accurate estimate of the population prevalence of autism spectrum disorder across the United States and non-U.S. countries?

  a 0.1%

  b 0.2%

  c Around 0.5%

  d Approaching 1%

  e Approximately 1.5%

25 Autism spectrum disorder is usually a lifelong disorder. Individuals with autism spectrum disorder may have different pathways, courses, and outcomes. All of the following statements regarding the development and course of autism spectrum disorder are correct *except*:

  a Onset of the symptoms is usually recognizable during the second year of life, but may be apparent earlier than 12 months if developmental delays are severe.

  b Most regression or deterioration occurs after the age of 2 years.

  c Initial symptoms frequently involve delayed language accompanied by lack of social interests or unusual social interactions.

  d Autism is not a degenerative disorder, and learning and compensation tend to continue to improve throughout life.

  e Autism spectrum disorder can be first diagnosed in adulthood.

26 About 70% of individuals with autism spectrum disorder may have one co-occurring mental disorder, and 40% of them may have two or more comorbid mental disorders. At times, differential diagnoses can be difficult and confusing. All of the following related statements are correct *except*:

  a In contrast to autism spectrum disorder, in selective mutism early development is usually not disturbed and social reciprocity is not usually impaired.

  b In contrast to autism spectrum disorder, in language disorder nonverbal communication is not usually impaired, and restricted, repetitive patterns of behavior are absent.

  c In intellectual disability without autism spectrum disorder, there is no apparent discrepancy between the level of social-communicative skills and other intellectual skills.

  d Stereotypic movement disorder diagnosis should be given when stereotypic movements exist in children who are diagnosed with autism spectrum disorder.

  e Comorbid diagnosis of ADHD should be given when inattention and hyperactivity exceed that typically seen in children of comparable mental age.

27 Which of the following tests does *not* specifically measure adaptive functioning during the process of assessing children who might have intellectual disability?

a Kaufman Assessment Battery for Children, 2nd Edition (K-ABC-II)

b Vineland Adaptive Behavior Scales, 2nd Edition

c Battele Developmental Inventory, 2nd Edition

d Scales of Independent Behavior-Revised (SIB-R0)

e Supports Intensity Scale (SIS)

28 Which of the following standardized tests of intelligence can be used with children who are nonverbal?

a Stanford-Binet Intelligence Scales, 5th Edition (SB5)

b Wechsler Preschool and Primary Scale of Intelligence (WPPSI)

c Kaufman Assessment Battery for Children, 2nd Edition (K-ABC-II)

d Differential Ability Scales, 2nd Edition (DAS-II)

e Leiter International Performance Scale-Revised (Leiter-R)

29 As with other neurogenetic syndromes, Angelman syndrome's clinical presentation can be varied. However, all of the following symptoms are commonly present in individuals with Angelman syndrome *except*:

a Severe speech delays

b Ataxia of gait and/or tremulous movements of limbs

c Frequent irritable and sad demeanor

d Short attention span

e Hand flapping

30 Which of the following is *not* a known genetic mechanism that causes Angelman syndrome?

a Maternal deletion of chromosome 15q11-q13

b Paternal chromosome 15 uniparental disomy

c UBE3A

d Imprinting defects

e Maternal chromosome 15 uniparental disomy

31 Which of the following is the *least* likely characteristic of Down syndrome?

a Triplication of chromosome 21 as a common genetic cause

b Increased risk of Alzheimer's dementia at an early age

c Physical findings including single palmar crease, hyperlax joints, and facial dysmorphisms

d Significant impairments in visual processing and strengths in language skills

e Relative strengths in social skills

32 All of the following statements regarding Fragile X syndrome are accurate *except*:

a As a leading cause of inherited intellectual disability, Fragile X syndrome has an incidence of 1/4,000 in males and 1/8,000 in females.

b Up to one-fourth of individuals with Fragile X syndrome meet criteria for autism spectrum disorder.

c Responsible gene: FMR1 is a mutation in the X-linked gene (Xq27.3).

d Females with the above gene are more likely to have intellectual disability than their male counterparts.

e Individuals with Fragile X syndrome show more impaired short-term memory and sequential information processing than long-term memory and theory of mind abilities.

33 All of the following statements concerning Rett syndrome are correct based on current knowledge and understanding of the condition *except*:

a Rett syndrome primarily affects females and rarely occurs in males.

b X-linked gene MECP2 mutations are responsible for all the cases.

c Mutations of MECP2 gene lead to inappropriate expression of the gene.

d Diagnosis is usually made based on clinical features, supported by identified genetic mutation.

e Rett syndrome is associated with a higher risk of developing scoliosis and arrhythmias with QTC prolongation.

34 Support services for families of individuals with intellectual disabilities are usually available through the Division of Developmental Disabilities of each state. All of the followings are useful resources more geared toward the families and individuals with intellectual disabilities *except*:

a American Association on Intellectual Disability and Developmental Disabilities (AAIDD)

b The ARC of the United States

c Division on Developmental Disabilities of the Council for Exceptional Children

d Wrightslaw Special Education Law and Advocacy

e National Alliance for the Mentally Ill (NAMI)

35 All of the following are common characteristics of fetal alcohol syndrome *except*:

a Microphthalmia (small eyeballs)

b Short palpebral fissures

c Midface hyperplasia

d Smooth or short philtrum

e Thin upper lip

36 All of the following statements regarding velocardiofacial syndrome are accurate *except*:

a Velocardiofacial syndrome is also known as DiGeorge syndrome, craniofacial syndrome, and 22q11 deletion syndrome.

b Deletion or mutations of the TBX1gene at 22q11 is believed to be responsible for the phenotypic features of the syndrome.

c Receptive language skills are more delayed than expressive language skills.

d The prevalence of this syndrome is between 1/10,000 and 1/4,000 in the United States.

e Up to 30% of people with this syndrome may develop major psychiatric disorders such as schizophrenia and bipolar disorder.

37 Williams syndrome is caused by a deletion on chromosome 7 and is characterized by distinct facial features, varied degree of intellectual disabilities, connective tissue abnormalities, failure to thrive, growth deficiency, cardiovascular diseases, and a unique cognitive profile. All of the following are accurate descriptions of Williams syndrome *except*:

a Deletions can occur to a number of genes at 7q11.23 on chromosome 7; thus it is one of the contiguous gene syndromes.

b Individuals with Williams syndrome have more delayed visuospatial construction whereas they have strengths in verbal short-term memory and language.

c Individuals with Williams syndrome may have excessively friendly and anxious personality traits.

d Prefrontal cortices are more impaired compared to the posterior structures.

e Some studies show deletion of the elastin gene may be responsible for certain characteristics of Williams syndrome.

38 There are no FDA-approved medications that are specifically indicated for individuals with intellectual disability. However, studies show that one-third of this population receives at least one psychotropic drug, which creates significant public concern for "overmedication." Based on the most recent studies, all of the following related statements regarding psychopharmacologic treatment in this population are correct *except*:

a Risperidone and aripiprazole are not FDA approved for intellectual disability but for the treatment of irritability in individuals with autism spectrum disorder.

b One recent survey in the United Kingdom showed risperidone was the most commonly prescribed medication by child and adolescent psychiatrists specializing in intellectual disability.

c Antipsychotics should be avoided in individuals with intellectual disability because most patients who receive treatment with antipsychotics for non-psychotic symptomologies receive little if any benefit and experience many side effects.

d Behavioral activation to selective serotonin reuptake inhibitors (SSRIs) occurs more often in children and in individuals with intellectual disability.

e Clonidine may have a role in treating impulsivity and hyperactivity in children with intellectual disability.

39 All of the following are considered as X-linked recessive disorders *except*:

a Fragile X syndrome

b Lesch-Nyhan syndrome

c Lissencephaly (double cortex)

d Spinobular muscular atrophy

e Wilson disease

40 All of the following statements concerning lissencephaly are accurate *except*:

a Lissencephalies consist of several syndromes such as isolated lissencephaly (ILS), Miller-Dicker syndrome (MDS), and X-linked lissencephaly (double cortex).

b Disruption of neuronal migration occurs in these conditions.

c Cortical surfaces have more gyri and sulci due to an increased number of layers.

d LIS-1 was identified in MDS and was believed to be associated with disruptions of cytoskeletal proteins.

e X-linked lissencephaly (double cortex) is associated with intellectual disability and epilepsy.

41 All of the following statements correctly describe the DSM-5 diagnostic criteria for Attention-Deficit/Hyperactivity Disorder *except*:

a ADHD is categorized under neurodevelopmental disorders and separated from oppositional and defiant disorder and conduct disorder (which are under "disruptive, impulse-control, and conduct disorders").

b Six of nine criteria have to be met for children under age 17.

c Five of nine criteria have to be met for individuals age 17 and older.

d Several of the symptoms have to be present prior to age 7.

e Specifiers can be used to distinguish different presentations (combined, predominantly inattentive, predominantly hyperactivity/impulsivity) and to describe severity (mild, moderate, and severe) and progress (in partial remission).

42 All of the following statements regarding ADHD are accurate *except*:

a Before age 4, ADHD symptoms are more difficult to distinguish from normative behaviors.

b Environmental risk factors may include extreme low birth weight, history of child abuse, neglect, multiple foster placements, neurotoxin exposure, infections, and prenatal alcohol exposure.

c African American children are more likely to be identified with ADHD than Caucasian populations in the United States.

d ADHD is highly heritable with elevated prevalence in first-degree relatives.

e ADHD occurs more frequently in males than in females (with a male:female ratio approximately of 2:1 in children).

43 Family adoption studies, twin studies, and molecular genetic studies on the genetics of ADHD indicate ADHD has a very high heritability. Many genes have been suspected to be related to ADHD and have been studied extensively. People who carry any of the following alleles increase the odds ratio for ADHD *except*:

a Catecholamine-O-methyl transferase (COMT) gene

b Dopamine D4 receptor, DRD4 7-repeat allele

c Dopamine D5 receptor, a dinucleotide repeat near the transcription start site

d Dopamine transporter, a 10-repeat sequence in the 3'untranslated region

e Dopamine beta-hydroxylase gene (DBH)

44 Numerous neuroimaging studies have been conducted to identify differences between people with ADHD and control groups. Some structural brain abnormalities were found in ADHD. Here is the list of brain regions that showed smaller volume in ADHD compared to that of control groups *with the exception of*:

a Prefrontal cortex

b Hippocampus

c Caudate

d Corpus callosum

e Cerebellum

45 Functional neuroimaging techniques such as single photon emission computed tomography (SPECT), positron emission tomography (PET), functional MRI (fMRI), and proton magnetic resonance spectroscopy (PMRS) can obtain dynamic measures of brain metabolisms at rest and during certain cognitive tasks. All of the following statements correctly describe the findings of the studies using these techniques in studying ADHD *except*:

a SPECT studies found hypoperfusion in various cortical areas such as the prefrontal cortex, striatum, and cerebellum.

b fMRI studies found decreased cerebral blood flow to the frontal cortex, prefrontal cortex, and basal ganglia, and decreased activation of these regions during certain cognitive tasks.

c PET studies found decreased glucose metabolism in the prefrontal/frontal and other cortical areas and reduced metabolic rates in the same areas during certain cognitive tasks.

d Some dopamine transporter (DAT) binding studies using SPECT and PET showed positive findings.

e PMRS studies found decreased glutamate in the right prefrontal cortex and left striatum.

46 Electroencephalogram (EEG) has been used to study ADHD for many years. All of the following related statements are correct *except*:

a Analytic approaches have been used including quantitative EEG studies, waveform amplitude studies, power studies, ratio coefficients studies, and coherence studies.

b Most studies find elevated levels of slow wave activity in children with ADHD compared to children without ADHD.

c Elevated relative theta power and reduced amounts of relative alpha and beta waves are seen in children with ADHD.

d Based on EEG studies, three models of ADHD are proposed including the maturational lag model, the developmental deviation model, and the hypoarousal model.

e These models successfully explain the electrophysiological endophenotypes of ADHD.

47 According to DSM-5, based on population surveys which pair of the following numbers reflects ADHD prevalence rates of children and adults respectively?

a 2% and 1%

b 5% and 2.5%

c 7.5% and 5%

d 10% and 7%

e 12% and 8%

48 Even though not diagnostic, some soft neurological signs and minor physical anomalies may increase confidence in the ADHD diagnosis. All of the following are such signs or anomalies *except*:

a Hypertelorism

b Highly arched palate

c Macrocephaly

d Deficits in balance and motor planning

e Deficits in sensory integration

49 Longitudinal studies on the course of ADHD show a variety of rates of ADHD continuing into adulthood from childhood. Adult samples show which of the following differences from children with ADHD?

a Exaggerated male>female predominance

b Greater homogeneity of symptoms

c Steady decrease in impulsivity across adolescence

d Hyperactivity being replaced by restlessness in adulthood

e Persistent inattentiveness

50 Which of the following psychotropic medications is *least* likely to be beneficial in the treatment of ADHD (without comorbidity)?

a Amphetamine (Adderall)

b Atomoxetine (Strattera)

c Clonidine (Catapres)

d Fluoxetine (Prozac)

e Bupropion (Wellbutrin)

51 Parent- and teacher-implemented behavior therapy is the only validated psychosocial intervention in managing ADHD. All of the followings are some of the key principles of parent/teacher behavior therapy in treating ADHD *except*:

a Learning information about the nature of ADHD

b Learning to attend more carefully to the child's misbehavior and to when the child complies

c Establishing a home token economy

d Identifying cognitive distortion

e Using daily school report card

52 All of the following statements regarding using stimulants to treat ADHD are correct *except*:

a Research data supports efficacy in both amphetamine agents and methylphenidate agents.

b Long-acting agents are found to have similar efficacies and safety compared to immediate-release counterparts.

c Preschool ADHD Treatment Study (PATS) showed preschoolers respond to amphetamine agents with lower dose than school-aged children.

d It is preferable to start with low dose and gradually titrate it up to optimal dosage.

e It is acceptable to initiate with a long-acting agent without establishing dose with immediate-release agents.

53 Among all of the following FDA-approved brand-name stimulant agents for ADHD which one is considered a prodrug?

a Daytrana

b Concerta

c Focalin

d Adderall

e Vyvanse

54 Based on DSM-5, all of the following statements regarding diagnosis of specific learning disorder are correct *except*:

a Criterion A lists a total of six symptoms describing difficulties in learning and using academic skills.

b To diagnose specific learning disorder, at least two of the six symptoms in Criterion A have to be present.

c Criterion B requests a documented history of impairing learning difficulties, which may be substituted for the standardized assessments for individuals age 17 and older.

d DSM-5 requires specifying all academic domains and subskills that are impaired by using different coding.

e Severity can be categorized into mild, moderate, and severe.

55 DSM-5 uses the term "dyslexia" to describe impairment in reading. Which of the following aspects should *not* be included under dyslexia?

a Problems with accurate word recognition

b Problems with fluent word recognition

c Problems with poor word decoding

d Problems with poor spelling abilities

e Problems with reading comprehension

56 DSM-5 uses the term "dyscalculia" to describe impairment in mathematics. Which of the following aspects should *not* be included under dyscalculia?

a Problems with processing numerical information

b Problems with learning arithmetic facts

c Problems with performing accurate calculations

d Problems with performing fluent calculations

e Problems with math reasoning

57 What is the prevalence of specific learning disorder across the academic domains in school-aged children across different languages and cultures?

a 1–2%

b 2–4%

c 5–15%

d 15–20%

e 20–25%

58 The Individuals with Disabilities Education Act (IDEA, Public Law 105–17) was amended in 2004. It recognizes all of the following categories as having a disability *except*:

a Autism

b Emotional disturbance

c Seizure disorders

d Specific learning disability

e Visual impairment

59 Based on the reauthorized and amended IDEA of 2004, local educational agencies can choose to use the responsiveness to intervention (RTI) model that has better evidence of support. All of the following are characteristics of the RTI model *except*:

a Severe discrepancy between IQ and achievement scores is required.

b Comparison of performance of the student in question with the performance of the student's peers on academic tasks is required.

c The model is structured primarily by individualized interventions and accommodations with a goal of maximizing the effectiveness of the learning environment.

d The model is multilayered/multitiered, with each layer/tier offering a chance for further differentiation and individualization of education for students in need.

e Special learning disability can be established only after these multilayered attempts are failed.

60 Which of the following is *not* one of the central features of the RTI model?

a High-quality classroom instruction

b Research-based instruction

c Classroom performance measures

d Universal screening

e Varied duration, time, and frequency of intervention

61 Based on DSM-5, which of the following terms is *not* used under the category of motor disorders?

a Developmental coordination disorder

b Stereotypic movement disorder

c Tourette's disorder

d Persistent (chronic) motor or vocal tic disorder

e Transient tic disorder

62 Developmental coordination disorder is *not* commonly diagnosed before which of the following ages?

a Age 1

b Age 3

c Age 5

d Age 7

e Age 9

63 All of the following statements regarding diagnosing stereotypic movement disorder based on DSM-5 are correct *except*:

a Repetitive, seemingly driven, and apparently purposeless motor behavior is present.

b The behavior interferes with social, academic, or other activities.

c The behavior is not attributable to the physiological effects of a substance or neurological condition.

d The behavior persists for four weeks or longer.

e When the stereotypic movement disorder co-occurs with another medical condition, both conditions should be coded.

64 Which of the following is the accurate cut-off duration to distinguish persistent (chronic) motor or vocal tic disorder from provisional tic disorder?

a Three months

b Six months

c One year

d Eighteen months

e Two years

65 All of the following statements regarding tics are correct *except*:

a Tics are involuntary yet can be suppressed with voluntary efforts at certain times.

b Tics can have a waxing and waning pattern with variable frequency and intensity throughout the day, across months, and even across years.

c Unlike other movement disorders, tics do not occur during sleep.

d Premonitory urges can precede tics.

e Persons with Tourette's disorder may have obsessions that are aggressive, sexual, and religious in nature.

66 During which of the following age groups do symptoms of Tourette's disorder peak?

a Ages of 2–3

b Ages of 3–5

c Ages of 5–8

d Ages of 8–12

e Ages of 12–14

67 All of the following statements regarding comorbid conditions with Tourette's disorder are correct *except*:

a Children with Tourette's disorder have a higher rate of comorbid obsessive-compulsive and related disorders and ADHD.

b Tics occur about two years prior to the onset of ADHD symptoms.

c Obsessive and compulsive symptoms commonly occur after the onset of tics around the ages of 12–13.

d Children with comorbid Tourette's disorder and obsessive-compulsive and related disorders have a higher rate of developing anxiety/mood disorders, oppositional defiant disorder, and conduct disorder.

e Compared to children with obsessive-compulsive and related disorders, children with Tourette's disorder usually have earlier onset of obsessive and compulsive symptoms.

68 All of the following statements regarding genetic etiological factors of Tourette's disorder and other tic disorders are correct *except*:

a Twin studies suggested a strong genetic component.

b Tourette's disorder may be caused by a single gene inherited with an autosomal dominant pattern.

c Sib-pair studies do not support association between some candidate genes such as DRD2 and DRD4 on chromosomal regions of 11q22 and 11p15, respectively.

d Incidence of male offspring of a parent with Tourette's disorder developing tic disorders is higher than female offspring.

e Frame-shift mutation of the SLITRK1 gene and a micro-RNA binding site variant were identified in certain people with Tourette's disorder.

69 All of the following statements regarding perinatal etiological factors for Tourette's disorder and other tic disorders are correct *except*:

a A study found children with tics were at 1.5 times higher risk to have mothers who experienced a complication during pregnancy.

b In monozygotic twin studies of Tourette's disorder, index twins had lower birth weights than unaffected twins.

c Potential risk factors may include maternal life stress during pregnancy and severe nausea/vomiting during the first trimester.

d Premature birth and low birth weight are risk factors.

e Few prenatal visits are associated with a higher risk.

70 All of the following statements regarding neuroanatomical etiological factors for Tourette's disorder and other tic disorders are correct *except*:

a Tics are associated with abnormal functioning in basal ganglia and cortico-striatal thalamo-cortical (CSTC) loop circuits.

b The basal ganglia can be viewed as a way station between intent and action in CSTC loops.

c Lower total neuron number was found in the globus pallidus pars interna (GPi) whereas a higher neuron number and density was found in the globus pallidus pars externa (GPe) and in the caudate nucleus.

d Effectiveness of dopamine-depleting agents (tetrabenazine and alpha-methyl-paratyrosine) and dopaminergic receptor antagonists (pimozide, haloperidol) in the reduction of tics provides support for the involvement of CSTC and basal ganglia.

e MRI studies show smaller caudate volumes in people with Tourette's disorder.

71 All of the following conditions share common anatomic targets (the basal ganglia and related cortical and thalamic sites) *except*:

a Sydenham's chorea (SC)

b Tourette's disorder (TS)

c Obsessive-compulsive and related disorders (OCD)

d ADHD

e Major depressive disorder (MDD)

72 There are some common differences between stereotypic movements/behaviors and complex motor tics. Which of the following is *not* characteristic of stereotypic movements/behaviors?

a An earlier age of onset (2 to 3 versus 6 years)

b Unilateral in nature

c More stable presentation over time

d Less waxing and waning course

e None of the above

73 According to DSM-5, which of the following diagnoses is *most* appropriately considered for a 20-year-old male who recently started experiencing symptoms characteristic of a tic disorder but the symptoms do not meet the full criteria for a tic disorder?

a Provisional tic disorder

b Other specified tic disorder

c Unspecified tic disorder

d Other specified neurodevelopmental disorder

e Unspecified neurodevelopmental disorder

74 All of the following statements regarding non-pharmacological interventions for tic disorders are correct *except*:

a Education is very important not only for family members, but also for teachers and peers.

b Advocacy organizations such as the TS Association, the Obsessive Compulsive Foundation, and the Children and Adults with Attention Deficit Disorder can be good resources for the families.

c Habit reversal training (HRT) is the first behavioral intervention with promising effectiveness.

d It is important for parents and teachers to consistently point out the child's tics so the child can try to stop the tic behaviors.

e Strong relationships between therapists and patients predict better outcome when using behavioral interventions.

75 Habit reversal training (HRT) has two main focuses: awareness training and competing response practice. All of the following are components of awareness training *except*:

a Response description

b Response detection

c Early warning procedure

d Situational awareness training

e Production of an incompatible physical response

76 Which of the following pharmacologic agents has the *least* evidence for benefit in the treatment of Tourette's disorder?

a Guanfacine

b Clozapine

c Risperidone

d Ziprasidone

e Olanzapine

77 M. S. Durkin et al. (2008) studied the relationship between advanced parental age and the risk of autism spectrum disorders in older parents' offspring. They found firstborn offspring of two older parents are more likely to develop autism. Which of the following numbers is the *closest* odds ratio indicated in the study?

a 1

b 3

c 6

d 9

e 12

78 Kabir et al. (2011) examined the association between second-hand smoke exposure (SHS) and parent-reported neurobehavioral disorders (ADHD, learning disabilities, conduct disorder, and oppositional defiant disorder) in youth. What is the percentage of increased odds for children exposed to SHS having two or more childhood neurobehavioral disorders compared to those who were not exposed to SHS?

a 20%

b 30%

c 40%

d 50%

e 60%

Matching

79–82 For each of the syndromes usually associated with intellectual disability listed below, select one description that fits it *best*:

a Diet prevents intellectual disability

b Obesity

c Microcephaly and medal epicanthal folds

d Long face and predominant chin

79 Prader-Willi syndrome

80 Down syndrome

81 Phenylketonuria

82 Fragile X syndrome

83–87 A number of neuropsychological tests can be used to measure different aspects of executive functioning. Please match the following specific functioning measured to the listed tests:

a Continuous Performance Test

b Wisconsin Card Sorting Test

   c Tower of Hanoi/London

   d Digits Backward Test

   e Self-Ordered Pointing Test

83 Spatial working memory

84 Working verbal memory

85 Planning ability

86 Set shifting

87 Response inhibition

88–90 Levy and Hyman (2008) reviewed existing literature and proposed a grade system to indicate the strength of evidence that supports or refutes particular complementary and alternative medicine treatments for children with autism spectrum disorders as grade A (randomized controlled trials, reviews, and/or meta-analysis), grade B (other evidence such as isolated well-designed controlled and uncontrolled studies), or grade C (case reports or theories). Please match the following specific therapies to the listed grades:

   a Grade A

   b Grade B

   c Grade C

88 Vitamin B6, magnesium, Vitamin C, melatonin, carnosine, dimethylglycine, fatty acids, gluten-free/casein-free diet, auditory integration, and music therapy

89 Yoga, amino acids, folate, oxidative stress, gastrointestinal medications, hyperbaric oxygen therapy, chelation, antibiotics, immune therapies, antifungal agents, chiropractic, craniosacral massage, and massage/therapeutic touch therapies

90 Secretin

ANSWERS AND EXPLANATIONS

1 **(d)** Reactive Attachment Disorder is included in the Trauma- and Stressor-Related Disorders chapter of DSM-5. *(Ref. 4, pp. 265–268)*

2 **(c)** Asperger's disorder was not singled out and was subsumed under autism spectrum disorder. The term itself was eliminated. Those individuals who were previously diagnosed with Asperger's disorder under DSM-IV should be diagnosed with autism spectrum disorder under DSM-5. Additional specifiers such as "without accompanying intellectual impairment" and "without accompanying language impairment" can be helpful in identifying the lack of deficits in such areas. Under DSM-5, both autism spectrum disorder and ADHD can be given to the same individual. *(Ref. 4, pp. 50–55)*

3 **(c)** DSM-5 does not call for a strict IQ score threshold to meet Criterion A (deficits in intellectual functions) for diagnosis. DSM-5 notes, "Individuals with intellectual disability have scores of approximately two standard deviations or more below the population mean, including a margin for measurement error (generally ± 5 points). On tests with a standard deviation of 15 and a mean of 100, this involves a score of 65–75 (70 ± 5). Clinical training and judgment are required to interpret test results and assess intellectual performance." *(Ref. 4, p. 37)*

4 **(c)** "Flynn effect" may artificially increase test scores because of out-of-date test norms and practice effects. Population mean IQ is 100, and 15 points is one standard deviation. Thus, two standard deviations lower than population mean is 70. Considering a margin of measurement error of five points, individuals with lower than 65–75 (70 ± 5) will meet Criterion A of intellectual disability. Because of a variety of factors that can influence test scores, clinical judgment is needed in interpreting the results of IQ tests. *(Ref. 4, p. 37)*

5 **(d)** Impairments in at least one of the three domains are needed to qualify for Criterion B, and they must be directly related to the intellectual deficits in Criterion A. Many factors (such as sensory and physical impairments, severe behavioral problems, locomotor disability, and co-occurring mental disorder, etc.) may make it difficult or impossible to administer standardized measures. In such cases, individuals can be diagnosed with unspecified intellectual disability. Clinicians should always use clinical judgment to interpret scores from standardized measures and interview sources. *(Ref. 4, pp. 37–38)*

6 **(d)** While overall general population prevalence of intellectual disability is approximately 1%, the approximate prevalence of severe intellectual disability is 6 per 1000 (about 0.6%). Individuals with severe intellectual disability have limited attainment of conceptual skills, have limited spoken language in terms of vocabulary and grammar, and require support for all activities of daily living. *(Ref. 4, pp. 36, 38)*

7 **(d)** Intellectual disability is generally nonprogressive although the course may be influenced negatively by many factors such as underlying medical or genetic conditions and other co-occurring conditions. Sanfilippo syndrome follows a progressive worsening course of intellectual disability whereas Rett syndrome may have periods of worsening followed by stabilization. On the other hand, early and ongoing interventions may improve adaptive functioning throughout the life span, which may also lead to improvement of intellectual functioning. If the improved adaptive skills result from a stable, generalized skill acquisition the diagnosis may no longer be appropriate, whereas the diagnosis is still appropriate if the improvement is contingent on the presence of supports and ongoing interventions. *(Ref. 4, pp. 38–39)*

8 **(e)** In general, males are more likely to be diagnosed with intellectual disability due to possible sex-linked genetic factors and male vulnerability to brain insult. The average male:female ratio is 1.6:1 for mild forms of intellectual disability and 1.2:1 for severe forms. Risk factors for intellectual disability include prenatal factors (genetic syndromes, inborn errors of metabolism, brain malformations, maternal diseases, and exposure to alcohol, drugs, or toxins), perinatal factors (various labor/delivery-related events, e.g. neonatal encephalopathy), and postnatal factors (hypoxic ischemic injury, traumatic brain injury, infections, seizures, and intoxications—lead, mercury). *(Ref. 4, p. 39)*

9 **(a)** A diagnosis of intellectual disability *cannot* be assumed because of the existence of a medical or genetic condition that commonly causes intellectual disability. Intellectual disability diagnosis should be made if Criteria A, B, and C are met, and the genetic or medical condition linked to intellectual disability should be noted as a concurrent diagnosis. Intellectual disability is distinct from neurocognitive disorders—for instance, children with Down syndrome who are diagnosed with intellectual disability may also develop dementia (Alzheimer's disease) later on, in which case both diagnoses of intellectual disability and neurocognitive disorder may be given. *(Ref. 4, pp. 39–40)*

10 **(b)** Anorexia nervosa is the least likely comorbidity compared to many other conditions such as ADHD, depressive and bipolar disorders, anxiety disorders, autism spectrum disorder, stereotypic movement disorder, impulse-control disorders, and major neurocognitive disorder. As a vulnerable population, people with intellectual disability may have limited awareness of risks, which may result in exploitation by others, victimization, fraud, unintentional criminal involvement, and false confessions. They are at risk for suicide and may also exhibit aggression and disruptive behaviors. *(Ref. 4, pp. 38–40)*

11 **(c)** Unspecified intellectual disability is used for children over the age of 5 years when assessment of the degree of the intellectual disability is difficult or impossible because of the existence of sensory or physical impairments, locomotor disability, severe behavioral problems, or severe co-occurring mental disorder. Prior to age 5, if the clinical severity of intellectual functioning cannot be reliably assessed (e.g., too young to participate in standardized testing), the global developmental delay diagnosis can be given to individuals who fail to meet expected developmental milestones in several areas of intellectual functioning. *(Ref. 4, p. 41)*

12 (b) In contrast to DSM-IV, in DSM-5 phonological disorder was eliminated and replaced by speech sound disorder, and expressive language disorder and mixed receptive-expressive language were replaced by language disorder. Stuttering was changed to childhood-onset fluency disorder (stuttering). In addition, social (pragmatic) communication disorder was added. *(Ref. 4, p. 41)*

13 (e) As a part of the criteria for diagnosing language disorder, impairment of discourse refers to the inability to put words and sentences together in a narrative way to explain/describe a topic or event(s) or to carry a conversation. Reduced vocabulary (word knowledge) and limited sentence structure (mostly refer to grammar and morphology difficulties) are other important deficits of language disorder. Children with language disorder may have discrepant expressive ability and receptive ability, referring to the production of vocal, gestural, or verbal signs, and ability in receiving and comprehending language signals, respectively. Both aspects should be assessed during the evaluation of children with a possible language disorder. *(Ref. 4, p. 42)*

14 (b) Onset of symptoms of language disorder must be in the early developmental period (a criterion based on DSM-5). Even though there are tremendous individual variations in early vocabulary acquisition and word combination, by age 4 such differences become stable. Diagnosis of language disorder obtained at age 4 is likely to be stable over time and to be persistent into adulthood. *(Ref. 4, p. 43)*

15 (a) Children with Williams syndrome may have various degrees of intellectual disability, more in the area of visual-spatial deficits, but usually have strength in language and speech such as vocabulary, auditory memory, and social use of language. Children with Landau-Kleffner syndrome may lose their ability for speech and language and become aphasic. All other syndromes/conditions such as autism spectrum disorder, Fragile X syndrome, and Down syndrome can be associated with difficulties in speech and language to various extents. *(Ref. 3, p. 207; Ref. 4, pp. 43–45)*

16 (c) Monosyllabic whole-word repetition (e.g., "I-I-I-I saw you") is a feature of childhood-onset fluency disorder (stuttering) among other features such as sound and syllable repetitions, sound prolongations of consonants and vowels, broken words, audible or silent blocking, circumlocutions, and words produced with excess physical tension. All other descriptions are deficits seen in children with social communication disorder, which reflect the pragmatic aspect of communicational difficulties (deficits in understanding and following social rules of verbal and nonverbal communications in real-world situations, changing language based on the needs of the listener and situation, and following rules for conversations and storytelling). *(Ref. 4, pp. 45–48)*

17 (a) Many studies showed strong evidence of the importance of neurobiological factors in the pathogenesis of autism spectrum disorder, but no specific bio markers or precise pathogenic mechanisms are identified. Statistically speaking, individuals with autism spectrum disorder showed increased peripheral serotonin level, persistent primitive reflexes, increased head size, changes in brain morphology/cytoarchitecture, more failure to activate the fusiform face region, and high rates of EEG abnormality/seizure disorder. *(Ref. 3, pp. 386–388)*

18 (e) Many studies show that people with autism spectrum disorder have reduced levels of responsivity to the human face and performance deficits in face and facial expression recognition, which was evidenced by difficulties in processing certain facial features/information and tendency of focusing on the mouth rather than the eyes when observing social interactions and facial emotional expressions. Typically developing individuals tend to focus on eyes in this situation. *(Ref. 3, pp. 387–388)*

19 (d) There are two predictive factors that are more consistently associated with the outcome of autism: (1) intellectual functioning and (2) communicative competence. Individuals with low IQ/low intellectual functioning have overall poorer outcomes. *(Ref. 1, p. 392)*

20 (a) Autism is found less frequently associated with Down syndrome than in the general population. It is observed more commonly in all of the other syndromes listed. However, these associations are by no means invariable. *(Ref. 3, p. 390)*

21 (a) Recent studies showed that 80% of patients with typical Rett syndrome carry one of six known mutations in the encoding region of the X-linked MECP2 gene, which has been considered as the genetic etiology of Rett syndrome. Mutation of the FMR1 gene, deletion of an elastin gene, deletion of chromosome 15p11q13, and Trisomy 21 are possible genetic etiologies of Fragile X syndrome, Williams syndrome, Angelman syndrome, and Down syndrome, respectively. *(Ref. 3, pp. 205–210)*

22 (a) Alternative treatments are often used by parents of children with autism spectrum disorder. Even with a lot of anecdotal successful case reports or stories, most such treatments were not rigorously studied or evaluated. However, a series of well-controlled trials of the gut hormone secretin were conducted. Unfortunately, they failed to show significant improvement compared to placebo groups. Evidence shows that appropriate educational interventions are critical, behavioral modification approaches are often helpful, and collaboration among providers is important. Psychotherapy is not usually indicated, but it may be considered in higher-functioning children, e.g. in those without accompanying intellectual or language impairment. At this time, there is no known pharmacological agent used in the treatment of autism spectrum disorder that is curative. However, some antipsychotics such as risperidone and aripiprazole are clinically effective in reducing irritability and aggression. *(Ref. 3, pp. 392–393)*

23 (b) Criterion A, describing deficits in social communication, contains three areas of deficit that must all be met for diagnosing autism spectrum disorder: social-emotional reciprocity, nonverbal communication, and social relationships. Criterion B, describing restricted and repetitive behavior, interests, and activities, contains four items, at least two of which must be present: stereotyped or repetitive movements, use of objects, or speech; insistence on sameness, inflexible routines, or ritualized behavior; restricted, fixated interests; and sensory hyper- or hyporeactivity. *(Ref. 4, pp. 50–51)*

24 (d) The population prevalence of autism spectrum disorder across the United States and non-U.S. countries has approached 1% based on reports in recent years. Although the reasons for the increased prevalence rate are still not fully understood, speculations include the expansion of the diagnostic criteria of

DSM-IV, increased awareness, study methodology differences, or a true increase in frequency of autism spectrum disorder. *(Ref. 4, p. 55)*

25 **(b)** Regression and deterioration of autism spectrum disorder usually occur between 12 and 24 months of age compared to that found in Rett syndrome, which occurs usually after the second birthday. During the regressive phase of Rett syndrome, a lot of young girls' presentations are consistent with autism spectrum disorder, but many of them may eventually improve their social communication skills to the point they may no longer meet criteria for autism spectrum disorder. The other condition, childhood disintegrative disorder (previously described in DSM-IV), also has regression that occurs after age 2. If there is evidence of poor social and communication skills in childhood, and the criteria are met based on current clinical observations, autism spectrum disorder diagnosis can be given to affected adults. *(Ref. 4, pp. 55–56)*

26 **(d)** A comorbid diagnosis of stereotypic movement disorder should *not* be given when stereotypic movements exist in children who are diagnosed with autism spectrum disorder routinely unless stereotypic movements or repetitive behaviors cause self-injury and become a focus of treatment. *(Ref. 4, pp. 57–59)*

27 **(a)** Kaufman Assessment Battery for Children is a standardized test of intelligence. It is not a test that specifically measures adaptive functioning. Adaptive functioning assessment is an important aspect of evaluating and diagnosing intellectual disability. In addition to all other tests listed in the question, Adaptive Behavior Assessment System, 2nd Edition (ABAS-II) is also a measure of adaptive functioning. The Vineland Adaptive Behavior Scales come with both a "teacher form" and "survey, caregiver, and expanded forms," which provide information from different settings. *(Ref. 1, Ch. 7, Assessment of Intellectual and Adaptive Function section)*

28 **(e)** As standardized tests of intelligence, both the Leiter International Performance Scale-Revised and the Universal Non-verbal Intelligence Test (UNIT) measure only nonverbal problem-solving and reasoning abilities. That is why they are especially useful for children who are nonverbal or have significant language delays. None of the other tests listed in the question or the Wechsler Intelligence Scale for Children, 4th Edition (WISC-IV) can be used for children who are nonverbal. *(Ref. 1, Ch. 7, Assessment of Intellectual and Adaptive Function section)*

29 **(c)** Frequent laughter and happy demeanor are common in the presentation of Angelman syndrome among other features such as severe developmental delays with severe speech impairment, ataxia and/or tremulous movements in limbs, excitable personality, hand flapping, and short attention span. Other less consistent signs and symptoms may include delayed head growth (microcephaly) by age 2, seizures, abnormal electroencephalography (EEG), feeding problems, drooling, sleep disturbance, hypopigmented skin, strabismus, and prognathia. *(Ref. 1, Ch. 7, Congenital Syndromes and Neurobehavioral Phenotypes section)*

30 **(e)** Maternal chromosome 15 uniparental disomy causes almost 30% of Prader-Willi syndrome, and the rest is mostly caused by paternal deletion on chromosome 15q11-q13, the same region implicated in Angelman syndrome. All other listed answers are the known genetic mechanisms that cause Angelman syndrome. In contrast to Angelman syndrome, Prader-Willi syndrome presents with unique clinical features such as hypotonia, early obesity, hypogonadism, sleep apnea, and compulsive food-seeking/hoarding behaviors. *(Ref. 1, Ch. 7, Congenital Syndromes and Neurobehavioral Phenotypes section)*

31 **(d)** Significant impairments in language and strengths in visual processing and social skills relative to communication and other adaptive behavior skill domains are observed in individuals with Down syndrome. *(Ref. 1, Ch. 7, Congenital Syndromes and Neurobehavioral Phenotypes section)*

32 **(d)** Males with the FMR1 gene are more likely to have intellectual disability than their female counterparts. Cognitive impairments are more in the areas of short-term memory, sequential information processing, and sustaining attention, whereas long-term memory, processing simultaneous information, and theory of mind abilities are relative strengths. Behavioral characteristics can include hyperarousal, hyperactivity, social anxiety, shyness, and gaze aversion. There are also increased risks for schizotypal disorder and ADHD. *(Ref. 1, Ch. 7, Congenital Syndromes and Neurobehavioral Phenotypes section)*

33 **(b)** X-linked gene MECP2 mutations are responsible for more than 80% of the Rett syndrome cases. However, discovery was made of mutations in two other genes, CDKL5 and NTNG1. Mutations of MECP2 are suspected of interfering with the transcription and expression of the gene, which is believed to result in the gradual production of toxic products during the developmental period, which also helps to explain the regressive pattern of the condition after initial unremarkable development. With the vast majority of cases occurring in females, it does rarely affect males. Individuals with Rett syndrome have increased risk of developing QTC prolongation, so caution should be made in prescribing certain medications that may exacerbate such a problem. In the middle 20s, they may develop scoliosis, which can limit mobility. *(Ref. 1, Ch. 7, Congenital Syndromes and Neurobehavioral Phenotypes section; Ref. 3, Ch. 3.3, Molecular Basis of Select Childhood Psychiatric Disorders section)*

34 **(e)** The National Alliance for the Mentally Ill (NAMI) is a foundation that offers an array of free education and support programs for individuals, family members, providers, and the general public, and helps build better lives for the millions of Americans with mental illness (but not specifically for people with intellectual disabilities). In addition to all other organizations or agencies listed in the question, the National Dissemination Center for Children with Disabilities (NICHCY) is a useful resource for individuals with intellectual disabilities and their families. Other support services may include respite care, in-home behavioral interventions, and crisis interventions. *(Ref. 1, Ch. 7, Educational and Community Services and Supports section)*

35 **(c)** Midface hypoplasia (underdevelopment) can be a common characteristic of fetal alcohol syndrome. Individuals with fetal alcohol syndrome can also have growth retardation of weight and height, microcephaly, and may suffer from hyperactivity, attention deficits, learning disabilities, intellectual deficits, and

seizures. *(Ref. 6, Ch. 2.1, Acquired Developmental Factors section)*

36 **(c)** Receptive language skills are usually less delayed than expressive language skills, although overall speech difficulty, defects in phonation, language acquisition, comprehension, and social communication are all significant concerns for children with the syndrome. *(Ref. 1, Ch. 7, Educational and Community Services and Supports section)*

37 **(d)** Frontal cortices and the limbic system are relatively more preserved compared to the posterior structures such as parietal and occipital cortices that are known to be involved in visual processing. Elastin is involved in development of skin, blood vessels, and lung tissues, and deletion of such a gene may explain the vascular abnormalities and special facial features of the syndrome. Studies also show the deletion of another gene named LIM kinase in this region which may cause abnormalities in synaptic morphology and deficits in learning. *(Ref. 1, Ch. 7, Genetic and Molecular Basis of Intellectual Disability section; Ref. 3, Ch. 3.3, Molecular Basis of Select Childhood Psychiatric Disorders section)*

38 **(c)** While the side-effect profile of antipsychotic medications warrants caution in their use and dosing and in this population, and continued assessment for side effects and ongoing need for the medication, they have the greatest evidence base in managing aggression, irritability, and problem behaviors in patients with intellectual disability. *(Ref. 1, Ch. 7, Pharmacological Treatment section)*

39 **(e)** Wilson disease is an autosomal recessive disorder, and is caused by point mutations and deletions (copper-transporting ATPase) at 13q14.21. In addition to the rest of the disorders listed in the question, Duchenne dystrophy, Becker dystrophy, and Rett syndrome are all X-linked recessive disorders. *(Ref. 3, Ch. 3.3, Molecular Basis of Select Childhood Psychiatric Disorders section)*

40 **(c)** The cortical surface is smoother with an abnormal pattern of gyri and sulci and decreased number of layers from six to four in affected individuals of lissencephaly. *(Ref. 3, Ch. 3.3, Molecular Basis of Select Childhood Psychiatric Disorders section)*

41 **(d)** In contrast to DSM-IV, which used age 7 as the cut-off age for which some of the ADHD symptoms have to be present, DSM-5 requires several symptoms be present prior to age 12. In DSM-5, ADHD is still separated into three types, but called "presentations" (combined presentation, predominantly inattentive presentation, and predominantly hyperactive/impulsive presentation). There are still a total of nine criteria in each category, and six of nine are required for children and young adolescents, but only five of nine are needed for older individuals (age of >17). Different specifiers are designed for different purposes. Again, autism spectrum disorder is no longer a mutually exclusive condition. *(Ref. 4, pp. 59–61)*

42 **(c)** African Americans and Latino Americans are *less* likely to be identified with ADHD than Caucasian populations in the United States. This might be related to cultural variations in attitudes toward or interpretations of children's behaviors. Because of highly variable normative behaviors of toddlers before age 4, ADHD symptoms are less stable. In preschool, hyperactivity and impulsivity are more dominant,

and inattention becomes more prominent during elementary school. In adolescence, whereas hyperactivity and impulsivity subside, inattention can be more persistent. *(Ref. 4, pp. 61–63)*

43 **(a)** Pooled data showed no association between catecholamine-O-methyl transferase (COMT) gene and ADHD. However, in addition to the other genes listed in the question, synaptosomal-associated protein (SNAP-25 gene), SLC6A4 serotonin transporter gene, and serotonin 1 B receptor (HTR1B) gene are associated with increased risk for ADHD. *(Ref. 1, Ch. 10, Etiology and Risk Factors section; Ref. 3, Ch. 5.1, Attention-Deficit Hyperactivity Disorder section)*

44 **(b)** Instead of associations with the decreased volumes of many different brain regions, the hippocampus showed increased volume bilaterally in a large sample of children with ADHD compared to the control group. *(Ref. 1, Ch. 10, Neurocircuitry section; Ref. 3, Ch. 5.1, Attention-Deficit Hyperactivity Disorder section)*

45 **(e)** PMRS studies found elevated glutamate in the right prefrontal cortex and left striatum. A few SPECT studies showed elevated DAT binding in ADHD subjects compared to controls, and a PET study also showed elevated DAT binding in the striatum in ADHD subjects compared to controls, which provides additional evidence supporting the role of dopamine in the etiology and treatment response of ADHD. Most studies consistently show hypoperfusion of frontal/prefrontal and striatal areas and reduced cerebral activation during certain cognitive tasks in children with ADHD. *(Ref. 3, Ch. 5.1, Attention-Deficit Hyperactivity Disorder section)*

46 **(e)** In an attempt to separate ADHD into different subtypes based on EEG studies, none of the models can account for the complex clinical presentation of ADHD. Attempts have been made to combine EEG and event-related potentials (ERPs) techniques to identify the electrophysiological endophenotypes of ADHD, but more studies are needed. *(Ref. 3, Ch. 5.1, Attention-Deficit Hyperactivity Disorder section)*

47 **(b)** Across different cultures, prevalence of ADHD is 5% and 2.5% in children and adults respectively. *(Ref. 4, p. 61)*

48 **(c)** Macrocephaly is not a physical anomaly commonly seen in children with ADHD. Children with autism spectrum disorder may have macrocephaly at times. Children with ADHD do commonly show difficulty in balance and motor control and deficits in sensory integration. Data suggest significant correlation between the soft neurological signs and decreased cerebral blood flow in frontal lobes in children with ADHD. Medical history and a physical exam may help to elicit such signs and anomalies. *(Ref. 3, Ch. 5.1, Attention-Deficit Hyperactivity Disorder section); Ref. 4, p. 62)*

49 **(b)** Compared to children with ADHD, adult samples of individuals with ADHD show a lower male:female ratio, approximating 2:1 or even 1:1; more heterogeneity and subtley of symptoms; waning hyperactivity being replaced by a feeling of restlessness; and persistent inattentiveness. Impulsivity also tends to wane but may have a spike in adolescence. *(Ref. 1, Ch. 7, Course and Prognosis section)*

50 **(d)** First-line treatments of ADHD are still stimulants or atomoxetine. Other alternatives may include Intuniv, Kapvay, clonidine, guanfacine (Tenex), bupropion (Wellbutrin), etc. However, SSRIs have not been found effective in treating core

symptoms of ADHD although they can be considered in the treatment of comorbid conditions such as depression and anxiety. *(Ref. 1, Ch. 7, Treatment section; Ref. 3, Ch. 5.1, Attention-Deficit Hyperactivity Disorder section)*

51 **(d)** Identifying cognitive distortion is a technique used in cognitive behavioral therapy (CBT). However, CBT has not been shown effective in treating children with ADHD. Behavior therapy is a mainstream validated treatment approach in which a number of key principles are applied: learning information about the nature of ADHD, learning to attend more carefully to the child's misbehavior and to when the child complies, establishing a home token economy, using timeout effectively, managing noncompliant behaviors in public settings, using a daily school report card, and anticipating future misconduct. *(Ref. 1, Ch. 7, Treatment section)*

52 **(c)** The Preschool ADHD Treatment Study (PATS) funded by NIMH showed preschoolers responded to methylphenidate agents with lower dose (0.7mg/kg/day) than school-aged children (in MTA study). *(Ref. 1, Ch. 7, Treatment section; Ref. 3, Ch. 5.1, Attention-Deficit Hyperactivity Disorder section)*

53 **(e)** Vyvanse (lisdexamfetamine dimesylate) is a d-amphetamine that is bound to the amino acid l-lysine. This is a nonactive compound until it is converted to d-amphetamine in the body after d-amphetamine broken apart from l-lysine results from enzymatic hydrolysis following oral administration. Speed of conversion of Vyvanse, the prodrug, to the active compound, d-amphetamine, is dependent on the rate-limited production of the appropriate enzyme (lysinase) that is responsible for the hydrolysis, which creates the long-acting fashion of this drug. *(Ref. 1, Ch. 34, Stimulants section)*

54 **(b)** To diagnose specific learning disorder, at least one of the six symptoms listed in Criterion A has to be present. Each two of six symptoms are used to describe difficulties in reading, written expression, and mathematics, respectively. Even when the onset of learning difficulties starts during the early school years, they may not become apparent or fully manifested until the academic demands exceed the individual's capacities to cope. DSM-5 also requires that the learning difficulties cannot be better explained by intellectual disabilities, uncorrected visual/auditory impairments, other mental or neurological conditions, psychosocial adversity, lack of proficiency in the language of academic instruction, or inadequate educational instruction. *(Ref. 4, pp. 66–67, 70–71)*

55 **(e)** Difficulty with reading comprehension is not included in dyslexia. Dyslexia refers to a pattern of learning difficulties and problems with accurate or fluent word recognition, poor decoding, and poor spelling abilities. Reading comprehension should be specified as additional difficulty, if applicable, if *dyslexia* is chosen to describe reading impairment. *(Ref. 4, p. 67)*

56 **(e)** Difficulty with math reasoning is not included in dyscalculia. Dyscalculia refers to a pattern of learning difficulties and problems with processing numerical information, learning arithmetic facts, and performing accurate or fluent calculations. Math reasoning should be specified as an additional difficulty, if applicable, if *dyscalculia* is chosen to describe mathematics impairment. *(Ref. 4, p. 67)*

57 **(c)** About 5–15% of school-aged children across different languages and cultures suffer from a specific learning disorder

across the academic domains of reading, writing, and mathematics. In the adult population, the prevalence is unknown with an estimation of 4%. *(Ref. 4, p. 70)*

58 **(c)** The Individuals with Disabilities Education Act (IDEA, Public Law 105–17) was amended in 2004, and it recognizes 13 categories under which a child can be identified as having disability including: "autism; deaf-blindness; deafness; emotional disturbance; hearing impairment; mental retardation; multiple disabilities; orthopedic impairment; other health impairment; traumatic brain injury; and visual impairment." Seizure disorders are not considered as one of the categories. *(Ref. 3, Ch. 5.2, Learning Disabilities section)*

59 **(a)** The most widely used model to identify special learning disabilities prior to the 2004 reauthorization of IDEA was the aptitude–achievement discrepancy model that required severe discrepancy between IQ and achievement scores (e.g., two standard deviations, two years of age equivalence). Since 2004, local educational agencies can choose to use different diagnostic models. RTI is considered an evidence-supported model that has a number of characteristics illustrated in answers (b) through (e). Answer (a) describes the characteristic of the discrepancy model. With the amendment of IDEA, local educational agencies find it really challenging to fully implement the RTI model. *(Ref. 3, Ch. 5.2, Learning Disabilities section)*

60 **(e)** Varied duration, time, and frequency of intervention is one of the common attributes of different RTI models, which are concepts of: (1) multiple tiers, (2) transition from instruction for all to increasingly intense interventions, (3) implementation of differentiated curricula, (4) instruction delivered by staff other than the classroom teacher, (5) varied duration, time, and frequency of intervention, and (6) categorical or noncategorical placement decisions. Eight central features of the RTI were identified including: (1) high-quality classroom instruction, (2) research-based instruction, (3) classroom performance monitoring, (4) universal screening, (5) continuous progress monitoring, (6) research-based intervention, (7) progress monitoring during intervention, and (8) fidelity measures. *(Ref. 3, Ch. 5.2, Learning Disabilities section)*

61 **(e)** In DSM-IV, there was only one disorder—developmental coordination disorder listed under "motor skills disorder"—and tic disorders were categorized separately, including Tourette's disorder, chronic motor or vocal tic disorder, and transient tic disorder. This latter category is largely preserved in DSM-5 under "motor disorders" with slight modification; that is, chronic motor or vocal tic disorder was changed to "persistent (chronic) motor or vocal tic disorder" with added specifiers to identify "with motor tics only" or "with vocal tics only." Further, transient tic disorder is no longer used in DSM-5 but is now referred to as "provisional tic disorder." In DSM-5, motor disorders include: developmental coordination disorder, stereotypic movement disorder, and tic disorders. *(Ref. 4, pp. 74–85)*

62 **(c)** According to the diagnostic criteria of DSM-5, the onset of symptoms of developmental coordination disorder should occur in the early developmental period. However, there is significant variation in the time frame when children acquire their different motor skills and there is a lack of stability of measurement in early childhood. Thus, it is uncommon that a developmental coordination disorder diagnosis is given to children under the age of 5 years. *(Ref. 4, pp. 74–75)*

63 **(d)** The criteria "the behavior persists for 4 weeks or longer" existed in DSM-IV and was eliminated in DSM-5. In DSM-5, stereotypic movement disorder is allowed to co-occur with other medical or neurogenetic disorders, such as Lesch-Nyhan syndrome, Rett syndrome, Fragile X syndrome, Cornelia de Lange syndrome, and Smith-Magenis syndrome, and both conditions are required to be coded. *(Ref. 4, pp. 77–80)*

64 **(c)** Both Tourette's disorder and persistent (chronic) motor or vocal tic disorder require at least one year duration of tics that can wax and wane in frequency, which is less than one year in the case of provisional tic disorder. DSM-5 eliminated other time duration requirements mentioned in DSM-IV—that is, not tic-free for more than three months in Tourette's disorder or chronic tic motor or vocal tic disorder, and at least for four weeks in transient tic disorder. Still, all the tic disorders require an age of onset before 18. *(Ref. 4, p. 81)*

65 **(c)** Unlike other movement disorders, tics *may* occur during sleep. About 75–80% of persons with persistent tic disorder or Tourette's disorder experience premonitory urges such as localized tingling, itch-like sensations, tensions in muscles, or ideation of making sounds, movements, or gestures preceding the tic events. Obsessions can be another type of mental event associated with tics. Compared to people with obsessive-compulsive and related disorders, people with persistent motor or vocal tics disorder and Tourette's disorder are more likely to have aggressive, sexual, and religious obsessions and less likely to have obsessions about contaminations, neatness, and cleanliness. Tics can be triggered by emotionally stimulating events, such as exciting, pleasuring, stressful, or distressing situations. *(Ref. 1, Ch. 20, Definition and Clinical Description section)*

66 **(d)** The severity of tics of Tourette's disorder tends to wax and wane throughout the course of the disorder, with high variability. Tics can also come in bouts or clusters. However, tic severity starts to dissipate with the onset of puberty and generally peaks at ages 8–12 even though a minority of cases can persist into adulthood. *(Ref. 3, Ch. 5.6, Clinical Course section)*

67 **(b)** When Tourette's disorder and ADHD are comorbid, the ADHD symptoms precede the onset of tics by about two years. Obsessive and compulsive symptoms tend to occur after the peak of tics around ages 12–13. However, children with obsessive-compulsive and related disorders without Tourette's disorder comorbidity tend to experience obsession and compulsion during late adolescence. *(Ref. 3, Ch. 5.6, Coexisting Conditions section)*

68 **(b)** Family and twin studies provide evidence that Tourette's disorder and other tic disorders are fundamentally genetic disorders with much higher concordance rates in monozygotic twins compared to those of dizygotic twins, and high recurrence rates among family members. Although a number of segregation analyses of large multigenerational families implicated the possibility of a single gene(s) inherited with an autosomal dominant pattern in Tourette's disorder, genetic screening of the entire genome through genetic linkage studies has eliminated the possibility of a single gene model of etiology for Tourette's disorder. *(Ref. 3, Ch. 5.6, Etiology section)*

69 **(e)** A case study showed that low Apgar score at five minutes and *more* prenatal visits were associated with a higher risk of Tourette's disorder. Limited evidence is available to show smoking and alcohol use or forceps delivery can predispose Tourette's disorder. *(Ref. 3, Ch. 5.6, Etiology section)*

70 **(c)** Higher total neuron number was found in the globus pallidus pars interna (GPi) whereas a lower neuron number and density was found in the globus pallidus pars externa (GPe) and in the caudate nucleus. At the cellular level in the striatum, medium-sized spiney neurons receive afferents using glutamate (excitatory), gamma-aminobutyric acid (GABA, inhibitory), dopamine (D_1 excitatory, D_2 inhibitory), and send inhibitory GABA efferent to the GPi. Dysfunction of spiney neurons caused by the impairment of these neurotransmitter systems causes tic movements. *(Ref. 3, Ch. 5.6, Neuroanatomical Factors section)*

71 **(e)** SC, TS, OCD, and ADHD but not MDD share common anatomic targets. Post-rheumatic fever (caused by group A beta hemolytic streptococci [GABHS]), results from central nervous system inflammatory lesions; people with SC often present with motor and vocal tics and obsessive-compulsive and ADHD symptoms, which indicates that these disorders may share a common etiology. *(Ref. 3, Ch. 5.6, Neuroanatomical Factors section)*

72 **(b)** It is often difficult to distinguish complex motor tics from other complex repetitive behaviors such as stereotypic movements and behaviors. However, compared to complex motor tics, stereotypic movements and behaviors tend to have earlier onset, occur bilaterally, stay more consistent over time, and usually do not have a waxing and waning course. *(Ref. 3, Ch. 5.6, Diagnostic Assessment section)*

73 **(b)** Other specified tic disorder is used when symptoms characteristic of a tic disorder cause clinically significant distress or impairment in social, occupational, or other important areas but do not meet full criteria for a tic disorder or any of the disorders in the neurodevelopmental disorders diagnostic class, and the clinician chooses to communicate the specific reasons for not meeting the full criteria. In this case, it should be coded as "other specified tic disorder" followed by the specific reason "with onset after age 18 years." If there was no age description in this case, the clinician may choose not to specify the reason that the criteria are not met, then the diagnosis of "unspecified tic disorder" should be given. *(Ref. 4, pp. 81–85)*

74 **(d)** Repeatedly calling attention to a child's tics in the home and classroom settings can be counterproductive. Building awareness of tics and the sensations that precede them (premonitory urges) is an important component of behavioral therapy for tics, such as habit reversal training, when facilitated by a trained therapist. *(Ref. 1, Ch. 20, Psychotherapeutic Interventions section; Ref. 3, Ch. 5.6, Treatment section)*

75 **(e)** Production of an incompatible physical response is used in "competing response practice" (one of the two focuses of HRT), which makes it impossible to produce the tic (e.g., isometric contraction of tic-opposing muscles). "Awareness training" has four components that were listed as answers (a) through (d). Tics with premonitory urges are good candidates for such intervention. *(Ref. 1, Ch. 20, Psychotherapeutic Interventions section; Ref. 3, Ch. 5.6, Treatment section)*

76 **(b)** Patients with Tourette's disorder in general respond to haloperidol, fluphenazine, and/or pemozide. α-adrenergic agonists, such as clonidine and guanfacine are especially helpful in mild cases. Some atypical neuroleptics (such as ziprasidone, olanzapine, and risperidone, but not clozapine) are shown to be efficacious in some studies. *(Ref. 1, Ch. 20, Pharmacological Treatment section; Ref. 3, Ch. 5.6, Treatment section)*

77 **(b)** M. S. Durkin et al. (2008) examined the age effects and birth order on the risk of autism spectrum disorders in ten U.S. study sites. They found that the firstborn offspring of two older parents (mother aged ≥35 and father aged ≥40) were three times (odds ratio: 3.1) more likely to develop autism than third or later-born offspring of younger parents. *(Durkin et al. 2008)*

78 **(d)** Z. Kabir et al. (2011) examined an association between second-hand smoke exposure (SHS) and parent-reported neurobehavioral disorders (ADHD, learning disabilities, conduct disorder, and oppositional defiant disorder) in youth. They found that children exposed to SHS at home had 50% increased odds of having two or more childhood neurobehavioral disorders compared to those who were not exposed to SHS. *(Kabir et al. 2011)*

Matching

79 **(b)** Prader-Willi syndrome, which is associated with the deletion of q11-q13 on chromosome 15 in 70% of cases, is characterized by hypotonia, obesity, small hands and feet, hyperphagia, narrow forehead, downward-slanted palpebral fissures, an IQ between 20 and 80, and frequent behavioral problems. *(Questions 79–82: Ref. 5, p. 3506)*

80 **(c)** Down syndrome, or Trisomy 21, is characterized by microcephaly, hypotonia, medial epicanthic folds, small ears, an IQ range of 25–50, and manifests early symptomatology of Alzheimer's disease.

81 **(a)** Phenylketonuria is a disorder of amino-acid metabolism in which the infant is normal at birth, but progresses to vomiting and irritability, and then to developmental delay, seizures, microcephaly, and spasticity. A phenylalanine-restricted diet prevents intellectual disability, and prenatal diagnosis is possible.

82 **(d)** Fragile X syndrome is the most common known inherited cause of intellectual disability. The responsible gene, FMR1, locates on the X chromosome containing CGG trinucleotide repeat (6 to 60 in unaffected individuals). Infants with Fragile X syndrome present with relative microcrania and facial edema, while older children and adults present with a long face and a prominent chin.

83 **(e); 84 (d); 85 (c); 86 (b); 87 (a)** Individuals with ADHD have been identified as having deficits in the executive functions, which refers to higher neurocognitive processes including response inhibition/execution, verbal and spatial working memory, set shifting/task switching, planning/organization, vigilance, and interference control. The Continuous Performance Test assesses response inhibition and vigilance. The Wisconsin Card Sorting Test and Trailmaking Test part B assess set shifting. The Tower of Hanoi/London Porteus Mazes assess planning ability. The Rey-Osterreith complex figure test assesses planning/organization. The Working Memory Sentence Span test and Digits Backward test assess working verbal memory. The Self-Ordered Pointing Test and CANTAB Spatial Working Memory Test assess spatial working memory. *(Ref. 3, Ch. 5.1, Attention-Deficit Hyperactivity Disorder section)*

88 **(b); 89 (c); 90 (a)** Levy and Hyman (2008) reviewed existing literature and proposed a grading system to indicate the strength of evidence that supports or refutes particular complementary and alternative medicine treatments for children with autism spectrum disorders as grade A (randomized controlled trials, reviews, and/or meta-analysis), grade B (other evidence such as isolated well-designed controlled and uncontrolled studies), or grade C (case reports or theories). As a gastrointestinal hormone, secretin is the one that has been most extensively studied for autism. Thus, it was listed under grade A. However, it was concluded that there is no evidence that single- or multiple-dose intravenous secretin is effective for the treatment of autism spectrum disorders, which rejected its use. According to Levy and Hyman, the therapies under grade B are: Vitamin B6, magnesium, Vitamin C, melatonin, carnosine, dimethylglycine, fatty acids, gluten-free/casein-free diet, auditory integration, and music therapy. Yoga, amino acids, folate, oxidative stress, gastrointestinal medications, hyperbaric oxygen therapy, chelation, antibiotics, immune therapies, antifungal agents, chiropractic, craniosacral massage, and massage/therapeutic touch therapies are under the category of grade C. *(Levy and Hyman 2008)*

References

Durkin, M. S. et al. (2008). Advanced Parental Age and the Risk of Autism Spectrum Disorder. *Am J Epidemiol, 168*, 1268–1276.

Levy, S. E. and Hyman, S. L. (2008). Complementary and Alternative Medicine Treatments for Children with Autism Spectrum Disorders. *Child Adolesc Psychiatric Clin N Am, 17*, 803–820.

Kabir, Z. et al. (2011). Secondhand Smoke Exposure and Neurobehavioral Disorders among Children in the United States. *Pediatrics, 128*, 263–270.

3

SCHIZOPHRENIA AND OTHER PSYCHOTIC DISORDERS

DOI: 10.4324/9781003308805-4

QUESTIONS

Directions: Select the best response for each of the questions 1–22.

1 Based on DSM-5, which of the following disorders should *not* be considered under the category of schizophrenia spectrum and other psychotic disorders?

   a Schizotypal (personality) disorder

   b Delusional disorder

   c Brief psychotic disorder

   d Schizoaffective disorder

   e None of the above

2 Which of the following terms describes a patient with schizophrenia experiencing decreased motivation of self-initiated purposeful activities?

   a Diminished emotional expression

   b Avolition

   c Alogia

   d Asociality

   e Anhedonia

3 Which of the statements regarding the DSM-5 diagnostic criteria for delusional disorder is *incorrect*?

   a Presence of one or more delusions for at least one month.

   b Never met Criterion A of schizophrenia.

   c Associated behavior can be odd or bizarre.

   d Specifier can be used to identify bizarre content.

   e Assessment measures can be used to specify current severity.

4 Delusional disorder can be categorized into different subtypes such as erotomanic type, grandiose type, jealous type, persecutory type, somatic type, mixed type, and unspecified type. Which of the following subtypes is *most* frequent?

   a Erotomanic type

   b Grandiose type

   c Jealous type

   d Persecutory type

   e Somatic type

5 The DSM-5 criteria for the diagnosis of schizophrenia in children and adolescents are the same as in adults *except for*:

   a Presence of hallucinations

   b Duration of at least six months

   c Level of functioning below the level previously achieved

   d Presence of delusions

   e Presence of negative symptoms

6 Development and course of psychosis can be variable, and onset can be abrupt or insidious, with the majority of cases having a slow and gradual development. Which of the following age groups represents the *peak age* at onset of the first psychotic episode?

   a Early teens

   b Late teens

   c Early to mid-20s for males and late 20s for females

   d Late 20s for males and early 30s for females

   e Early 30s for both males and females

7 Which of the following features is *more* common in children with schizophrenia compared to their adult counterparts?

   a Erotomanic delusion

   b Persecutory delusion

   c Auditory hallucination

   d Visual hallucination

   e Thought insertion

8 Which of the following genetic syndromes/conditions is *most* likely to develop schizophrenia-like psychotic disorder?

   a DiGeorge syndrome

   b Williams syndrome

   c Fragile X syndrome

   d Down's syndrome

   e Angelman syndrome

9 There are some similarities and differences in terms of phenomenology and neurobiology of childhood-onset schizophrenia (COS) compared to adult-onset schizophrenia (AOS). All of the following related statements are correct *except*:

   a COS has a higher rate of early language, social, and motor developmental abnormalities and premorbid impairments.

   b There is an association of COS with advanced paternal age.

   c Studies show more striking abnormalities in smooth pursuit eye movement (SPEM) in COS than in AOS.

   d Higher rates of familial schizophrenia spectrum disorders were found for COS than for AOS.

   e Abnormalities found in neuropsychological testing for COS are not significantly higher than those found for AOS.

10 Based on recent studies comparing individuals with COS comorbid with autism spectrum disorders (ASDs) to those without ASDs, which of the following is *different*?

   a Age of onset

   b IQ

   c Response to medications

   d Rate of familial schizotypy

   e Rate of gray matter loss

11 Based on studies by Asarnow and colleagues, which aspect of the following neurocognitive functioning in COS probands is *not* significantly impaired?

a Rote language skills

b Fine motor coordination

c Attention

d Short-term memory

e Learning and abstraction

12 Comorbid psychiatric conditions are common in children with COS. Which of the following conditions is the *most* common one?

a Depression

b Obsessive-compulsive disorder

c Generalized anxiety disorder

d Attention-deficit/hyperactive disorder

e Eating disorder

13 Based on recent imaging studies, all of the following statements regarding brain morphology and functioning in youths with schizophrenia are correct *except*:

a They show increasing ventricular volume.

b They show decreasing total cortical, frontal, medial, temporal, and parietal gray matter.

c They show shape abnormalities of the anterior hippocampus.

d They have larger overall brain volume.

e They show abnormal neural circuitry in the cerebellum.

14 Based on recent genetic studies, all of the following candidate genes were found to be associated with early onset of schizophrenia (EOS) *except*:

a Dysbindin gene

b Neuregulin gene

c 22q11 deletion

d DAOA/G72 gene

e MECP2 gene

15 All of the following statements regarding clinical presentation of schizophrenia in youth are correct *except*:

a Hallucinations, disorganized thought, and affective flattening are common in EOS.

b Complex delusions and catatonia occur more frequently in EOS.

c Loose associations and illogical thinking are commonly seen in EOS.

d COS tends to have chronic onset with signs in early childhood.

e Compared to adult-onset schizophrenia, EOS commonly presents four phases: prodromal, acute, recovery, and residual. The majority of youth with EOS present with ongoing chronic impairment to a certain degree during the residual phase.

16 Acute hallucinations in young children can be the result of all of the following *except*:

a Delirium

b Seizure disorders

c Attention deficits and hyperactivity

d AIDS

e Meningitis

17 All of the following statements regarding relationships of psychosocial factors and schizophrenia are correct *except*:

a By themselves, psychosocial factors do not cause schizophrenia, but they may interact with biological factors to mediate the onset, course, and severity of the disorder.

b Family interactions influence the course and morbidity of illness.

c Criticism and high expressed emotion in families can be associated with worse outcomes.

d Positive remarks from caregivers are associated with decreased positive symptoms in adolescents and young adult patients.

e Greater deficits in peer relations and social relatedness predict a poorer outcome.

18 All of the following represent higher risk factors for the development of schizophrenia *except*:

a Pregnancy and birth complications

b Female gender

c Winter/early spring birth in some locations

d Maternal stress and malnutrition

e Maternal infections and diabetes

19 All of the following statements regarding treatment of EOS are correct *except*:

a A comprehensive, integrated approach combining medication therapies with psychosocial interventions is required for the treatment of EOS.

b Recent studies show the newer atypical antipsychotic agents are superior to the traditional ones in regard to long-term response and side-effect profiles.

c Short-term controlled trials support the efficacy of some traditional and second-generation antipsychotic agents.

d Clozapine has been shown superior to treat treatment-resistant schizophrenia, but its side-effect profile limits its use.

e Family psycho-educational therapy is associated with lower relapse rates and improved global functioning.

20 All of the following antipsychotic agents are FDA approved for the treatment of adolescents with schizophrenia *except*:

a Aripiprazole (Abilify)

b Olanzapine (Zyprexa)

c Quetiapine (Seroquel)

d Risperidone (Risperdal)

e Ziprasidone (Geodon)

21 All of the following are true *except*:

   a A child who is hearing voices most likely has COS.

   b Imaginary friends are normal in children.

   c Flashbacks due to trauma can look like hallucinations.

   d Children with OCD can present with obsessions that may be mistaken for delusions.

   e Adolescents with autism may appear "internally preoccupied."

22 Which of the following cause catatonia?

   a Schizophrenia

   b Autoimmune encephalitis

   c Bipolar disorder

   d Homocystinuria

   e All of the above

ANSWERS AND EXPLANATIONS

1 **(e)** According to the DSM-5, schizotypal (personality) disorder is under "schizophrenia spectrum and other psychotic disorders" and its full description is under the chapter "personality disorders." In the DSM-IV, all the personality disorders were under Axis II. Because DSM-5 has eliminated the axis system, none of the disorders listed in the question should be excluded. Here are all the disorders under this category: schizotypal (personality) disorder, delusional disorder, brief psychotic disorder, schizophreniform disorder, schizophrenia, schizoaffective disorder, substance/medication-induced psychotic disorder, psychotic disorder due to another medical condition, catatonia, other-specified schizophrenia spectrum and other psychotic disorder, and unspecified schizophrenia spectrum and other psychotic disorder. *(Ref. 4, pp. 87–122)*

2 **(b)** Negative symptoms can be a part of schizophrenia and interfere with overall functioning and cause impairments. All of the listed terms are negative symptoms seen in people with schizophrenia. Diminished emotional expression is presented as decreased facial expression, eye contact, prosody of speech, and facial/body gestures that normally give emotional emphasis of speech. *Avolition* refers to reduction of self-motivated or initiated purposeful activities, e.g. lack of motivation to get up, to go to work, or to participate in social activities. *Alogia* refers to diminished speech output. *Anhedonia* refers to the inability or decreased ability to experience pleasure or difficulty in recalling pleasure experienced in the past. This is also seen in people with depressive disorders. *Asociality* refers to the lack of interest in engaging in social activities or the lack of opportunities of social interactions. *(Ref. 4, p. 88)*

3 **(c)** Delusion-associated behavior should not be obviously bizarre and overall functioning is not markedly impaired except for the impact of the delusion(s) or its ramifications; otherwise, Criterion A of schizophrenia might be met. However, the content of delusion can be bizarre in nature, which can be specified as "with bizarre content." Delusional disorder does not have other characteristic symptoms of the active phase of schizophrenia. Clinicians can use clinician-rated dimensions of psychosis symptom severity from the chapter "assessment measures" in DSM-5 to specify current severity of delusional disorder. *(Ref. 4, pp. 90–91)*

4 **(d)** Among all the subtypes of delusional disorder, the most frequent one is persecutory type. Jealous type is more prevalent in males than in females. The lifetime prevalence of delusional disorder is around 0.2%. *(Ref. 4, p. 92)*

5 **(c)** According to the DSM-5, there are hallucinations, delusions, and thought disturbances, and negative symptoms during the active phase. Continuation signs of illness must be at least six months, which may include prodromal or residual symptoms. However, while functioning below the highest level previously achieved is a criterion for adults, in children or adolescents, "failure to achieve the expected level of interpersonal, academic, or occupational functioning" is the diagnostic criterion. *(Ref. 4, p. 99)*

6 **(c)** Early onset of schizophrenia is rare, and the psychotic features of schizophrenia usually emerge between the late teens and mid-30s. The peak age at onset for the first psychotic episode is in the early to mid-20s for men and in the late 20s for women. Positive psychotic symptoms are more likely to diminish over the life course, whereas negative symptoms are more persistent and more reliable poor prognostic predictors. Cognitive deficits associated with schizophrenia are hard to improve. *(Ref. 4, p. 102)*

7 **(d)** It is difficult to diagnose schizophrenia in children and childhood-onset schizophrenia is very rare. With essentially the same features of schizophrenia, positive symptoms of schizophrenia seen in children are less elaborate than those seen in adults and *visual hallucinations* are more common. Childhood-onset cases commonly have poorer outcome with gradual onset and prominent negative symptoms. *(Ref. 4, pp. 102–103)*

8 **(a)** Individuals with DiGeorge syndrome (also called velo-cardio-facial or 22q11.2 deletion syndrome) tend to develop comorbid mental illness, and 10–30% of them develop schizophrenia-like psychotic disorders. *(Ref. 3, Ch. 5.3, Genetic Studies section)*

9 **(b)** Contrary to findings in adult-onset schizophrenia, no correlation was found between COS and maternal or paternal age. All other statements are correct. *(Ref. 3, Ch. 5.3, Phenomenology section)*

10 **(e)** An MRI brain imagining study showed the rate of gray matter loss is more significant in the COS-ASDs group than in the COS without ASDs group. Premorbid social impairment was more common in the COS-ASDs group as well. However, the two groups did not show differences in age of onset, IQ, response to medications, or rate of familial schizotypy. *(Ref. 3, Ch. 5.3, Pervasive Developmental Disorder section)*

11 **(a)** Neuropsychological functioning in COS has been studied in the outpatient setting by Asarnow and colleagues (1994–1995). Rote language skills and simple perceptual processing are found not impaired. But fine motor coordination, learning and abstraction, attention, and short-term memory are impaired. *(Ref. 3, Ch. 5.3, Neurocognitive Functioning section)*

12 **(a)** Based on some NIMH studies, the most frequent comorbid condition was depression (54%), followed by OCD (21%), GAD (15%), and ADHD (15%). Forty-two percent of COS subjects had one of the following: GAD, OCD, separation anxiety, PTSD, and panic disorder. The studies also showed the comorbid anxiety disorders lasted longer and were more resistant to treatment than depression, suggesting the possible close association between anxiety and core pathology of schizophrenia. *(Ref. 3, Ch. 5.3, Comorbid section)*

13 **(d)** Brain structural and functional abnormalities are found in adults with schizophrenia. Researchers have made efforts to examine the brain morphology and functioning in children with schizophrenia. Even though replication studies are needed, preliminary results indicate several significant differences between children with schizophrenia and control subjects. All of the listed structural and functional differences are found in recent studies except for answer (d). As a matter of fact, overall brain volume is smaller in children with schizophrenia. *(Ref. 3, Ch 5.3, Brain Imaging section)*

14 **(e)** Mutation of the X-linked MECP2 gene is found to be involved in the etiology of Rett syndrome (not schizophrenia). Whereas causal relationships between candidate genes and early-onset schizophrenia are difficult to establish, recent genetic studies show a positive association between EOS and candidate genes such as dysbindin gene, neuregulin gene, DAOA/G72, GAD1, Prodh2/DGCR6, DISC1, and 22q11.2 deletion. *(Ref. 3, Ch. 5.3, Genetic Studies section)*

15 **(b)** Complex delusions and catatonia occur less frequently in EOS. All other statements in the question are correct. In addition, many children with COS have a history of premorbid issues, such as cognitive delays, learning difficulties, social withdrawal, and odd behaviors. Some of them (about 10–20%) have borderline IQ or intellectual disabilities, whereas many have other comorbid psychiatric conditions, such as ADHD, disruptive disorders, and anxiety/mood disorders. *(Ref. 1, Ch. 18, Clinical Presentation section)*

16 **(c)** ADHD symptoms of inattention and hyperactive symptoms or even the diagnosis can precede the appearance of psychotic symptoms. However, acute hallucinations are not usually the results of attention deficits and hyperactivity. Other conditions/disorders should be considered in the differential diagnoses, such as mood disorders, schizoaffective disorder, posttraumatic stress disorder, obsessive-compulsive disorder, autism spectrum disorders, some psychosocial stress situations, underlying medical conditions, such as seizure disorders, central nervous system lesions, delirium, metabolic and endocrine disorders, neurodegenerative disorders, toxic encephalopathies, infectious diseases, autoimmune disorders, etc. *(Ref. 1, Table 18-1)*

17 **(d)** Positive remarks from caregivers are associated with decreased *negative* symptoms in adolescents and young adult patients. Different studies show conflicting findings regarding whether high expressed emotion is a predictor of worse outcomes and future relapse of the illness, which indicates that cultural context influences how patients perceive and react to their families' behaviors and interactions with other family members. *(Ref. 1, Ch. 18, Family Influence section)*

18 **(b)** Either an equal or a predominant male gender ratio is found in clinical studies of schizophrenia in child and adolescent

populations. Perinatal stress and obstetrical complications are more common in the histories of patients with schizophrenia than in those of controls. In addition to pubertal development, infectious disease and immunological factors, other medical conditions, and genetic factors all can be potential risk factors of developing schizophrenia. *(Ref. 1, Ch. 18, Environmental Factors section; Ref. 4, p. 103)*

19 **(b)** Comparative studies found that the newer atypical antipsychotic agents are not superior to first-generation antipsychotics in regards to long-term response or side-effect profiles. There are short-term controlled trials that support the efficacy of some traditional agents (e.g., haloperidol, loxapine, thioridazine, and thiothixene) and a number of second-generation agents (e.g., risperidone, aripiprazole, quetiapine, and olanzapine). Clozapine is not FDA approved for the treatment of adolescents with schizophrenia, but it was found superior to both haloperidol and olanzapine in youth who have treatment-resistant schizophrenia. Unfortunately, its side-effect profile limits its use. *(Ref. 1, Ch. 18, Treatment section)*

20 **(e)** All the listed antipsychotic agents are FDA approved for the treatment of adolescents (age 13–17) with schizophrenia except for ziprasidone. In addition, paliperidone (Invega) was FDA approved for the treatment of adolescents (age 12–17) with schizophrenia. Haloperidol is FDA approved for the treatment of children older than 3 with "psychosis," "Tourette syndrome," and "severe behavioral disorders." *(Ref. 1, Ch. 18, Treatment section; please visit The U.S. Food and Drug Administration [FDA] website at www.fda.gov for updated drug label information of each medication)*

21 **(a)** COS is extremely rare. Children sometimes describe "hearing voices" as a way to express shameful or uncomfortable thoughts and is not necessarily pathologic. Careful diagnostic assessment is needed to distinguish psychosis from normal phenomena such as imaginary friends and other psychiatric symptoms such as OCD obsessions and PTSD flashbacks. *(Ref. 5, p. 3444)*

22 **(e)** A wide variety of psychiatric and medical conditions are associated with catatonia including bipolar, depression, schizophrenia, and ASD, neurologic (seizures, encephalitis, paraneoplastic encephalopathy, etc.), metabolic (pellagra, porphyria, homocystinuria, uremia, hepatic dysfunction, etc.), autoimmune (lupus, NMDAR encephalitis, etc.), and endocrine (diabetic ketoacidosis, hyperthyroidism, Addison disease, etc.) disorders, infection, and drug intoxication. *(Ref. 3, Ch. 5.11, Catatonia section)*

4

BIPOLAR AND RELATED DISORDERS AND DEPRESSIVE DISORDERS

DOI: 10.4324/9781003308805-5

QUESTIONS

Directions: Select the best response for each of the questions 1–30.

1 According to DSM-5, all of the following statements regarding disruptive mood dysregulation disorder are correct *except*:

  a This disorder was categorized under bipolar and related disorders.

  b Children with this disorder present with severe recurrent temper outbursts that are inconsistent with developmental level.

  c The temper outbursts are frequent and the mood between temper outbursts is persistently irritable or angry in nature.

  d The mood symptoms and temper outbursts present at least two settings, and are present for more than 12 months.

  e Onset of these symptoms has to be before the age of 10 years.

2 According to DSM-5, the diagnosis of disruptive mood dysregulation disorder cannot be made prior to which of the following ages:

  a 3 years

  b 4 years

  c 6 years

  d 8 years

  e 10 years

3 Prevalence of major depressive disorder in children is lower (about 2%) than in adolescents (about 4–8%). What is the male to female ratio during childhood?

  a 1:1

  b 1:2

  c 1:3

  d 1:4

  e 1:5

4 Which of the following conditions is the *most* frequent comorbid diagnosis with major depressive disorder in youth?

  a ADHD

  b Anxiety disorders

  c Substance-related and additive disorders

  d Persistent depressive disorder (dysthymia)

  e Psychotic disorders

5 Based on DSM-5, all of the following statements regarding diagnosing major depressive disorder in youth are correct *except*:

  a Almost identical DSM-5 criteria are used in diagnosing major depressive disorder in both youth and adults.

  b In children and adolescents, depressed mood can be replaced by anhedonia.

  c In children, failure to make expected weight gain can be considered significant weight loss.

  d Adolescents with initial onset of major depressive disorder may later present a bipolar disorder.

  e For those with adolescent onset, psychotic features, a family history of bipolar illness, and presence of a "with mixed features" specifier have an increased risk for bipolar diagnosis.

6 All of the following statements regarding diagnosing persistent depressive disorder (dysthymia) are correct *except*:

  a Duration of symptoms can be longer in children for dysthymic disorder.

  b Depressed mood can be irritable mood.

  c Early onset is before age 21 and later onset is at age 21 or older.

  d The absence or presence of coexisting major depressive episodes should be indicated with specifiers.

  e Specifiers include "with mood-congruent psychotic features" and "with mood-incongruent psychotic features."

7 Based on DSM-5, which of the following is the key diagnostic difference for cyclothymic disorder in children/adolescents compared to adults?

  a Onset of symptoms

  b Duration of the symptoms required

  c Severity of the symptoms required

  d Number of the symptoms required

  e Specifier used

8 Based on DSM-5, children and adolescents who experience multiple episodes of hypomanic symptoms that do not meet criteria for a hypomanic episode and multiple episodes of depressive symptoms that do not meet criteria for a major depressive episode that persist less than 12 months, but have no symptom-free periods longer than two months, should be diagnosed with which of the following diagnoses?

  a Cyclothymic disorder

  b Disruptive mood dysregulation disorder

  c Other specified bipolar and related disorder

  d Unspecified bipolar and related disorder

  e Mood disorder, not otherwise specified

9 In a large randomized controlled trial (RCT), Treatment of Adolescents with Depression Study (TADS) 2004, which of the following type of psychotherapies showed no difference compared to placebo in treating adolescents with MDD?

  a Interpersonal psychotherapy (IPT)

  b Cognitive behavioral therapy (CBT)

c Family therapy

d Group therapy

e Supportive therapy

10 A meta-analysis by Cipriani et al. (2016) found the strongest association with increased risk of suicidality for children and adolescents given which of the following antidepressants?

a Fluoxetine (Prozac)

b Citalopram (Celexa)

c Escitalopram (Lexapro)

d Sertraline (Zoloft)

e Venlafaxine (Effexor)

11 Based on a meta-analysis of published and unpublished pharmacological RCTs for MDD in youth (Bridge et al. 2007), which pair of the following numbers *most* closely reflects the "number needed to treat" compared to the "number needed to harm"?

a 2 vs. 70

b 4 vs. 80

c 6 vs. 90

d 8 vs. 100

e 10 vs. 110

12 Interpersonal psychotherapy for depressed adolescents (IPT-A), adapted from interpersonal therapy for adults, is based on the principle that depression occurs within an interpersonal context and that symptoms can improve by focusing on current interpersonal relationships and communication patterns. Which of the following is *not* an accurate statement regarding the empirical support for IPT-A?

a IPT-A leads to improvements in depressive symptoms, social functioning, and global functioning.

b IPT-A is particularly effective for adolescents with high levels of parent–adolescent conflict.

c IPT-A is significantly more effective than control conditions but less effective than cognitive behavioral therapy (CBT).

d A modified version of IPT-A has been demonstrated to be effective as a prevention intervention.

e The American Psychological Association's Clinical Practice Guideline for the Treatment of Depression recommends IPT-A as an option for the initial treatment of depression in adolescents.

13 Based on data from clinical trials, which of the following antidepressants has shown the *largest* response rate in treating MDD in children and adolescents?

a Citalopram (Celexa)

b Escitalopram (Lexapro)

c Fluoxetine (Prozac)

d Paroxetine (Paxil)

e Sertraline (Zoloft)

14 Which of the following medical conditions should be the *least* considered in the differential diagnosis of major depressive disorder?

a Hyperthyroidism

b Mononucleosis

c Brain tumor

d Premenstrual dysphoric disorder

e Chronic fatigue syndrome

15 Which of the following rating scales is the *least* useful as a screening instrument when evaluating youth with possible bipolar disorder?

a Child Behavior Checklist (CBCL)

b Child Symptom Inventory (CSI-4)

c Parent-completed versions of the General Behavioral Inventory (P-GBI)

d Vanderbilt Rating Scale

e Youth Mania Rating Scale (YMRS)

16 Which of the following antipsychotics does *not* have an FDA-approved indication for treating youth with bipolar I disorder?

a Aripiprazole (Abilify)

b Olanzapine (Zyprexa)

c Quetiapine (Seroquel)

d Risperidone (Risperdal)

e Ziprasidone (Geodon)

17 Based on new research findings, regarding treatment of ADHD in children with possible or definite mania, which of the following statements is *more* accurate?

a Typical ADHD medications always should be avoided before stabilizing mood symptoms.

b Treating ADHD symptoms is always considered a higher priority than treating mood symptoms.

c Outcomes of treatment are the same for youth with bipolar disorders alone compared to youth with bipolar disorder comorbid with ADHD.

d Treating ADHD symptoms can start prior to treating mood symptoms.

e Apparent return of worse ADHD symptoms at the end of day has diagnostic implications.

18 Which of the following agents has an FDA-approved indication for treating bipolar I disorder acute depression in children?

a Lithium

b Lamotrigine (Lamictal)

c Olanzapine/fluoxetine (Symbyax)

d Quetiapine (Seroquel)

e Risperidone (Risperdal)

19 Which of the following statements is *least* accurate regarding the use of antidepressants in children and adolescents with bipolar disorder?

   a The risk of precipitating a manic or hypomanic episode with an antidepressant may average 10–20%.

   b Antidepressant-induced activation in children is more common than "switching" to mania.

   c The risk of antidepressant-induced mania appears to be higher with SSRIs and SNRIs than with bupropion.

   d If a manic episode emerges during antidepressant treatment, a bipolar I diagnosis should be given if it persists at a fully syndromal level beyond the physiological effect of the medication.

   e Antidepressants, alone or in combination with mood stabilizers, appear to be less useful for children than adults with bipolar disorder.

20 All of the following statements about the epidemiology of depressive disorders in children and adolescents are accurate *except*:

   a Point prevalence of depressive disorder is lower in prepubertal children than in adolescents.

   b In adolescents, the rate of depressive disorders in females is three times more than in males.

   c Pre-pubertal depressive disorder shares similar risk factors and course with conduct disorder.

   d Pre-pubertal onset depressive disorder is more likely to lead to recurrent episodes in adulthood.

   e Early onset of puberty is a risk factor for girls to develop depression.

21 Based on meta-analysis of pediatric bipolar disorder, which of the following symptoms is the *least* frequent?

   a Increased energy

   b Distractibility

   c Euphoria/elation

   d Flight of ideas

   e Hypersexuality

22 Based on comparative studies on the phenomenology of bipolar disorder and ADHD in youth, which of the following symptoms was found significantly *more* frequently in bipolar disorder?

   a Irritability

   b Accelerated speech

   c Distractibility

   d Unusual energy

   e None of the above

23 In the study "Pediatric Bipolar Spectrum Disorder and ADHD: Comparison and Comorbidity in the LAMS Clinical Sample" (Arnold et al. 2011), the authors proposed four hypotheses, two of which were supported, one partially supported, and one rejected. All of the following statements are consistent with their results *except*:

   a Children with comorbid bipolar spectrum disorder (BPSD)+ADHD showed younger age of onset of BPSD symptoms than those with BPSD alone.

   b Parent ratings of ADHD symptoms were higher for comorbid ADHD+BPSD than for ADHD or BPSD alone.

   c Teacher ratings of both ADHD and BPSD symptoms were more severe for comorbid ADHD+BPSD than BPSD alone, but not ADHD alone.

   d Children with comorbid BPSD+ADHD have more impaired global functioning than those with either diagnosis alone.

   e Rates of other comorbid diagnoses were greater in the children with comorbid ADHD+BPSD.

24 According to the "Four-Year Longitudinal Course of Children and Adolescents with Bipolar Spectrum Disorders: The Course and Outcome of Bipolar Youth (COBY) Study" (Birmaher et al. 2009), during syndromal periods, compared to those with bipolar I disorder or bipolar disorder not otherwise specified (bipolar NOS), youth with bipolar II disorder spent *more* time experiencing which of the following symptoms?

   a Aggression/agitation

   b Hypomania

   c Major depression

   d Mania

   e Psychosis

25 According to the "Four-Year Longitudinal Course of Children and Adolescents with Bipolar Spectrum Disorders: The Course and Outcome of Bipolar Youth (COBY) Study" (Birmaher et al. 2009), which of the following pairs of numbers reflects conversion rates of bipolar II to bipolar I and bipolar NOS to either bipolar I or bipolar II, respectively?

   a 20% and 48%

   b 25% and 38%

   c 30% and 32%

   d 32% and 28%

   e 38% and 20%

26 According to "Switching to Another SSRI or to Venlafaxine With or Without Cognitive Behavioral Therapy for Adolescents With SSRI-Resistant Depression: The TORDIA Randomized Controlled Trial" (Brent et al. 2008), all of the following statements reflect the findings *except*:

   a Cognitive behavioral therapy plus a switch to venlafaxine showed a higher response rate than a medication switch alone.

   b Cognitive behavioral therapy plus a switch to another SSRI showed a higher response rate than a medication switch alone.

c   The response rate of venlafaxine is statistically significantly lower than that of a second SSRI.

d   No differential treatment effects on change in the CDRS-R, self-rated depressive symptoms, suicidal ideation, or the rate of harm-related or any other adverse events were found.

e   A greater increase in diastolic blood pressure and pulse was found more frequently during venlafaxine treatment than during SSRI treatment.

27   According to "Treatment of Resistant Depression in Adolescents (TORDIA): Week 24 Outcomes" (Emslie et al. 2010), out of 334 adolescents enrolled in the study, approximately which percent of youth achieved remission by 24 weeks?

a   24%

b   29%

c   32%

d   39%

e   45%

28   According to "Long-Term Outcome of Adolescent Depression Initially Resistant to SSRI Treatment" (Vitiello et al. 2011), the depressive symptom trajectory of the remitters diverged from that of non-remitters by the end of which of the following weeks of treatment?

a   Six weeks

b   Eight weeks

c   Ten weeks

d   Twelve weeks

e   Twenty weeks

29   According to "Treatment of Selective Serotonin Reuptake Inhibitor–Resistant Depression in Adolescents: Predictors and Moderators of Treatment Response" (Asarnow et al. 2009), all of the following are predictors of poorer treatment response *except*:

a   Higher baseline depression severity

b   Greater impairment

c   Higher baseline levels of suicidal ideation and hopelessness

d   More severe family conflict

e   More months of pre-enrollment SSRI medication treatment

30   Klomek et al. (2007) studied the relationships of "Bullying, Depression, and Suicidality in Adolescents." They found approximately 9% of the sample (2,342 9th through 12th grade students) reported being victimized frequently and 13% reported bullying others frequently. All of the following statements reflect their findings *except*:

a   Bullying was more prevalent in the school setting than away from school settings.

b   Compared to boys who were never victimized, frequently victimized boys were more likely to be depressed, to have serious suicidal ideation (SSI), and to attempt suicide.

c   Compared to boys who never bullied others, boys who frequently bullied others were more likely to die by suicide.

d   Compared to girls who were never victimized, victimized (either frequently or infrequently) girls were more likely to be depressed, to have SSI, and to attempt suicide.

e   Compared to girls who never bullied others, girls who bullied (either frequently or infrequently) others were more likely to be depressed, to have SSI, and to attempt suicide.

Matching

31–35 Match each definition of treatment outcome of depression to the following descriptions:

a   Emergence of symptoms of depression during the period of recovery (a new episode)

b   An episode of depression meeting DSM criteria during the period of remission

c   Absence of significant symptoms of depression (e.g., no more than one to two)

d   A period of at least two weeks and less than two months with no or very few depressive symptoms

e   No symptoms or a significant reduction in depressive symptoms for at least two weeks

31   Response

32   Remission

33   Recovery

34   Relapse

35   Recurrence

ANSWERS AND EXPLANATIONS

1 (a) Disruptive mood dysregulation disorder is a brand-new diagnosis in DSM-5 under the category of depressive disorders. The intention of adding this diagnosis was to address the concerns about the potential for overdiagnosing of and overtreating for bipolar disorder in children. The disorder refers to a pattern of mood dysregulation, chronic and persistent irritability, and frequent extreme behavioral dyscontrol in children who do not present with typical, classic, distinct episodes of mania or hypomania. In DSM-5, the term "bipolar disorder" is explicitly reserved for the episodic nature of bipolar manifestations. Studies show that children with chronic irritability are at risk to develop unipolar depression and/or anxiety disorders in adulthood with a low rate of conversion to bipolar disorders. *(Ref. 4, pp. 156–157)*

2 (c) Based on DSM-5, the diagnosis of disruptive mood dysregulation disorder should not be made for the first time before age 6 years or after age 18 years. However, by history or observation, the onset of symptoms of temper outbursts and chronic irritable/angry mood has to be before age 10 years. *(Ref. 4, p. 156)*

3 (a) Prevalence of major depressive disorder in children is lower (approximately 2%) than in adolescents (approximately 4–8%). The male-to-female ratio during childhood is 1:1, but 1:2 during adolescence, with increased prevalence by twofold to fourfold after puberty, especially in females. *(Ref. 1, Ch. 13, Epidemiology section)*

4 (b) About 40–90% of youth with depressive disorders have other psychiatric disorders, anxiety disorders being the most frequent comorbid diagnoses, followed by disruptive disorders, ADHD, and, in adolescence, substance-related and addictive disorders. Major depressive disorder and persistent depressive disorder (dysthymia) can co-occur, which is called "double depression." *(Ref. 1, Ch. 13, Comorbidity section)*

5 (b) In DSM-5, there is only one set of criteria for major depressive disorder, with only two *notes* to specify the different manifestations between children/adolescents and adults: (1) in children and adolescents, depressed mood can be irritable mood; (2) in children, consider failure to make expected weight gain, referring to significant weight loss when not dieting. Any existing manic or hypomanic episodes will exclude major depressive disorder diagnosis. A substantial portion of people with bipolar illnesses initially present with a major depressive episode, and those who have adolescent onset, family history of bipolar illness, or the presence of a "with mixed features" specifier have increased risk for future bipolar disorders. *(Ref. 4, pp. 160–165)*

6 (a) In children and adolescents, duration can be *shorter* (must be at least one year) and mood can be irritable. Sharing with major depressive disorder, it can be specified by the specifiers: with anxious distress, with mixed features, with melancholic features, with atypical features, with mood-congruent psychotic features, with mood-incongruent psychotic features, with peripartum onset, mild, moderate, severe, in partial remission, and in full remission. Four specifiers are also used to describe whether there is ever a major depressive episode coexisting within two years preceding the persistent depressive disorder, and how these major depressive episodes (if there is one) are related to the dysthymic syndrome. *(Ref. 4, pp. 127, 162, 168–169)*

7 (b) Similar to persistent depressive disorder (dysthymia), duration of the symptoms required for children and adolescents is *shorter* (one year) compared to for adults (two years) in making a diagnosis of cyclothymic disorder in DSM-5. *(Ref. 4, p. 139)*

8 (c) DSM-5 recognizes that many people, especially children and adolescents, experience bipolar-like phenomena that do not meet the criteria for bipolar I, II, or cyclothymic disorder. Other specified bipolar and related disorder was designed for clinicians to communicate the specific reason that the presentation does not meet the criteria for any specific bipolar and related disorder. In this question, a case of a "short-duration cyclothymia" (less than 24 months for adults/less than 12 months for children or adolescents) was described. "Mood disorder, NOS" was eliminated from DSM-5. *(Ref. 4, pp. 123, 148)*

9 (b) In TADS, combination of CBT and fluoxetine showed the best outcome with a rapid decline in depressive symptoms. However, it did not show a significant difference compared to fluoxetine alone at endpoint. These two treatment groups were better compared to either CBT alone or placebo during acute treatment. CBT did not show statistically significant differences compared to the placebo group. CBT is the most widely studied psychotherapy for the treatment of youth with MDD. Even with some conflicting data, CBT appears to be more efficacious in treating depression with comorbidity, suicidal ideation, and hopelessness. But it appears less efficacious when there is a history of sexual abuse or when one of the parents is depressed. IPT is another psychotherapy that has evidence of efficacy based on RCTs, especially for older adolescents with moderate or severe depression. Data supports that IPT is at least as efficacious as CBT. *(Ref. 1, Ch. 13, Pharmacotherapy section)*

10 (d) A network meta-analysis of RTCs for acute treatment of major depressive disorder in children and adolescents was conducted with primary outcomes of efficacy and tolerability. Thirty-four eligible trials were found, which included 5,260 participants. Only fluoxetine was found to be statistically significantly more effective than placebo. Imipramine, venlafaxine, and duloxetine were associated with more discontinuations than placebo due to adverse events. Venlafaxine was associated with a significantly increased risk of suicidal behavior or ideation compared to placebo and five other antidepressants. *(Cipriani et al. 2016)*

11 (e) Based on a meta-analysis of published and unpublished pharmacological RCTs for MDD in youth (Bridge et al. 2007), the "number needed to treat" was 10 and the "number needed to harm" was 112. *(Ref. 1, Ch. 13, Pharmacotherapy section)*

12 (c) Interpersonal psychotherapy for adolescents (IPT-A) has been shown in clinical trials to lead to decreased depressive symptoms, better social functioning, and better global functioning, and has been demonstrated to be particularly effective for adolescents with high parent–adolescent conflict. IPT-A has been shown in a meta-analysis to have a larger effect size than that of cognitive behavioral therapy (CBT). The American Psychological Association's Clinical Practice Guideline for the Treatment of Depression recommends the use of either IPT-A or CBT for the initial treatment of depression in adolescents *(Ref. 1, Ch. 42, Empirical Support section)*

13 (c) Based on data from clinical trials, fluoxetine (Prozac) showed the largest response rate in treating MDD in children and adolescents compared to other antidepressants. It has been speculated that this may be due to the actual differences in the effect of the medication or because the clinical trials that studied fluoxetine included more severely depressed patients and were better designed and conducted. *(Ref. 1, Ch. 13, Pharmacotherapy section)*

14 (a) Hypothyroidism (*not* hyperthyroidism) is more likely to manifest with symptoms similar to those of major depressive disorders. Thus, it should be considered as one of potential medical differentials along with certain cancers, autoimmune diseases, anemia, multiple sclerosis, stroke, and others listed in the question when evaluating major depressive disorder. Hyperthyroidism, on the other hand, should be considered as one of medical conditions that may manifest with symptoms similar to those of anxiety disorders. *(Ref. 1, Ch. 13, Evaluation section; Ref. 4, p. 167)*

15 (d) Vanderbilt Rating Scales are more useful in screening youth with possible ADHD, oppositional defiant disorder (ODD), and conduct disorder (CD). Similar to the Conners' scales, Vanderbilt Rating Scales come with both parent-report and teacher-report versions. The scales are free online (www.nichq. org), and the items cover symptoms of ADHD, ODD, and CD, as well as some symptoms of anxiety and depression. In addition, they have subscales to assess school behavioral and academic performance. All other listed instruments are more useful in screening mood symptoms, especially manic and hypomanic symptoms. *(Ref. 1, Ch. 4, Assessment Tools section; Ref. 1, Ch. 10, Clinical Evaluation section)*

16 (e) Ziprasidone (Geodon) does not have any FDA-approved indications for children or adolescents at this time. The remainder of the listed antipsychotics all have FDA-approved indications for treating bipolar I disorder in youth. Quetiapine (Seroquel) has an indication for bipolar I disorder and acute mania. Aripiprazole (Abilify), risperidone (Risperdal), and olanzapine (Zyprexa) all have an indication for bipolar I disorder, acute manic, and mixed episodes for youth as young as 10 years old. Olanzapine (Zyprexa) approved age range is from 13 to 17 for acute manic and mixed episodes. The earliest second-generation antipsychotic, clozapine (Clozaril), does not have any indications for children or adolescents either. *(Ref. 1, Ch. 14, Pharmacological Treatment section)*

17 (d) Consensus documents recommended stabilizing mood symptoms first, then treating the comorbid disorder. However, some new data suggested treating ADHD symptoms either with or without first stabilizing mood can be considered for children with ADHD along with possible or definite mania. If children become more irritable or aggressive with ADHD treatment, usage of an antipsychotic or a mood stabilizer should be definitely considered. Youth with bipolar disorder alone have better treatment responses than those with comorbid ADHD. Apparent return of worse ADHD symptoms at the end of day, also known as "rebound," has no diagnostic implications. *(Ref. 1, Ch. 14, Mania and ADHD section)*

18 (c) Olanzapine/fluoxetine (Symbyax) has an FDA-approved indication for treating acute depression in children ages 10 to 17 with bipolar disorder (lurasidone is the other medication that has an FDA approval for bipolar depression in this age group). Quetiapine (Seroquel) and Olanzapine/fluoxetine (Symbyax) both have FDA indications for bipolar I disorder, acute depression. Lithium and lamotrigine (Lamictal) have an FDA indication for bipolar disorder, maintenance treatment in adults, but not for youth. Lithium also has an FDA-approved indication for bipolar disorder in adolescents. *(Ref. 1, Ch. 14, Pharmacological Treatment section)*

19 (b) The risk of antidepressant-induced mania has not been fully clarified in youth. The risk of antidepressant-induced activation, however, is common and may average 10–20%. Average rate of switching by SSRIs is 10%. Treatment-emergent mania/hypomania must be carefully differentiated from antidepressant-induced activation, but if symptoms persist at a fully syndromic level beyond the physiological effects of the treatment, a bipolar diagnosis should be assigned accordingly. *(Ref. 1, Ch. 14, Pharmacological Treatment section; Ref. 1, Ch. 35, Safety and Tolerability section)*

20 (d) Adolescent-onset depression is more likely to lead to recurrent episodes in adulthood. The point prevalence of depressive disorder is lower in children (1–2%) than in adolescents (3–8%). Female predominance in depression emerges after onset of puberty, possibly due to hormonal changes, higher comorbid anxiety, and increased interpersonal conflicts in females. Pre-pubertal depression seems to follow a course of conduct disorder, along with other behavioral problems, but does not typically predict depression in adulthood. Early onset of puberty in girls is a risk factor of developing depression. *(Ref. 3, Ch. 5.4.1, Descriptive Epidemiology section)*

21 (e) Based on a meta-analysis of studies of pediatric bipolar disorder, the frequency of the symptoms follows the this order (from the most frequent to the least frequent): increased energy, distractibility, pressured speech, irritability, grandiosity, racing thoughts, decreased need for sleep, euphoria/elation, poor judgment, flight of ideas, and hypersexuality. *(Ref. 3, Ch. 5.4.2, Clinical Characteristics section)*

22 (e) With significant overlap of symptoms shared between bipolar disorder and other common psychiatric conditions, especially ADHD, none of the symptoms listed in the question is specific to mania. The lack of specificity of symptomology of bipolar disorder makes it challenging and problematic to diagnose bipolar disorder simply based on the particular symptoms being present or not. Some researchers advocate that two of the symptoms are more specific to mania—elated/elevated mood

and grandiosity—and consider them as "cardinal" or "hallmark" symptoms. *(Ref. 3, Ch. 5.4.2, Clinical Characteristics section)*

23 **(a)** The authors of the study proposed four hypotheses; two of which were supported, one partially supported, and one rejected. The first hypothesis, "children with BPSD+ADHD show younger age of onset of BPSD symptoms than those with BPSD alone," was not supported by their findings. The authors found that children with BPSD+ADHD had onset of mood symptoms at 6.7 years and those with BPSD alone had onset at 6.9 years (p = 0.8). However, they found the age of their first visit to the LAMS-site clinic was statistically significantly younger (9.6 vs. 10.5 years, p < 0.01). Their second hypothesis, "children with BPSD+ADHD have more severe ADHD symptoms than those with ADHD alone and more severe bipolar symptoms than those with BPSD alone," was partially supported—see the answers (b) and (c). The answers (d) and (e) reflect hypotheses 3 and 4, which were supported by their findings. *(Arnold et al. 2011)*

24 **(c)** According to the study, during syndromal periods, youth with bipolar II disorder manifest with less frequent manic symptoms. Instead, they are more likely to present with major depression. *(Birmaher et al. 2009)*

25 **(b)** According to the study, 25% of youth with bipolar II converted to bipolar I, whereas 38% of those with bipolar disorder, NOS, converted to either bipolar I or II. *(Birmaher et al. 2009)*

26 **(c)** According to the study, CBT plus a switch to a medication regimen (either venlafaxine or another SSRI) showed a higher response rate than a medication switch alone. However, no statistically significant difference in response rate between venlafaxine and a second SSRI (48.2%; 95% CI, 41%–56% vs. 47.0%; 95% CI, 40%–55%; P = 0.83) was found. *(Brent et al. 2008)*

27 **(d)** According to the study, out of 334 adolescents enrolled in the study, 38.9% achieved remission by 24 weeks. Initial treatment assignment did not affect treatment remission rates. The study also found that, at week 12, the positive predictors of higher remission included lower depression, hopelessness, anxiety, suicidal ideation, family conflict, and absence of comorbid dysthymia, anxiety, and drug/alcohol use and impairment. *(Emslie et al. 2010)*

28 **(a)** According to the study, the depressive symptom trajectory of remitters diverged from that of non-remitters by the first six weeks of treatment. They also found that by 72 weeks, approximately 60% of the randomized youth had reached remission, but one-fourth of remitted youth experienced a relapse. The youth who were assigned to SSRIs had a faster decline in self-reported depressive symptoms and suicidal ideation than those assigned to venlafaxine (p < 0.05). *(Vitiello et al. 2011)*

29 **(e)** According to the study, "fewer months" of pre-enrollment SSRI medication treatment is one of the poor response predictors among the others listed in the answers. The authors also found that by using logistic regression, adjusting for site, age, sex, and race, the decreased scores on baseline Beck Depression Inventory (BDI), Suicidal Ideation Questionnaire-JR (SIQ), Beck Hopelessness Scale (BHS), or Conflict Behavior Questionnaire-Adolescent Report (CBQ-A) and Children's

Global Adjustment Scale (CGAS) impairment levels significantly increased the likelihood of response. The authors found the statistically significant positive response *moderators* to combination treatment (CBT+medication) compared to medication alone were the absence of abuse histories and the presence of more comorbid disorders, with a marginally significant effect for comorbid ADHD. *(Asarnow et al. 2009)*

30 **(c)** Compared to boys who never bullied others, boys who frequently bullied others were not more likely to die by suicide, but were more likely to be depressed and to have SSI. Bullying was more prevalent in the school setting than away from school settings. However, regardless of settings, students who were involved in bullying behaviors (either as victims or bullies) were at overall higher risk for depression, SSI, and suicide attempts compared with students who were not involved in such behaviors. There were some gender-specific differences (see the answers in the question). *(Brunstein Klomek et al. 2007)*

Matching

31 **(e)**; 32 **(d)**; 33 **(c)**; 34 **(b)**; 35 **(a)** In general, three phases are involved in the treatment of depression: acute, continuation, and maintenance, with a primary goal of achieving response and ultimately full remission during the acute phase. The goal of the continuation phase is to solidify the response to treatment and avoid relapses, whereas the goal of the maintenance phase is to prevent recurrence or new episodes. *(Ref. 1, Ch. 13, Treatment section)*

References

Arnold, L. E. et al. (2011). Pediatric bipolar spectrum disorder and ADHD: comparison and comorbidity in the LAMS clinical sample. *Bipolar Disorders*, 13(5–6), 509–521. https://doi.org/10.1111/j.1399-5618.2011.00948.x

Asarnow, J. R. et al. (2009). Treatment of selective serotonin reuptake inhibitor-resistant depression in adolescents: predictors and moderators of treatment response. *Journal of the American Academy of Child and Adolescent Psychiatry*, 48(3), 330–339. https://doi.org/10.1097/chi.0b013e3181977476

Birmaher, B. et al. (2009). Four-year longitudinal course of children and adolescents with bipolar spectrum disorders: The Course and Outcome of Bipolar Youth (COBY) study. *The American Journal of Psychiatry*, 166(7), 795–804. https://doi.org/10.1176/appi.ajp.2009.08101569

Brent, D. et al. (2008). Switching to another SSRI or to venlafaxine with or without cognitive behavioral therapy for adolescents with SSRI-resistant depression: The TORDIA randomized controlled trial. *JAMA*, 299(8), 901–913. https://doi.org/10.1001/jama.299.8.901

Brunstein Klomek, A., Marrocco, F., Kleinman, M., Schonfeld, I. S., & Gould, M. S. (2007). Bullying, depression, and suicidality in adolescents. *Journal of the American Academy of Child and Adolescent Psychiatry*, 46(1), 40–49. https://doi.org/10.1097/01.chi.0000242237.84925.18

Cipriani, A. et al. (2016). Comparative efficacy and tolerability of antidepressants for major depressive disorder in children and adolescents: a network meta-analysis. *Lancet (London, England)*, *388*(10047), 881–890. https://doi.org/10.1016/S0140-6736(16)30385-3

Emslie, G. J. et al. (2010). Treatment of Resistant Depression in Adolescents (TORDIA): Week 24 outcomes. *The American Journal of Psychiatry*, *167*(7), 782–791. https://doi.org/10.1176/appi.ajp.2010.0904055228

Vitiello, B. et al. (2011). Long-term outcome of adolescent depression initially resistant to selective serotonin reuptake inhibitor treatment: A follow-up study of the TORDIA sample. *The Journal of Clinical Psychiatry*, *72*(3), 388–396. https://doi.org/10.4088/JCP.09m05885blu

5

DISRUPTIVE, IMPULSE-CONTROL, AND CONDUCT DISORDERS

DOI: 10.4324/9781003308805-6

QUESTIONS

Directions: Select the best response for each of the questions 1–20.

1 Based on DSM-5, which of the following conditions is *not* considered under the category of disruptive, impulse-control, and conduct disorders (CD)?
a Oppositional defiant disorder (ODD)
b Intermittent explosive disorder (IED)
c Conduct disorder
d Pyromania
e Pathological gambling

2 All of the following statements regarding disruptive, impulse-control, and conduct disorders are accurate *except*:
a Most of them tend to be male predominant.
b They tend to have childhood or adolescence onset.
c Most youth with CD met criteria for ODD previously.
d Most youth with ODD develop CD eventually.
e Youth with ODD have high risk for eventually developing anxiety and depressive disorders.

3 In the DSM-5 diagnostic criteria for ODD, a "Note" was added indicating different frequencies of defiant behaviors required for children younger versus older than 5 years. How frequently do children younger than 5 years need to show the behaviors to meet the criteria for ODD (unless otherwise noted in Criterion A8)?
a Once per week for at least 12 months
b Once per week for at least six months
c Twice per week for at least six months
d Four times per week for 12 months
e Most days for at least six months

4 A minimal age requirement was added to the DSM-5 diagnostic criteria for intermittent explosive disorder (IED). What is the *minimal* chronological age required to diagnose youth with IED?
a 3 years
b 6 years
c 9 years
d 12 years
e 15 years

5 In the DSM-5 diagnostic criteria for conduct disorder (CD), a specifier "with limited prosocial emotions" was added. All of the following characteristics reflect the aspects of this specifier *except*:
a Heightened irritability
b Lack of remorse or guilt
c Callous—lack of empathy
d Unconcerned about performance
e Shallow or deficient affect

6 Conduct disorder is influenced by genetic, physiological, and environmental factors. All of the following statements correctly reflect such risk factors *except*:
a The risk increases in youth with either a biological or an adoptive parent with CD.
b The risk increases in youth with biological parents who have severe alcohol use disorder, depressive and bipolar disorders, schizophrenia, or a history of ADHD/conduct disorder.
c The risk increases in youth with faster resting heart rates.
d The risk increases in youth with reduced autonomic fear conditioning.
e The risk increases in youth who experience parental rejection, neglect, inconsistent child-rearing practices, harsh discipline, and abuse.

7 Which of the following is the correct female-to-male prevalence ratio for kleptomania?
a 3:1
b 6:1
c 1:1
d 1:2
e 1:3

8 Based on teachers' reports of the most common oppositional symptoms, such as arguing, screaming, disobedience, and defiance, the peak presentation is at which of the following age groups?
a Between 3 and 5 years
b Between 4 and 7 years
c Between 5 and 9 years
d Between 8 and 11 years
e Between 10 and 13 years

9 Which of the following is a correct estimated heritability of antisocial behavior?
a 30%
b 40%
c 50%
d 60%
e 70%

10 Interactions between genetic and environmental risk factors for conduct disorder are very complicated. All of the following statements are accurate *except*:
a Accumulation of risk may act not only additively but also multiplicatively.
b Genetic influence is important, but it can also be modified by environmental variables.
c Genetic influences are the same in children from poor families compared to those from rich ones.

d   Genes may influence individuals' choices and shape their environment.

e   The same risk factor may lead to different outcomes depending on other circumstances.

11 Studies show that it is not uncommon that youth with ODD or CD present with out-of-control behaviors and aggression and need crisis interventions in the emergency department (ED). All of the following statements are general management principles to follow in this kind of situation *except*:

a   Crisis intervention strategies should be implemented before using psychotropic medications to control behavior.

b   Physical restraint and seclusion should be considered as first-line options.

c   Usage of emergency medications should correspond to the risk for potential injury.

d   Staff members in the ED should be knowledgeable of the risks and side effects of acute sedation and follow the appropriate protocols.

e   Physicians may consider a standing psychotropic medication order in case PRN medication is needed multiple times a day.

12 Which of the following psychosocial treatment modalities is *not* a recommended treatment for conduct problems in youth?

a   Parent management training (PMT)

b   Multisystemic therapy (MST)

c   Therapeutic foster care

d   Families and schools together (FAST Track)

e   Wildness programs and boot camps

13 There are a few principles and recommendations clinicians may want to follow when using psychotropic drugs for youth with aggression in nonemergency situations. Which of the following statements is *incorrect?*

a   Start with a low dose, titrate up slowly, and taper off slowly.

b   Cautiously prescribe stimulants to adolescents with CD because of the high comorbidity with substance abuse.

c   Routinely and systematically monitor adherence, side effects, and drug interactions.

d   An adequate trial combined with psychosocial interventions is completed prior to consideration of switching, augmenting, combining, or discontinuation.

e   Polypharmacy is encouraged because of overall better efficacy.

14 Which of the following is *false* regarding treatment of ODD?

a   Treatment should involve parents.

b   Comorbid conditions should be identified and treated.

c   Medication should be used as a first-line treatment.

d   Increasing compliance and reducing conflict is the main goal of treatment.

e   Parent management training can reduce oppositional symptoms.

15 Among all of the following treatment modalities for youth with fire-setting behavior, which of them showed an accumulating evidence of efficacy?

a   Fire safety skills training (FSST)

b   Self-monitoring

c   Parent–child communication

d   Parental psychoeducation

e   Restitution for damages

16 Based on human studies, in which of the following ways is the serotonin system *most* likely affected in individuals with aggressive behaviors?

a   Increased sensitivity of the serotonin 1A receptor (5-HT$_{1A}$)

b   Decreased sensitivity of the serotonin 1A receptor (5-HT$_{1A}$)

c   Increased sensitivity of the serotonin 2 C receptor (5-HT$_{2C}$)

d   Decreased sensitivity of the serotonin 2 C receptor (5-HT$_{2C}$)

e   Decreased sensitivity of the serotonin 2A receptor (5-HT$_{2A}$)

17 Investigations of developmental psychopathology find that adult antisocial behaviors may have important roots in childhood. A subgroup of youth possess callous-unemotional traits, noted by the DSM specifier "with limited prosocial emotions." Which of the following is *not* one of the characteristics?

a   Shallow emotions and low anxiety

b   Inability to feel guilt or remorse

c   Lack of empathy

d   Deficits in information processing

e   Lack of concern about performance

18 Risk and prognostic factors that are associated with a poorer outcome from conduct disorder include all of the following *except*:

a   Lower-than-average intelligence (especially low verbal IQ)

b   Large family size

c   Adolescent onset of conduct-disordered behavior

d   Peer rejection and association with a delinquent peer group

e   Comorbid with ADHD

19 Based on the study "Differentiating Early-Onset Persistent Versus Childhood-Limited Conduct Problem Youth" by

E. Barker and B. Maughan (2009), the predictors that increase risk of persistent conduct problem trajectory for both girls and boys include all of the following *except*:

a High practical support for the mother

b Higher levels of undercontrolled temperament

c Anxiety during pregnancy

d Harsh parenting

e Partner cruelty toward the mother

20 Based on the study "Agitation Treatment for Pediatric Emergency Patients" by R. J. Hilt and T. A. Woodward (2008), all of the following are recommended non-pharmacological and calming interventions for clinicians' use *except*:

a Use simplified language and soft voice

b Reduce environmental simulation

c Remove distracting toys

d Remove breakable objects/equipment

e Allow space for pacing

ANSWERS AND EXPLANATIONS

1 (e) Pathological gambling (previously under "impulse-control disorders not elsewhere classified" in DSM-IV-TR) was renamed "gambling disorder" and is currently under the category of "substance-related and addictive disorder" in DSM-5. Trichotillomania (new name: hair-pulling disorder) was recategorized under "obsessive-compulsive and related disorders" in DSM-5. ADHD was recategorized under neurodevelopmental disorders; on the other hand, ODD and CD appear under "disruptive, impulse-control, and conduct disorders" along with IED, pyromania, kleptomania, antisocial personality disorder (which can be also found under "personality disorders" in DSM-5), other specified disruptive, impulse-control, and conduct disorder, and unspecified disruptive, impulse-control, and conduct disorder. *(Ref. 4, pp. 461–489)*

2 (d) Even though most youth with CD met criteria for ODD previously, youth with ODD do not always develop CD. Although most of the disorders under this category have a male predominance, the relative degree of such predominance varies both across disorders and within a disorder at different ages. *(Ref. 4, pp. 461–464)*

3 (e) In DSM-5 diagnostic criteria for ODD, a "Note" was added indicating different frequencies of defiant behaviors required for children younger versus older than 5 years. For children younger than 5 years, the behaviors need to occur *most days* for at least six months to meet criteria for ODD, unless otherwise noted (Criterion A8: "has been spiteful or vindictive at least twice within the past 6 months"). For children older than 5 years, the behaviors have to occur at least *once a week* for at least six months, unless otherwise noted (Criterion A8). *(Ref. 4, p. 462)*

4 (b) Onset of IED-associated behaviors is commonly in later childhood or early adolescence, and the behaviors rarely start for the first time after age 40 years. DSM-5 requires the minimal chronological age of six years or equivalent developmental level to diagnose youth with IED. *(Ref. 4, pp. 466–467)*

5 (a) In DSM-5 diagnostic criteria for conduct disorder (CD), a specifier "with limited prosocial emotions" was added, but heightened irritability was not one of the characteristics that reflect the core pattern of such a specifier. To qualify for this specifier, at least two of the characteristics (answers b. through e.) have to present persistently over more than 12 months in multiple relationships and settings. *(Ref. 4, pp. 469–471)*

6 (c) Even though nondiagnostic, *slower* resting heart rates and reduced autonomic fear conditioning are unique psychophysiological markers found in individuals with CD. *(Ref. 3, Ch. 5.1.2, Neuropsychological section; Ref. 4, pp. 473–474)*

7 (a) With variable onset, kleptomania often starts in adolescence, and may also begin in childhood and adulthood. In the general population, it has a very low prevalence rate: approximately 0.3% to 0.6%. It is a female predominant disorder at a ratio of 3:1. *(Ref. 4, p. 478)*

8 (d) Based on teachers' reports, the frequency of oppositional behaviors peaks between 8 and 11 years, and then declines over time. However, available data show that symptoms of conduct disorder are more persistent with a higher resistance to change compared to oppositional behaviors. *(Ref. 3, Ch. 5.1.2, Validity section)*

9 (c) Even though it is not diagnosis specific, the estimated heritability of antisocial behavior is 50%. It applies to the population at large, not to a particular individual. *(Ref. 3, Ch. 5.1.2, Etiology section)*

10 (c) It has been shown that genetic influences are stronger in children from more disadvantaged families than those from affluent ones. *(Ref. 3, Ch. 5.1.2, Etiology section)*

11 (b) Acute situations can happen both at the ED and the inpatient setting. Physical restraint and seclusion should be considered as last resorts after all other approaches have failed. *(Ref. 3, Ch. 5.1.2, Treatment section)*

12 (e) Based on social learning theory, PMT is the most extensively studied in this field. It encourages parents to use positive reinforcement, to adopt more effective discipline strategies, and to learn how to negotiate with their children, and it also shows indirect effectiveness in improving sibling behavior, maternal psychopathology, marital satisfaction, and family cohesion. MST has variable, moderate effectiveness in reducing offending depending on the skills of the treatment team. Therapeutic foster care demonstrates some evidence of reducing youths' criminal activities. With less rigorous data to support it, FAST Track demonstrates some improvements in social coping skills, more positive peer relations, improved academic performance, and social competency. Research shows conflicting results for the effectiveness of wildness programs, boot camps, and other residential treatments due to the poor quality of the studies, and there are concerns about exposure to deviant peers and limited generalization beyond the treatment setting. *(Ref. 3,Ch. 5.1.2, Treatment section)*

13 (e) Polypharmacy should be avoided as much as possible, especially with concerns of potential drug–drug interactions, a higher risk of adverse reactions, side effects, and long-term negative consequences. *(Ref. 3, Ch. 5.1.2, Treatment section)*

14 (c) Psychosocial and behavioral interventions such as parent management training are the first-line treatment for ODD. Medication should only be considered for treatment of comorbidities with better evidence for pharmacologic treatment such as ADHD or depression, or in cases of ODD with severe aggression that hasn't responded to psychosocial treatments. *(Ref. 3, Ch. 5.1.2, Treatment section)*

15 (a) Fire safety skills training (FSST) as well as CBT showed an accumulating evidence of efficacy in treating fire-setting behavior in youth, and fire safety education remains a core component. *(Ref. 3, Ch. 5.1.4, Treatment section)*

16 (b) Decreased sensitivity of the serotonin 1A receptor (5-HT$_{1A}$) is found to be associated with increased aggression in human and animal studies. The atypical anxiolytic agent buspirone acts as an agonist at the 5-HT$_{1A}$ receptor and has been reported to have anti-aggressive effects. Decreased antagonistic effect of

5-HT$_{1B}$ and abnormalities in the dopaminergic/noradrenergic neural system are found to be linked to impulsive aggression. When exposed to frustration or provoking events, children with disruptive behavior disorders have lower cortisol levels than the control group. The 5-HT$_{2A}$ receptor plays an important role in perception (evidenced by the agonist effect of lysergic acid diethylamide—LSD). Some neuroleptics (such as risperidone, ziprasidone, and olanzapine) have antagonistic effects on 5-HT receptors, and their antipsychotic effects are at least partially mediated at cortical 5-HT$_{2A}$ receptors. The 5-HT$_{2C}$ receptor may be associated with the increased appetite and weight gain side effects of certain neuroleptics. *(Ref. 3, Ch. 6.1.1, Serotonergic section; Ref. 5, p. 3615)*

17 **(d)** Deficits in information processing (such as low verbal intelligence) is not found in youth with conduct disorder with limited prosocial emotions. They lack guilt and empathy, are unconcerned about performance, and have shallow affect. *(Ref. 5, p. 3608)*

18 **(c)** Childhood-onset CD (with at least one symptom prior to age 10) predicts a worse prognosis along with the others listed. *(Ref. 4, pp. 473–474)*

19 **(a)** Multivariate predictions analysis indicated that low practical support for the mother was a risk factor for girls only (not for boys). All other listed factors increase risks for both boys and girls to follow a persistent conduct problem trajectory relative to the childhood-limited conduct problem trajectory. *(Barker & Maughan 2009)*

20 **(c)** Offering distracting toys or other sensory modalities is recommended. In addition, other interventions are suggested: clear self-introduction, slow movements, explanation of what will happen in the ED, offering food or drink of the child's choice, honoring the child's reasonable requests, clarification of the child's goal, remaining engaged with the child, and not taking the child's anger personally. *(Hilt & Woodward 2008)*

References

Barker, E. & Maughan, B. (2009). Differentiating Early-Onset Persistent Versus Childhood-Limited Conduct Problem Youth. *Am. J. Psychiatry*, *166*, 900–908.

Hilt, R. J. & Woodward, T. A. (2008). Agitation Treatment for Pediatric Emergency Patients. *JAACAP*, 47, 132–138.

6

ANXIETY DISORDERS, OBSESSIVE-COMPULSIVE AND RELATED DISORDERS, TRAUMA- AND STRESSOR-RELATED DISORDERS, AND DISSOCIATIVE DISORDERS

DOI: 10.4324/9781003308805-7

QUESTIONS

Directions: Select the best response for each of the questions 1–40.

1 Which of the following best describes the DSM-5 characterization of separation anxiety disorder (SAD)?

a Excessive anxiety and apprehensive expectations, which are difficult for the child to control

b Consistent pattern of inhibited, emotionally withdrawn behavior toward caregivers

c Excessive anxiety about being apart from the individuals to whom the individual is most attached

d A maladaptive response to an identifiable stressor

e Significant anxiety provoked by social or performance situations

2 Manifestations of separation anxiety disorder (SAD) vary with age, and adults with SAD may not recall a childhood onset, although they may recall symptoms. What is the *minimal* required length of symptoms presented in youth versus in adults respectively?

a Two weeks vs. three months

b Four weeks vs. six months

c Six weeks vs. nine months

d Two months vs. ten months

e Four months vs. 12 months

3 All of the following statements regarding school refusal (school phobia) are correct *except*:

a School refusal is classified under anxiety disorders in DSM-5.

b There are three subtypes of school refusal in a community sample: anxious school refusers, truants, and mixed school refusers.

c There are significant gender differences in prevalence.

d Comorbid conditions include separation anxiety disorder, social anxiety disorder, specific phobia, panic disorder, and depression.

e Multimodal treatment approach is recommended.

4 Which of the following conditions is the *most* common comorbid condition associated with selective mutism (SM)?

a Communication disorders

b Depression

c ODD

d Separation anxiety disorder

e Social anxiety disorder (social phobia)

5 According to the study "Behavioral and Emotional Adjustment, Family Functioning, Academic Performance, and Social Relationships in Children with Selective Mutism," authors

(C. E. Cunningham et al., 2004) reached all of the following conclusions *except*:

a Selective mutism is associated with more anxious behaviors than oppositional behavior based on both parents' and teachers' reports.

b Teachers rate more ODD (and ADHD) symptoms in the selective mutism group at school.

c No differences are found in the marital status, economic resources, or support networks of families regardless of whether children have or have no selective mutism.

d Academic performance on math and reading of children with selective mutism do not differ from the control group.

e Overall children with selective mutism are not victimized more than the control group.

6 There has been a concern about overdiagnosing selective mutism in bilingual minority children who are recent immigrants. Which of the following criteria are necessary for a diagnosis of selective mutism in such populations?

a The duration of disturbance is longer than one month.

b The child is between the ages of 3 and 8 years.

c The child is younger than age 3 years.

d The child cannot speak his or her first language at home or in familiar settings.

e Comprehension of the new language is adequate, but the child persistently refuses to speak in unfamiliar settings.

7 Based on DSM-5, children with specific phobia are *more* likely to manifest their fear or anxiety as any of the following *except*:

a Crying

b Clinging

c Freezing

d Rapid speech

e Tantrums

8 How much more likely are individuals with specific phobia to make suicide attempts than those without the diagnosis?

a 20%

b 30%

c 40%

d 50%

e 60%

9 To meet the DSM-5 criteria for a social anxiety disorder (social phobia), children *must* invariably demonstrate anxiety in which of the following situations?

a Interactions with parents

b Interactions with other relatives

c Giving testimony in a church setting

d In peer settings, such as school

e Eating in front of people

10 What is the overall prevalence rate of panic disorder in children under the age of 14 years?

a < 0.1%

b < 0.4%

c About 1%

d Between 2–4%

e > 4%

11 Based on DSM-5, all of the following statements regarding agoraphobia are correct *except*:

a Agoraphobia is not itself a diagnosis, but rather a specifier for panic disorder.

b Agoraphobia's core symptom is marked fear or anxiety about certain situations (e.g., using public transportation, being in open or enclosed spaces, standing in line or being in a crowd, and being outside of the home alone).

c At least two of the above five fear- or anxiety-provoking situations need to be present to be considered agoraphobia.

d The situations almost always provoke fear or anxiety and lead to avoidance behaviors.

e Agoraphobia is diagnosed irrespective of the presence of panic disorder.

12 The core manifestation of generalized anxiety disorder (GAD) is frequent excessive anxiety and worry that are difficult for the patient to control, which is associated with a list of symptoms including restlessness, fatigue, poor concentration, irritability, muscle tension, and sleep disturbance. For children, what is the *minimal* number of the previously listed symptoms that have to be present for more days than not for the past six months to meet the criteria for GAD?

a One

b Two

c Three

d Four

e Five

13 Compared to adults, youth with GAD may be more likely to worry about all of the following or show all of the following characteristics *except*:

a Worry about performance or competence

b Worry about catastrophic events

c Worry about the whereabouts of things

d Being overly conforming and perfectionist

e Being overzealous in seeking reassurance

14 All of the following statements correctly describe some of the unique characteristics of children and adolescents with obsessive-compulsive disorder (OCD) *except*:

a Young children may not be able to articulate the aims of their compulsive behaviors or mental acts.

b Females are affected at a higher rate than males in the child population.

c Mean age at onset of OCD is 19.5 years, but one-fourth of cases begin by age 14 years.

d 40% of youth with childhood or adolescent onset of OCD may experience remission by early adulthood, but many of them can have a lifetime illness.

e Pattern of OCD symptoms is more variable in children and there are higher rates of harm obsessions in youth than in adults.

15 All of the following statements correctly describe risk and prognostic factors of OCD *except*:

a Behavioral disinhibition in childhood is a possible temperamental risk factor.

b Physical and sexual abuse during childhood increases risk for developing OCD.

c Some environmental factors (such as certain infectious agents and a post-infectious autoimmune syndrome) may trigger sudden onset of OCD symptoms.

d The rate of OCD among first-degree relatives of individuals with childhood or adolescence onset OCD is ten times more than that among first-degree relatives of those without the disorder.

e Concordance rate for monozygotic twins is 0.57 vs. 0.22 for dizygotic twins.

16 Individuals with OCD commonly have comorbid conditions. Which of the following is a more common *triad* seen in children?

a OCD, ODD, and ADHD

b OCD, tic disorder, and MDD

c OCD, tic disorder, and ADHD

d OCD, ADHD, and GAD

e OCD, ODD, and GAD

17 What is the most common age at onset of body dysmorphic disorder?

a 12–13 years

b 14–15 years

c 16–17 years

d 18–19 years

e 20–21 years

18 Which of the following body areas/regions is the *most* commonly affected by trichotillomania (hair-pulling disorder)?

a Axillary

b Eyelids

c Facial

d Pubic

e Peri-rectal

19 Which of the following estimated ratios *more* accurately reflects the gender difference (girls vs. boys) in the prevalence of trichotillomania (hair-pulling disorder) among children?

a 10:1

b 5:1

c 1:1

d 1:5

e 1:10

20 Which of the following is the *least* common functional consequence of excoriation (skin-picking) disorder?

a Missing school

b Difficulties managing responsibilities at school

c Difficulties studying due to skin picking

d Tissue damage, scarring, and infection

e Synovitis of the wrists

21 Which of the following statements does *not* reflect the current understanding, diagnosis, and categorization of reactive attachment disorder (RAD) under DSM-5?

a RAD represents a pattern of significant inhibited, emotionally withdrawn behavior toward adult caregivers.

b RAD represents a pattern of significant reduced or absent reticence in approaching and interacting with unfamiliar adults.

c There must be a history of experiencing a pattern of extremely insufficient care.

d The disturbance has to be evident prior to the age of 5 years.

e The developmental age has to be at least 9 months.

22 Posttraumatic stress disorder (PTSD) has two separate sets of criteria depending on the age of the individual. Which of the following is the *correct* age cut-off for these two sets of diagnostic criteria?

a Age of 3 years

b Age of 6 years

c Age of 8 years

d Age of 10 years

e Age of 12 years

23 All of the following statements regarding diagnosing PTSD in young children are correct *except*:

a Learning traumatic events that occurred to a parent or caregiving figure can be qualified as one of the symptoms listed in Criterion A (exposure).

b Witnessing events in electronic media, television, movies, or pictures can be qualified as one of the symptoms listed in Criterion A (exposure).

c Intrusive memories may not seem distressing but may be expressed as play reenactment.

d Dissociative reactions such as flashbacks may occur as reenactment in play.

e Irritability and angry outbursts may present as extreme temper tantrums.

24 The psychotherapy with the strongest evidence base for the treatment of PTSD in children and adolescents is:

a Eye movement desensitization and reprocessing (EMDR)

b Trauma-focused cognitive-behavioral therapy (TF-CBT)

c Child–parent psychotherapy (CPP)

d Trauma grief component therapy for Adolescents (TGCT-A)

e Trauma Affect Regulation: Guidelines for Education and Therapy (TARGET)

25 All of the following statements regarding dissociative identity disorder (DID) are accurate *except*:

a Individuals with DID may experience altered perceptions, such as hearing a child's voice.

b Individuals with DID may report their bodies feel different, such as feeling like a small child.

c In children, symptoms cannot be better explained by imaginary friends or other fantasy play.

d Full-blown DID may first present at almost any age, from early childhood to late adulthood.

e Females with DID predominate in both adults and children in clinical settings.

26 What is the mean age at onset of depersonalization/derealization disorder?

a 6 years

b 12 years

c 16 years

d 20 years

e 24 years

27 All of the following statements regarding the differential diagnoses and specific features of separation anxiety disorder and social anxiety disorder (social phobia) are correct *except*:

a Increased sensitivity to carbon dioxide (CO_2) exposure is found in children with separation anxiety disorder but not in children with social anxiety disorder (social phobia).

b School refusal in children with social anxiety disorder is due to the fear of being negatively judged by others, not due to worries about being separated from attachment figures.

c Children with separation anxiety disorder are generally comfortable in social settings as long as they are accompanied by the attachment figures.

d Children with separation anxiety disorder may show temperamental characteristics of behavioral inhibition to the unfamiliar as young as 21 months.

e Children with social anxiety disorder (not with separation anxiety disorder) exhibit increased fear response when challenged in the laboratory with social stressors.

28 In youth with any anxiety disorder, among all of the following listed conditions, which is the *most* common comorbid condition?

a Another anxiety disorder

b Depression

c ADHD

d ODD

e CD

29 Which of the following neurotransmitter systems has been shown to be an important genetic contributor for generalized anxiety disorder (GAD)?

a Serotonin transporter genes

b Serotonin receptor genes

c Dopamine transporter genes

d Noradrenergic receptor genes

e None of the above

30 Which of the following brain structures/regions are *most* likely implicated in children with anxiety disorders?

a Caudate of basal ganglia

b Putamen of basal ganglia

c Dorsal prefrontal cortex

d Inferior occipital cortex

e Amygdala

31 Which of the following best describes the evidence for the use of N-acetyl cysteine (NAC) for trichotillomania?

a There have been no RCTs evaluating NAC for trichotillomania in adults or children.

b RCT evidence has shown benefit of NAC for trichotillomania in both adults and children.

c RCT evidence has shown benefit of NAC for trichotillomania for adults, but there have been no RCTs in children.

d RCT evidence has shown benefit of NAC for trichotillomania in adults, but an RCT in children showed no benefit over placebo.

e RCT evidence has shown benefit of NAC for trichotillomania in children, but an RCT in adults showed no benefit over placebo.

32 Which of the following categories of psychopharmacological therapies should be considered as the first-line choice for treating children with social anxiety disorder, separation anxiety disorder, and OCD?

a Benzodiazepines

b Beta-blockers

c Buspirone

d Selective serotonin reuptake inhibitors (SSRIs)

e Tricyclic antidepressants

33 Which of the following statements is *least* accurate regarding psychiatric comorbidity in children and adolescents with OCD?

a Comorbid psychiatric disorders are present in more than half of children with OCD..

b Male gender and earlier age at onset of OCD are associated with increased likelihood of comorbid ADHD.

c Male gender and earlier age at onset of OCD are associated with increased likelihood of comorbid Tourette's disorder.

d Average age of onset for OCD is older than for each of the comorbid anxiety disorders.

e Children with OCD who have comorbid tic disorders differ from those without tic disorders in OCD symptoms, course, and response to treatment.

34 Which of the following is *least* associated with overall poorer prognosis of OCD?

a Comorbid psychiatric illness

b Poor initial treatment response

c Younger age at onset

d Longer duration of illness

e Positive first-degree family history of OCD

35 Based on clinical trials data using single-drug (serotonin reuptake inhibitors) treatment, which of the following numbers reflect the accurate proportion of drug-naïve patients with OCD that experience reduction of 25% to 40% severity in symptoms?

a 20–30%

b 30–40%

c 40–50%

d 50–60%

e 60–70%

36 Based on the pediatric OCD treatment study (POTS) randomized controlled trial (2004), the authors reached the following conclusion regarding the first line of intervention:

a Start CBT alone with addition of medication if CBT is unsuccessful.

b Start either CBT alone or CBT plus medication.

c Use medication alone and avoid CBT regardless of response.

d Use CBT alone and avoid medication regardless of response.

e Start both CBT and medication together regardless of severity of the symptoms.

37 All of the following statements regarding the study "Altering the Trajectory of Anxiety in At-Risk Young Children" by R. M. Rapee et al. (2010) are correct *except*:

a Authors evaluated the three-year effects of parent-focused intervention for anxiety in inhibited children aged 36 to 59 months (mean age of 46.5 months).

b Outcome measures included diagnostic interview of children and parents, objective measures of anxiety symptoms, and children's/parents' reported temperament assessment battery.

c The parent intervention program was compared to control group: monitoring-only condition.

d The intervention program is relatively expensive, being delivered in various community settings, such as pre-schools, parent–child centers, and health clinics.

e The intervention showed the potential of altering the trajectory of anxiety and related disorders in young inhibited children.

38 All of the following are the stages of systematic desensitization *except*:

a Relaxation training

b Constructing the anxiety hierarchy

c Desensitization in imagination

d Self-talk

e In vivo desensitization

39 Which of the following physical conditions is *least* likely to mimic PTSD-like symptoms?

a Asthma

b Caffeinism

c Hypothyroidism

d Migraine

e Seizure disorder

40 All of the following statements regarding trauma-focused psychotherapies are correct *except*:

a Trauma-focused psychotherapies should be the first-line treatment for youth with PTSD.

b Parents' participation in treatment improves resolution of children's trauma-related symptoms.

c Lower level of parental distress and stronger parental support is associated with better treatment response of PTSD symptoms in children receiving trauma-focused CBT.

d Empirical evidence supports that addressing the child's traumatic experiences using trauma-focused therapies is superior to nonspecific or nondirective therapies.

e Clinical worsening during the trauma-focused therapies warrants stopping the treatment and considering other options.

ANSWERS AND EXPLANATIONS

1 **(c)** Answer (a) characterizes generalized anxiety disorder; answer (b) characterizes reactive attachment disorder or autism spectrum disorders; answer (d) characterizes adjustment disorder; and answer (e) characterizes social anxiety disorder. *(Ref. 4, pp. 190–191, 202, 222, 265, 286)*

2 **(b)** In DSM-5, the fear, anxiety, or avoidance associated with separation anxiety disorder has to persist for more than four weeks in youth, and six months or longer in adults (age > 18 years). *(Ref. 4, pp. 191–193)*

3 **(a)** Defined as difficulty attending school associated with emotional distress (anxiety and depression), school refusal (school phobia) is *not* a DSM-5 diagnosis. It occurs in approximately 1% of all youth and 5% of all clinical-referred youth, with two peaks of onset: 5–6 years and 10–11 years of age (coinciding with starting kindergarten and the transition into middle school). An individualized multimodal approach is most beneficial for school refusal, and CBT and pharmacological therapy can both play effective roles. *(Ref. 3, pp. 331–334)*

4 **(e)** Among anxiety disorders that are common comorbid conditions with selective mutism, social anxiety disorder is the most common. A study shows nearly all children with selective mutism also meet criteria for social anxiety disorder. *(Ref. 1, Ch. 15, Diagnostic criteria section; Ref. 4, p. 197)*

5 **(b)** In contrast to parents' report at home, at school, teachers report fewer ODD or ADHD symptoms in children with selective mutism group than controls. *(Cunningham et al. 2004)*

6 **(e)** While acquiring a second language, immigrant children may normally undergo a "silent period" or nonverbal period. Such periods are typically shorter than six months with variations, are more common in 3- to 8-year-olds, and are usually longer in younger children. Selective mutism should not be diagnosed during the period while they are acquiring the new language. Children's ability to learn a second language easily, quickly, and automatically is a common myth. Based on DSM-5, "if comprehension of the new language is adequate but refusal to speak persistent, a diagnosis of selective mutism may be warranted." If children cannot speak in their first language in familiar settings, they may have speech delays or language disorders. *(Toppelberg et al. 2005)*

7 **(d)** Core symptoms of specific phobia are marked fear or anxiety about a specific object or situation, such as heights, animals, flying, exposure to needles or blood, enclosed places, loud sounds, etc. In children, the anxiety or fear is often manifested as crying, tantrums, freezing, and clinging. *(Ref. 4, p. 197)*

8 **(e)** There is up to 60% more likelihood for individuals with specific phobia to make suicide attempts than for those who are not diagnosed with the disorder, which could be due to its high comorbidity with personality disorders and other anxiety disorders. *(Ref. 4, p. 201)*

9 **(d)** Social anxiety disorder (social phobia) is involved with significant fear or anxiety about one or more social situations where patients worry about being exposed to possible scrutiny by others. Anxiety can be triggered by many different situations in different settings. However, in children, the anxiety must also occur in peer settings, not just during interactions with adults. Again, similar to specific phobia, children may also present their anxiety by crying, tantrums, freezing, clinging, shrinking, or failing to speak. *(Ref. 4, pp. 202–204)*

10 **(b)** Panic disorder (attacks) can occur in children, but rarely. The estimated overall prevalence rate of panic disorder is lower than 0.4% for children younger than 14 years old. The prevalence rates increase over time, especially during adolescence, with more female than male cases, and the rate increases seem to follow the onset of puberty, peak during adulthood (with a median age at onset of 20–24 years), and then decline after age 64. Overall, the female to male ratio is 2:1, and the prevalence rate for adults and adolescents is about 2–3%. *(Ref. 4, p. 210)*

11 **(a)** In contrast to DSM-IV-TR, in DSM-5 agoraphobia is a codable disorder, and can be diagnosed irrespective of the presence of panic disorder. In other words, if panic disorder and agoraphobia coexist, both diagnoses should be given. However, if the avoidance behaviors associated with the panic attacks do not extend to avoidance of two or more agoraphobic situations, only the diagnosis of panic disorder is assigned. *(Ref. 4, pp. 217–221)*

12 **(a)** Only one of the listed symptoms is required in children to meet criteria for GAD in contrast to three or more that are required for adults. *(Ref. 4, p. 222)*

13 **(c)** Elderly people with cognitive impairment may present their anxiety as worrying about the whereabouts of things, which should be regarded as more realistic given the cognitive impairment. The frail elderly person's worry about safety and falls may limit their daily activities. In children and adolescents with GAD, the anxiety and worries tend to be related to their performance or competence at school/in sports and to punctuality and catastrophic events. They tend to doubt themselves and need more reassurance and approval. *(Ref. 4, pp. 223–224)*

14 **(b)** Males are affected at a higher rate than females in the child population. Boys also have an earlier age of onset than girls, with almost 25% of boys having an onset prior to age 10 years. In general, the onset of symptoms is gradual. There are higher rates of sexual and religious obsessions in adolescents than in children, whereas there are higher rates of harm obsessions (such as fears of catastrophic events) in both children and adolescents than in adults. *(Ref. 4, pp. 237–239)*

15 **(a)** Temperamental factors such as greater internalizing symptoms, higher negative emotionality, and behavioral inhibition in childhood are possible risk factors for developing OCD. *(Ref. 4, pp. 239–240)*

16 **(c)** Up to 30% of people with OCD may also suffer from a lifetime tic disorder, which seems to be more common in males with a childhood-onset OCD. They seem to represent a separate population in terms of their manifestation of OCD symptoms, comorbidity, course, and pattern of familial transmission. A triad of OCD, tic disorder, and ADHD can be seen in children. *(Ref. 4, p. 242)*

17 (a) The most common age at onset of body dysmorphic disorder is 12–13 years, whereas the mean age at onset is 16–17, and the median age at onset is 15 years. Two-thirds of patients have onset prior to the age of 18 years. In DSM-5, body dysmorphic disorder is under the category of obsessive-compulsive and related disorders, along with hoarding disorder, trichotillomania (hair-pulling disorder), and excoriation (skin-picking) disorder, etc. The clinical features of body dysmorphic disorder are largely similar in youth and in adults. Early onset (prior to the age of 18 years) is associated with higher risk of suicide, more comorbidity, and gradual progression. *(Ref. 4, p. 244)*

18 (b) Hair pulling can occur anywhere hair grows. However, the *most* common sites are the eyebrows, eyelids, and scalp, followed by less common sites, such as axillary, facial, peri-rectal, and pubic regions. *(Ref. 4, p. 251)*

19 (c) Girls and boys with trichotillomania are more equally represented compared to adults where many more females are affected than males at a ratio of approximately 10:1. Onset of puberty often coincides with the onset of hair pulling in trichotillomania. Trichotillomania follows a usual chronic course with some waxing and waning if the disorder is untreated. To differentiate it from other causes of alopecia, skin biopsy and dermoscopy (or trichoscopy) can be used. Most common comorbid conditions with trichotillomania are major depressive disorder and excoriation (skin-picking disorder). *(Ref. 4, pp. 252–254)*

20 (e) Synovitis of the wrists due to chronic picking can occur, but rarely. Because of tissue damage, scarring, and infections, requirements for antibiotics to treat infections can frequently occur, along with occasional need for surgery. *(Ref. 4, p. 256)*

21 (b) Reactive attachment disorder is characterized by a pattern of inhibited, emotionally withdrawn behavior toward adult caregivers with impairments in seeking and responding to comfort when distressed. A pattern of behavior that involves culturally inappropriate, overly familiar behaviors with relative strangers is the core feature of disinhibited social engagement disorder (DSED). *(Ref. 4, pp. 265–270)*

22 (b) Two separate sets of criteria are used for either individuals who are adults, adolescents, and children older than the age of 6 years, or children who are younger than the age of 6 years. *(Ref. 4, pp. 271–274)*

23 (b) Witnessing events only in electronic media, television, movies, or pictures cannot be qualified as one of the symptoms listed in Criterion A (exposure). In adults, the exposure through electronic media, television, movies, or pictures can be counted as such traumatic events only if the exposure is work related (such as first responders collecting human remains or police officers/CPS social workers repeatedly exposed to details of child abuse). *(Ref. 4, pp. 271–274)*

24 (b) Trauma-focused cognitive-behavioral therapy (TF-CBT) has the strongest evidence base among psychotherapy modalities for treating children with PTSD, with 23 published RCTs including more than 2,000 children. The other answer choices have smaller evidence bases. Child–parent psychotherapy (CPP), for very young children, is delivered in joint child–parent treatment sessions. Trauma grief component therapy for adolescents (TGCT-A) is a cognitive-behaviorally based group treatment model typically provided in school settings. Eye

movement desensitization and reprocessing (EMDR) has been adapted for children, and Trauma Affect Regulation: Guidelines for Education and Therapy (TARGET) is a treatment for youth with complex trauma. *(Ref. 1, Ch. 16, Psychotherapeutic Treatments section)*

25 (e) Females with DID predominate in adults but not children in clinical settings. With DID, males may deny their trauma histories and associated symptoms whereas females are more likely to present with acute dissociative states. In contrast, males with DID are more likely to exhibit criminal or violent behavior with common triggers such as combat, prison conditions, and assaults. *(Ref. 4, pp. 292–295)*

26 (c) With a mean age at onset of 16 years, depersonalization/derealization disorder can start in early or middle childhood, with less than 20% of individuals having onset after age 20 years and only 5% after age 25 years. It is highly unusual to have the onset later than the fourth decade of life. The lifetime prevalence ranges from 0.8% to 2.8% with a gender ratio of 1:1. The onset can be either sudden or gradual, with variable length of episodes (from brief to prolonged). The disorder is often persistent, one-third of cases have distinct episodes, and the intensity of symptoms may wax and wane. *(Ref. 4, pp. 302–304)*

27 (d) Children with social anxiety disorder (*not* separation anxiety disorder) may show temperamental characteristics of behavioral inhibition to the unfamiliar as young as 21 months. Social skill impairments can be found both in children with social anxiety disorder and in children with autism spectrum disorders. The former usually results from delayed learning and refinement of social skills due to anxiety, whereas the latter more likely results from neuropsychiatric impairments. *(Ref. 3, Ch. 5.5.1, Etiology section; Ref. 4, pp. 194, 206)*

28 (a) Next to being comorbid with another anxiety disorder, depression is the most commonly reported comorbid condition among youth who suffer from anxiety disorders. ADHD is also one of the common comorbid conditions, and children with ADHD may also have a high comorbidity with anxiety disorder. *Ref. 3, Ch. 5.5.1, Comorbidity section)*

29 (e) Several studies have investigated the role of the serotonin transporter gene promoter (5-HTTLPR) in anxiety, but findings have been equivocal. 5-HTTLPR genotype has been associated with amygdala reactivity and cortisol stress reactivity. Further research is needed to clarify a potential role of 5-HTTLPR in anxiety. *(Ref. 3, Ch. 5.5.1, Etiology section)*

30 (e) Studies in both animal subjects and humans show significant evidence of the important role that the amygdala plays in fear conditioning and is considered as a critical element of the neural circuitry underlying anxiety disorders. The orbitofrontal cortex (OFC) and anterior cingulate cortex (ACC) are also implicated in emotion processing and regulation, and are thus likely to be involved in the neuronal circuitry of anxiety. *(Ref. 3, Ch. 5.5.1, Etiology section)*

31 (d) A randomized double-blind placebo-controlled add-on study of N-acetyl cysteine (NAC) for trichotillomania in adults showed significant improvement with few ill effects. However, an RCT in children showed differences between drug and placebo, demonstrating the importance of using caution in generalizing evidence in adults to children *(Ref 3, Ch. 5.5.3, Trichotillomania section)*

32 **(d)** Considering overall efficacy and safety, clinicians should use SSRIs as the first-line pharmacological therapies to treat social anxiety disorder, separation anxiety disorder, and GAD. Benzodiazepines have shown mixed results, and buspirone and beta-blockers have shown little or no evidence of efficacy. The only tricyclic antidepressant that has shown convincing evidence of efficacy is clomipramine for pediatric OCD. Placebo-controlled trials show efficacy of both fluvoxamine and fluoxetine in treating pediatric separation anxiety disorder, social phobia, and GAD. Other placebo-controlled trials also show efficacy of sertraline in treating pediatric GAD, as well as paroxetine in treating pediatric social anxiety disorder. *(Ref. 3, Ch. 5.5.1, Pharmacologic section)*

33 **(d)** A majority of children with OCD have comorbid psychiatric disorders, including tic disorders, mood, anxiety, and disruptive behavior disorders, ADHD, and developmental disorders. Male gender and earlier age of onset are associated with increased likelihood of comorbid ADHD and Tourette's disorder. OCD occurring in children with tic disorders has differences in its pattern of symptoms, course, and treatment response, warranting a specifier in the DSM-5 diagnostic criteria for OCD. OCD has an earlier average age of onset than most comorbid anxiety disorders but not separation anxiety disorder. *(Ref. 1, Ch. 17, Comorbidity section; Ref. 4, p.237–238, 242)*

34 **(c)** While very early age of onset may be an adverse prognostic factor, overall, pediatric OCD has a better long-term prognosis than adult-onset OCD. The other answers are all more clearly associated with poorer prognosis. *(Ref. 1, Ch. 17, Course and Prognosis section)*

35 **(c)** Only about 40–50% of drug-naïve patients with OCD experience 25–40% reduction of severity in symptoms responding to a single serotonin reuptake inhibitor. Thus, the choice of agents should take into account not only OCD itself, but also other possible comorbid conditions, such as panic disorder, depression, tic disorders, and psychotic disorders, etc. For the non-responders to SSRIs, augmentation strategies may be needed. *(Ref. 3, Ch. 5.5.2, Treatment section)*

36 **(b)** Investigators of POTS conclude that the first-line treatment for OCD is to start CBT alone or CBT plus an SSRI. *(Pediatric OCD Treatment Study (POTS) Team 2004)*

37 **(d)** The intervention program is brief and relatively low cost and delivered in various community settings, such as preschools, parent–child centers, and health clinics. The study showed lower frequency and severity of anxiety disorders and lower levels of anxiety symptoms in children whose parents received the intervention. Level of reduction of inhibition was noticed in both groups but no significant between group difference was observed. *(Rapee et al. 2010)*

38 **(d)** Self-talk is one of the cognitive strategies that can be used to treat children with anxiety disorders in that they identify maladaptive thoughts in order to correct their misinterpretations and biases. Relaxation training, constructing the anxiety hierarchy, desensitization in imagination, and in vivo desensitization are the stages of systematic desensitization. *(Ref. 3, Ch. 6.2.2, CBT Techniques section)*

39 **(c)** Many physical conditions can mimic PTSD-like symptoms, such as hyperthyroidism, caffeinism, migraine, asthma, seizure disorder, and catecholamine- or serotonin-secreting tumors. Some prescription medications and even some OTC medications may have similar effects, such as antiasthmatics, sympathomimetics, steroids, SSRIs, antipsychotics, diet pills, antihistamines, and cold medicines. *(Practice Parameter for the Assessment and Treatment of Children and Adolescents with Posttraumatic Stress Disorder 2010)*

40 **(e)** Using a more directive approach to address the child's traumatic experience is superior in reducing or resolving PTSD symptoms to nondirective or nonspecific approaches. Timing and pace depends on children's responses, and clinical worsening may indicate the need to strengthen mastery of previously learned interventions to enhance functioning and resiliency, rather than abandoning such an approach. *(Practice Parameter for the Assessment and Treatment of Children and Adolescents with Posttraumatic Stress Disorder 2010)*

References

Cunningham, C. E., McHolm, A., Boyle, M. H., & Patel, S. (2004). Behavioral and emotional adjustment, family functioning, academic performance, and social relationships in children with selective mutism. *Journal of Child Psychology and Psychiatry, and Allied Disciplines*, 45(8), 1363–1372. https://doi.org/10.1111/j.1469-7610.2004.00843.x

Pediatric OCD Treatment Study (POTS) Team (2004). Cognitive-behavior therapy, sertraline, and their combination for children and adolescents with obsessive-compulsive disorder: The Pediatric OCD Treatment Study (POTS) randomized controlled trial. *JAMA*, 292(16), 1969–1976. https://doi.org/10.1001/jama.292.16.1969

Practice Parameter for the Assessment and Treatment of Children and Adolescents with Posttraumatic Stress Disorder. *Journal of the American Academy of Child and Adolescent Psychiatry, 49*: 414–430, 2010.

Rapee, R. M., Kennedy, S. J., Ingram, M., Edwards, S. L., & Sweeney, L. (2010). Altering the trajectory of anxiety in at-risk young children. *The American Journal of Psychiatry*, 167(12), 1518–1525. https://doi.org/10.1176/appi.ajp.2010.09111619

Toppelberg, C. O., Tabors, P., Coggins, A., Lum, K., & Burger, C. (2005). Differential diagnosis of selective mutism in bilingual children. *Journal of the American Academy of Child and Adolescent Psychiatry*, 44(6), 592–595. https://doi.org/10.1097/01.chi.0000157549.87078.f8

7

FEEDING AND EATING DISORDERS, ELIMINATION DISORDERS, AND OBESITY

DOI: 10.4324/9781003308805-8

QUESTIONS

Directions: Select the best response for each of the questions 1–48.

1 Based on DSM-5, which of the following conditions is *not* under the category of feeding and eating disorders?

  a Pica

  b Obesity

  c Rumination disorder

  d Avoidant/restrictive food intake disorder

  e Binge-eating disorder

2 All of the following statements regarding pica are correct *except*:

  a The onset of the disorder has to be before the age of 18 years.

  b The symptoms have to persist longer than one month.

  c The prevalence of pica is unclear and it is highly comorbid with autism spectrum disorders and intellectual disability.

  d The "nonfood" does not include diet products that have minimal nutritional content.

  e Medical complications can result from pica, and pica can be potentially fatal.

3 All of the following statements correctly describe rumination disorder *except*:

  a With unclear prevalence, its onset can be at any age although in infants it usually starts between the ages of 3 and 12 months.

  b Repeat regurgitation can be attributable to associated medical conditions, such as gastro-esophageal reflux and pyloric stenosis.

  c Medical evaluation and laboratory tests can be warranted, such as esophageal pH monitoring, scintigraphic gastro-esophageal reflux scan, endoscopy, and gastric emptying studies.

  d It should be differentiated from anorexia nervosa and bulimia nervosa.

  e Position of straining and arching back and making movements with the tongue can be characteristics of rumination disorder in infants.

4 All of the following statements regarding avoidant/restrictive food intake disorder (ARFID) in DSM-5 are correct *except*:

  a Criteria can be met even if there are no weight concerns or nutritional deficiencies, if the eating disturbance impairs psychosocial functioning.

  b In children and adolescents, failure to maintain weight or height increases along with their developmental trajectory fulfills the criteria of weight loss.

  c Malnutrition can be life threatening, especially in infants.

  d Fear of gaining weight or getting fat can be a driving force behind avoidance.

  e Heightened sensory difficulty is a driving force of avoidance in some cases.

5 All of the following statements regarding diagnosing anorexia nervosa based on DSM-5 are correct *except*:

  a In children and adolescents, significantly low weight refers to less than that minimally expected.

  b Amenorrhea for at least three consecutive cycles is required for post-menarcheal females.

  c Two subtypes, restricting type and binge-eating/purging type, can be distinguished using different ICD-10 codes.

  d Disturbance of self-perceived body weight and shape and failure to recognize seriousness of low body weight are required.

  e DSM-5 uses body mass index (BMI) to specify severity of the disorder.

6 Patients with anorexia nervosa (AN) exhibit a number of neuroendocrine abnormalities. All of the following hormonal abnormalities have been found in emaciated patients with AN *except*:

  a Increased corticotropin-releasing hormone (CTRH)

  b Increased triiodothyronine (T3)

  c Blunted diurnal cortisol levels

  d Decreased estrogens

  e Decreased luteinizing hormone-releasing hormone (LHRH)

7 The symptoms of eating disorder tend to fluctuate and may show diagnostic crossovers between the anorexia nervosa (AN) subtypes and from AN to bulimia nervosa. Which of the following is a *correct* approximate rate of such crossovers during the course of the disorder?

  a 5%

  b 10%

  c 25%

  d 50%

  e 60%

8 Which of the following conditions is *least* likely to occur in patients with bulimia nervosa?

  a Hyperkalemia

  b Hypochloremia

  c Hyponatremia

  d Metabolic alkalosis

  e Metabolic acidosis

9 Based on DSM-5, on average how many episodes of inappropriate compensatory behaviors per week have to occur that will specify the severity of bulimia nervosa as "severe"?

a 1–3

b 4–7

c 8–13

d 14–18

e > 18

10 All of the following are risk factors for developing bulimia nervosa *except*:

a Low self-esteem, depression, and anxiety in childhood

b Internalization of a thin body ideal

c Underweight childhood

d Early pubertal maturation

e Familial transmission

11 All of the following statements correctly describe the characteristics of binge-eating disorder (BED) *except*:

a Excess eating occurs in a discrete period of time, with a sense of lack of control.

b Binge-eating episodes can be associated with eating too fast, eating too much, eating alone, and feeling disgusted and guilty afterward.

c Marked distress results from the presence of binge eating.

d Binge eating occurs at least once a week for three months on average.

e Binge eating may be accompanied by recurrent inappropriate compensatory behavior.

12 At which of the following *minimal* chronological ages (or equivalent developmental level) can a child be diagnosed with enuresis?

a 2 years

b 3 years

c 4 years

d 5 years

e 6 years

13 A diagnosis of enuresis can be made in the presence of which of the following situations?

a Neurogenic bladder

b Polyuria secondary to diabetes mellitus

c Polyuria secondary to diabetes insipidus

d Acute urinary tract infection

e Regular presence of incontinence prior to the onset of the above conditions

14 All of the following statements regarding *primary* encopresis are accurate *except*:

a Children must be older than 4 years of age to receive the diagnosis.

b Frequency must be more than once a month for three months.

c Children develop this condition after a period of fecal continence.

d Constipation and overflow incontinence are very common.

e Constipation may be complicated by anal fissure and painful defecation.

15 The *peak* time for the onset of bulimia nervosa is:

a Preadolescence

b Early adolescence

c Middle adolescence

d Late adolescence

e Middle adulthood

16 All of the following statements regarding comorbidity of anorexia nervosa (AN) and bulimia nervosa (BN) are accurate *except*:

a Both AN and BN have a high comorbidity with mood disorders.

b Comorbid anxiety disorders are commonly seen both in patients with AN and those with BN.

c Patients with AN are more commonly involved with alcohol and drug abuse than those with BN.

d Some researchers described three personality subtypes in patients with eating disorders: high-functioning and perfectionistic type, more constricted and over-controlled type, and more emotionally dysregulated and undercontrolled type.

e Adolescents with AN tend to show a more avoidant, inhibited, and constricted personality compared to those with BN, who tend to show more affective lability and an undercontrolled personality.

17 All of the following instruments are helpful in screening and assessing individuals with possible eating disorders *except*:

a Eating Disorder Examination (EDE)

b Eating Disorder Inventory (EDI)

c Eating Attitudes Test (EAT)

d Kids Eating Disorder Survey (KEDS)

e None of the above

18 Which therapeutic modality has the most evidence for treating adolescents with anorexia nervosa?

a Individual CBT

b Family-based treatment (FBT)

c Group therapy

d Individual interpersonal therapy (IPT)

e Individual psychodynamic psychotherapy

19 Which of the following associated conditions in adolescents with anorexia nervosa warrants pediatric inpatient care?

a Weight < 75% of ideal body weight

b Unresponsive to outpatient treatments

c Amenorrhea

d   Presence of comorbid psychiatric disorders

e   Hypercholesterolemia

20   There is limited data to support a role of psychopharmacological interventions for anorexia nervosa. Which of the following agents have shown benefits in decreasing anxiety around eating, improving sleep, and decreasing rumination about food and body concerns based on recent studies?

a   Lithium

b   Haloperidol

c   Olanzapine

d   Risperidone

e   Ziprasidone

21   Which of the following medications has shown *strong* evidence of efficacy in treating youth with bulimia nervosa?

a   Fluoxetine

b   Citalopram

c   Escitalopram

d   Sertraline

e   None of the above

22   Ipecac abuse in youth with eating disorders is *specifically* associated with which of the following conditions?

a   Periodontitis

b   Esophageal or gastric rupture

c   Renal failure

d   Cardiomyopathy

e   Seizure

23   Some chronic medical illnesses may cause weight loss. Thus, such illnesses should be considered in the differential diagnoses of anorexia nervosa. Which of the following is *least* likely to cause weight loss?

a   Crohn's disease

b   Diabetes mellitus

c   Addison's disease

d   Hyperthyroidism

e   Kleine-Levin syndrome

24   All of the following statements accurately describe the developmental course and outcome of anorexia nervosa (AN) based on up-to-date research data *except*:

a   Long-term studies show less than 50% of patients with AN achieve full recovery.

b   One-third of the patients partially remit, and one-fifth of the patients remain chronically ill.

c   Adolescents seem to have more favorable outcomes than adults.

d   Mortality risk is increased in bulimia nervosa (BN) but not AN.

e   Youth participating in family-based intervention for AN achieve substantial improvement and recovery.

25   Which of the following is *least* likely to be a personality characteristic of patients with anorexia nervosa?

a   Perfectionism

b   Competitiveness

c   Avoidant traits

d   Obsessional traits

e   Interpersonal security

26   All of the following neuroendocrine changes can be found in patients with anorexia nervosa *except*:

a   Decreased corticotrophin-releasing hormone (CRH)

b   Hyposecretion of GnRH

c   Reduced serotonin functioning

d   Low level of leptin

e   Increased adiponectin

27   All of the following statements regarding the epidemiology of anorexia nervosa (AN) and bulimia nervosa (BN) accurately reflect current knowledge *except*:

a   AN occurs about ten times more frequently in females than males.

b   AN is less common than BN.

c   AN is prevalent across different ethnic and socioeconomic groups.

d   AN is less prevalent in Asian American women.

e   BN is less common in African American women.

28   Individuals with bulimia nervosa are *least* likely to rate their families' dynamics as which of the following?

a   Disengaged

b   More controlling

c   Conflictive

d   Disorganized

e   Non-cohesive

29   All of the following are common laboratory findings with binging and purging behavior *except*:

a   Hypokalemia

b   Hypochloremic alkalosis

c   Decreased serum amylase

d   EKG—QT and T wave changes

e   Reduced bone density

30   Which of the following numbers correctly reflects the prevalence of obesity in children and adolescents based on data from the 2011–2014 National Health and Nutrition Examination Survey (NHANES)?

a   7%

b   10%

c   17%

d   46%

e   58%

31 Which of the following is the *least* likely comorbid medical condition of obesity?

a   Metabolic syndrome

b   Hyperthyroidism

c   Constipation

d   Obstructive sleep apnea

e   Pseudotumor cerebri

32 Which of the following distinguishes bulimia nervosa from anorexia nervosa?

a   Undue concern about body shape and weight

b   Normal weight

c   Binge eating

d   Self-induced vomiting

e   Excessive exercise

33 What is the first-line treatment for binge-eating disorder (BED)?

a   CBT

b   Dieting

c   Supportive psychotherapy

d   Lisdexamfetamine

e   Atomoxetine

34 Which of the following is *least* likely to influence hunger, satiety, and fat distribution?

a   Adiponectin

b   Ghrelin

c   Insulin

d   Leptin

e   Melatonin

35 Which is *not* a core part of CBT for avoidant/restrictive food intake disorder (ARFID)?

a   Increasing volume of food for low weight patients

b   Increasing variety of food for non-low-weight patients

c   Systemic desensitization to target sensory sensitivity

d   Handing control of eating back to the patient

e   Interoceptive exposures to address lack of interest

36 Which of the following defines childhood obesity?

a   BMI ≥ 25

b   BMI ≥ 30

c   BMI percentile ≥ 85th

d   BMI percentile ≥ 90th

e   BMI percentile ≥ 95th

37 All of the following statements regarding treatment of obesity are correct *except*:

a   The primary goal is to improve long-term physical health through a permanent healthy lifestyle.

a   Weight loss is another important goal.

c   Good sleep hygiene is encouraged as poor sleep is associated with overeating.

d   Physical activity interventions focus on increasing physical activity and/or reducing sedentary behaviors.

e   Parents' involvement in behavioral modification is very important.

38 An overweight patient has lost significant weight by restricting her food intake, going from obese to normal weight range. She feels that she needs to lose more weight and is fearful of regaining weight. What is the best diagnosis?

a   Healthy weight loss

b   AN

c   BN

d   Atypical AN

e   ARFID

39 Which of the following is *not* accurate regarding presurgical evaluation for bariatric surgery?

a   It typically includes a psychosocial interview.

b   Rates of psychiatric disorders are low in bariatric surgery patients.

c   Evaluation should include assessment of motivation.

d   Active bulimia is a contraindication.

e   Behavioral health specialists can help optimize patients for surgery by treating comorbid psychiatric conditions.

40 Based on epidemiological studies of enuresis, which of the following pairs of numbers reflects the rates of male:female 14-year-old adolescents respectively who are still wetting at least once a week?

a   6.2% vs. 3%

b   3% vs. 1.5%

c   1.1% vs. 0.5%

d   0.8% vs. 0.4%

e   0.5% vs. 0.1%

41 All of the following statements regarding the etiology, mechanism, and risk factors for enuresis are correct *except*:

a   Enuretic events can occur during all phases of the sleep cycle.

b   Efficacy of imipramine in treating bed wetting is related to its peripheral anticholinergic effects.

c   Studies show no difference of plasma atrial natriuretic peptide (ANP) in children with nocturnal enuresis versus without.

d   Secreted in pulsatile manner, low nocturnal arginine vasopressin (AVP) may represent a subgroup of enuresis.

e   Functional bladder capacity and thickness of bladder wall may be related to the response to desmopressin acetate (DDAVP).

42 All of the following statements regarding using imipramine to treat enuresis in children are correct *except*:

a   Drug overdose can be potentially lethal.

b   Cardiac monitoring is not routinely required.

c   Periodic determination of a blood level is needed.

d   A 25 mg starting dose and slow titration with 25 mg increment per week to a dose range of 75–125 mg is recommended.

e   Withdrawing the medication every three months to detect possible remission is recommended.

43   Which of the following is the *least* likely side effect of the DDAVP nasal inhaler?

a   Abdominal pain

b   Epistaxis

c   Headache

d   Hypernatremia

e   Nasal stuffiness

44   Which of the following factors is associated with a better treatment response of enuresis to DDAVP?

a   Older age

b   Higher frequency of baseline enuretic events

c   Smaller bladder capacity

d   Increased urinary osmolality

e   Nocturnal polyuria

45   All of the following statements regarding using the bell and pad alarm system to treat enuresis are correct *except*:

a   The bell and pad alarm system has an initial response rate of approximately 75%.

b   The sustained remission rate of the bell and pad alarm system is about 50%.

c   There are two subgroups of children associated with remission: those who learn to wake up to urinate and those who sleep through dry.

d   Decreased vasopressin explains the mechanism of the efficacy.

e   It can be considered as a first-line choice.

46   What is the approximate prevalence rate of encopresis in children between 7 and 8 years of age?

a   0.5%

b   1.5%

c   3%

d   5%

e   8%

47   Which of the following is *more* likely to have an elevated postprandial plasma level in children with encopresis?

a   Cholecystokinin

b   Estrogen

c   Gastrin

d   Pancreatic polypeptide

e   Motilin

48   Which of the following is *least* likely to be a medical cause of encopresis?

a   Hirschsprung's disease

b   Hemorrhoids

c   Hypocalcaemia

d   Lactase deficiency

e   Spina bifida

Matching

49–51   There are three phases of family-based treatment of anorexia nervosa. Match each phase listed with the following treatment that *best* describes it:

a   Discussion of adolescent development

b   Handing control over eating back to the adolescent

c   Restoring the adolescent's weight

49   Phase 1

50   Phase 2

51   Phase 3

ANSWERS AND EXPLANATIONS

1 **(b)** Even with robust association between obesity and a range of mental disorders (such as binge eating, depressive and bipolar disorders, schizophrenia, etc.), and side effects from many psychotropic medications, obesity is not included as a mental disorder in DSM-5 because it is such a diverse disorder and many etiologic factors are involved such as genetic, physiological, behavioral, and environmental factors. In addition to all the listed conditions, anorexia nervosa, bulimia nervosa, other specified feeding or eating disorder, and unspecified feeding or eating disorder are all under the category of feeding and eating disorders in DSM-5. *(Ref. 4, pp. 329–354)*

2 **(a)** With the usual onset in childhood, pica can also start in adolescence and adulthood. The core symptom of pica is a persistent pattern of eating nonnutritive, nonfood substances longer than one month, which is inappropriate to the developmental age, and is not within a culturally supported or socially normative practice. With unclear prevalence, it is highly comorbid with autism spectrum disorders and intellectual disability. The term "nonfood" does not include diet products with minimal nutritional value. Medical complications may bring attention to the disorder, including some serious ones, such as mechanical bowel problems, intestinal obstruction, and intestinal perforation, which can be potentially fatal. Pregnant women may crave nonnutritive and nonfood substances. The diagnosis of pica cannot be given unless ingestion of such substances poses potential medical risks to the pregnant woman. *(Ref. 4, pp. 329–331)*

3 **(b)** Under DSM-5, by definition the symptom of repeated regurgitation of food cannot be attributed to an associated gastrointestinal or other medical condition. Rumination disorder can lead to severe malnutrition and can be potentially fatal, especially in infants. Appropriate medical evaluation and laboratory tests may be warranted to rule out medical conditions that can mimic the symptoms. Psychologically, it is believed to be associated with the inability to regulate the internal state of satisfaction, a physical propensity to regurgitate, and a learned behavior to relieve the internal state of dissatisfaction. It is suggested that the treatment should focus on the learned aspect of rumination, using aversive and non-aversive behavioral reinforcement techniques. *(Ref. 3, Ch.5.7.2, Rumination section; Ref. 4, pp. 332–333)*

4 **(d)** Avoidant/restrictive food intake disorder (ARFID) should be differentiated from anorexia nervosa (AN), which is characterized by a core feature of restriction of energy intake for fear of gaining weight or getting fat. The eating disturbance in ARFID does not occur exclusively during the course of AN or bulimia nervosa, and is not due to the fear of gaining weight or getting fat. In some cases, sensory issues play an important role in food avoidance and restriction, especially to certain types of food. *(Ref. 4, pp. 334–338)*

5 **(b)** Amenorrhea for at least three consecutive cycles was required for post-menarcheal females as one of the diagnostic criteria of AN in DSM-IV-TR. But it was eliminated from DSM-5 even though amenorrhea can be commonly present as an indicator of physiological dysfunction. The severity of the disorder was measured by using BMI in adults and BMI percentile in children and adolescents. Specifiers include mild: BMI ≥ 17; moderate: BMI 16–16.99; severe: BMI 15–15.99; and extreme: BMI < 15. *(Ref. 4, pp. 338–343)*

6 **(b)** Except for answer b (should be decreased T3), all of the hormonal abnormalities listed, among others such as increased fasting and impaired growth hormone secretion response, uncoupled vasopressin secretion from osmotic challenge, and decreased testosterone in males, can be found in emaciated patients with anorexia nervosa. Other laboratory findings may include anemia, leukopenia with relative lymphocytosis, hypercarotenemia, hypoproteinemia, hypercholesterolemia, low basal metabolic rate, and reduced bone density. EKG may show sinus bradycardia, and occasionally QTc prolongation in certain patients. *(Ref. 3, Table 5.7.1.5; Ref. 4, pp. 342–343)*

7 **(d)** The symptoms of eating disorders tend to fluctuate and may show diagnostic crossovers between the AN subtypes and from AN to BN, which occur in approximately 50% of patients. Crossover from BN to AN occurs less frequently— about 15%—with the majority of them crossing back to BN or experiencing multiple back-and-forth crossovers between the two disorders. *(Ref. 1,Ch.19, Developmental Course section; Ref. 4, p. 347)*

8 **(a)** Hypokalemia is one of the common electrolyte abnormalities found in patients with BN as a consequence of purging. Metabolic alkalosis can occur because of loss of gastric acid through vomiting whereas metabolic acidosis can also occur because of frequent self-induced diarrhea or dehydration via abusing laxatives and diuretics. *(Ref. 4, p. 348)*

9 **(c)** Based on DSM-5, on average 8–13 episodes of inappropriate compensatory behaviors per week have to occur to specify the severity of a BN as "severe." "Mild" categorization needs on average 1–3 episodes per week; "moderate" needs 4–7 per week; and "extreme" needs more than 14 episodes per week. *(Ref. 4, p. 345)*

10 **(c)** Childhood obesity is one of the risk factors for the development of BN. *(Ref. 4, p. 348)*

11 **(e)** Binge eating cannot be accompanied by recurrent inappropriate compensatory behavior as seen in BN. In contrast to BN, patients with binge-eating disorder do not usually use marked or sustained dietary restriction to control body shape or weight in between the episodes but may attempt frequent dieting. Meeting criteria for BN is an exclusion criterion for binge-eating disorder. The treatment response and prognosis of binge-eating disorder is better than that of BN. *(Ref. 4, pp. 350–352)*

12 **(d)** The minimum chronological age or equivalent developmental level to diagnose someone with enuresis is 5 years. If urinary continence has never been established, it is called "primary" type; otherwise, it is called "secondary" if symptoms reemerge after a period of established urinary continence.

Thus, primary type only can start after age 5 years, whereas secondary type starts between ages 5 and 8 years in general. The rate of spontaneous remission is 5–10% per year after the age of 5 years. Most children with the disorder are continent by adolescence, but about 1% continue to be incontinent into adulthood. *(Ref. 4, pp. 355–357)*

13 **(e)** A diagnosis of enuresis *cannot* be made in the presence of neurogenic bladder, polyuria secondary to diabetes mellitus or diabetes insipidus, or acute urinary tract infection unless regular incontinence is present prior to the onset of these conditions or the symptoms persist after receiving appropriate interventions for the medical conditions. *(Ref. 4, p. 357)*

14 **(c)** Encopresis is the repeated passage of feces into places inappropriate for that purpose, occurring after age 4 when bowel control is expected. Children with primary encopresis have never developed fecal continence. Constipation and overflow incontinence can be associated with both primary and secondary encopresis and may lead to anal fissure and painful defecation. *(Ref. 3, Ch. 5.12, Encopresis section; Ref. 4, pp. 357–359)*

15 **(d)** The peak time of onset of BN is late adolescence or early adulthood. The 12-month prevalence of BN among young females is 1–1.5%, whereas the prevalence of AN is about 0.4%, with far less prevalence for both conditions in males (with approximate female to male ratio of 10:1). *(Ref. 4, pp. 341, 347)*

16 **(c)** Patients with BN are more commonly involved with alcohol and drug abuse than those with AN. *(Ref. 1, Ch.19, Developmental Course section)*

17 **(e)** All the listed are valid psychometric assessment instruments that can be used to screen and assess individuals with possible eating disorders. The EDE has both an adult version and a version for children and young adolescents. The EDI is a self-report measure that can be used for individuals as young as 14 years old. The EAT has a version specific for school-aged children, while the KEDS can be applied to elementary and middle school-aged children. *(Ref. 1, Ch. 19, Psychometric section)*

18 **(b)** FBT has the most evidence for treatment of adolescent AN. FBT is also recommended for treatment of adolescents with BN although it has been less well studied than in AN. CBT is the most effective treatment of adult BN. CBT can be considered for adolescent AN or BN if FBT is not available or appropriate for a specific family, but further studies are needed. *(Ref. 1, Ch 19, Psychotherapy section)*

19 **(a)** Medical complications of AN can be persistent and life threatening. Admission to a pediatric medical inpatient unit is warranted with the presence of medical instability, such as lower than 75% of ideal body weight, hypoglycemic syncope, fluid and electrolyte imbalance, cardiac arrhythmia, and severe dehydration, etc. Unresponsiveness to outpatient treatment and having serious comorbid psychiatric conditions may not necessarily warrant pediatric medical inpatient care but may warrant admission to a psychiatric facility that specializes in the treatment of eating disorders. *(Ref. 1, Ch. 19, Inpatient section)*

20 **(c)** Several recent case reports and open-label trials showed benefits from using olanzapine in the treatment of youth with AN in helping their anxiety around eating, improving sleep, and decreasing rumination about food and body concerns. *(Ref. 1, Ch. 19, Pharmacotherapy section)*

21 **(e)** There was only one open-label trial combining fluoxetine with supportive psychotherapy in treating adolescents with BN, which showed some impressive improvements. However, a paucity of systematic data exists to show any strong support for any medications in the treatment of either AN or BN. In adults, randomized, controlled clinical trials show evidence of using antidepressants in reducing binge frequency in patients with BN. *(Ref. 1, Ch. 19, Pharmacotherapy section)*

22 **(d)** Ipecac abuse may cause cardiomyopathy, which can potentially lead to cardiac failure and death. Pericardial pain, dyspnea, generalized muscle weakness with hypotension, tachycardia, and electrocardiogram abnormalities could be signs of ipecac intoxication. Periodontitis, dental enamel erosion and caries, perioral dermatitis, subconjunctival hemorrhage, esophageal or gastric rupture, metabolic alkalosis with hypokalemia, cardiac arrhythmia, renal failure, and seizure can all be potential complications of binging and purging behavior. *(Ref. 3, Ch. 5.7.1, Clinical section)*

23 **(e)** Kleine-Levin syndrome (a rare condition) is associated with hyperphagia and periodic hypersomnia lasting for several weeks at a time. Another condition named Klüver-Bucy syndrome presents with overeating episodes along with visual agnosia, compulsive licking and biting, and hypersexuality. These two conditions do not usually cause weight loss. On the other hand, Crohn's disease, diabetes mellitus, colitis, brain tumors, hyperthyroidism, and Addison's disease can all mimic the weight loss that is seen in AN. *(Ref. 3, Ch. 5.7.1, Differential section)*

24 **(d)** Mortality rate is increased in those with AN; adults with AN are five times more likely to die prematurely and 18 times more likely to die by suicide. Mortality rates are not increase in those with BN. *(Ref. 1, Ch. 19, Developmental Course section)*

25 **(e)** Studies found people with AN have greater obsessive-compulsive traits, tend to show perfectionism, and have high harm avoidance. *(Ref. 3, Ch. 5.7.1, Psychological section)*

26 **(a)** Increased corticotrophin-releasing hormone (CRH) secretion and decreased GnRH can be found in patients with AN. Functional disturbance of serotonin neurotransmission, mostly reduced serotonin function, is found in patients with AN. Cyproheptadine, a serotonin antagonist, demonstrates effects in facilitating weight gain in patients with AN. Clomipramine and fluoxetine have been useful in preventing weight relapse in patients with AN and OCD behaviors. Emaciated patients with AN have very low serum level of leptin (a product of an obesity gene). As a protein released from adipose tissue, adiponectin, with effects on enhancing insulin sensitivity, is increased in patients with AN. *(Ref. 3, Ch. 5.7.1, Neuroendocrine section)*

27 **(e)** Although more prevalent in industrialized societies, AN occurs across ethnicity and socioeconomic status. In the United States, AN is similarly prevalent in African Americans, Latinos, Asians, and non-Latino Whites. BN is more prevalent among African Americans and Latinos compared to non-Latino Whites. *(Ref. 3, Ch. 5.7.1, Social section; Ref. 5; p. 2069)*

28 **(b)** Studies of family dynamics of patients with BN uncovered lack of parental affection, negative, hostile, and disengaged interactions within the families, parental impulsivity, and family alcoholism and obesity. Patients with BN tend to rate their families as conflictive, disorganized, non-cohesive, and having

a lack of nurturance, which is quite different from those with AN (rating their family as more controlling, non-conflictive, cohesive with adequate nurturance). *(Ref. 1, Ch. 19, Etiology section)*

29 (c) Elevated serum amylase is more common laboratory finding in patients with binging and purging behavior. *(Ref. 3, Table 5.7.1.6)*

30 (c) The 2011–2014 NHANES found that 17% of children and adolescents were obese. *(Ref. 2, Ch. 16, Obesity section)*

31 (b) Obesity places the individual at risk of developing a series of medical comorbidities, including metabolic syndrome, diabetes mellitus, inflammation, polycystic ovary syndrome, hypothyroidism, hypertension, lipid abnormalities, nonalcoholic fatty liver disease, gallstones, gastric reflux, constipation, obstructive sleep apnea, asthma, pseudotumor cerebri, slipped capital femoral epiphysis, and increased injury rates. Psychological comorbidities may include depression, eating disorders, diminished self-esteem, body dissatisfaction, peer victimization and stigmatization, and decreased quality of life, etc. *(Ref. 5, p. 2211)*

32 (b) All of the answers can be seen in either BN or AN except normal weight. Patients with BN can be normal weight or overweight. If a patient is below 15% of the normal weight range and engages in binging and purging, the diagnosis is AN binge-purge subtype. *(Ref. 3, Ch. 5.7.1, Clinical Description section)*

33 (a) CBT is the first-line treatment for BED as there is the most evidence for its efficacy. Interpersonal psychotherapy and dialectical behavior therapy have also demonstrated efficacy. While there is some evidence that medications, including lisdexamfetamine, atomoxetine, citalopram, escitalopram, sertraline, desipramine, imipramine, topiramate, and zonisamide, can treat BED, they are less effective than psychotherapy. Lisdexamfetamine is the only medication FDA approved for treatment of BED. *(Ref. 3, Ch. 5.6.1, Treatment section)*

34 (e) Adiponectin, ghrelin, insulin, leptin, and plasma glucose all play important roles in hunger, satiety, and fat distribution. Adiponectin, a protein released from adipose tissue, can enhance insulin sensitivity. Ghrelin, a peptide released from endocrine cells in the stomach, acts in the hypothalamus to result in increased meal size. Leptin, an obesity gene product, is found to be associated with increased BMI and the amount of adipose tissue in the patients with AN. Insulin regulates glucose metabolism. *(Ref. 3, Ch. 5.7.1, Biologic Factors section)*

35 (d) There are both CBT and FBT treatment approaches to ARFID. CBT for ARFID has four stages consisting of (1) psychoeducation and early change with increases in volume or variety of food, (2) treatment planning, (3) addressing maintain mechanisms with systemic desensitization, exposures to foods, and interoceptive exposures, and (4) relapse prevention. Handing control of eating back to the patient is a phase of FBT for AN. *(Ref. 1, Ch. 19, Treatment section)*

36 (e) In children, BMI percentile ≥95th is considered obesity and between the 85th and 95th percentiles is considered overweight. In adults, overweight, obesity, and extreme obesity is measured by BMI ≥ 25, ≥ 30, and ≥ 40, respectively. *(Ref. 2, Ch. 16, Obesity section; Ref. 5, p. 2210–2211)*

37 (b) The primary goal of treatment should be increasing healthy behaviors using a family-based approach. Weight stabilization rather than loss is the goal, as BMI will decrease as children grow taller. *(Ref. 2, Ch. 16, Obesity section)*

38 (d) Patients with atypical AN meet criteria for AN except that, despite significant weight loss, their weight is not below the normal range. *(Ref. 5, p. 2076)*

39 (b) Bariatric surgery patients have a high rate of psychiatric disorders with a lifetime incidence of about 68%. Presurgical evaluation includes psychological testing and a psychosocial interview ideally conducted by an integrated behavioral health professional. The assessment includes patient's motivation, understanding of surgery, commitment to lifestyle changes, mental health, substance use, social supports, stressors, and eating patterns. *(Ref. 5, p. 2222)*

40 (c) Epidemiological studies of enuresis show a higher prevalence rate in males than females, and by the age of 14 years, approximately 1.1% of boys versus 0.5% of girls still wet the bed at least once a week. In general, the prevalence rates are 5–10% for 5-year-olds and 3–5% by age 10. *(Ref. 1, Ch. 21, Enuresis section)*

41 (b) Efficacy of imipramine in treating bed wetting is more likely to be related to its central effects than periphery effects, and it has an impact on decreasing osmolar clearance and urinary output. The notion of enuresis as a willful expression of anger or resentment has been largely abandoned. Whereas old sleep studies used to focus on "deep sleep," newer studies with larger sample sizes indicate that enuretic events occur during each phase of the sleep cycle. Enuresis is not found to be related to the level of ANP, which would indicate a possible abnormal tubular factor. Studies on AVP have not achieved consistent results. However, a subgroup of children with enuresis with lower AVP seems to be more responsive to DDAVP. *(Ref. 1, Ch. 21, Etiology section)*

42 (b) Cardiac monitoring, such as baseline EKG, is required prior to starting the treatment. Some children may decide to take a few more tablets to achieve full effects, which may result in overdose that can be potentially lethal. The starting dose of imipramine is 25 mg/night, but it is unlikely to be effective if 75–125 mg per night does not produce any positive response. With significant variation of serum levels of imipramine, a periodic blood level test is recommended to guard against toxicity. Withdrawing the medication every three months is recommended to determine whether there is a remission because spontaneous remission is not uncommon. *(Ref. 1, Ch. 21, Pharmacological section)*

43 (d) Hyponatremia and related seizures can be a serious potential side effect of DDAVP, especially intranasal preparation. Thus, the FDA provides a warning that the intranasal preparation of DDAVP should not be used for the treatment of primary nocturnal enuresis. In the presence of acute medical illnesses that can produce fluid or electrolyte imbalance, DDAVP should be interrupted. *(Ref. 1, Ch. 21, Pharmacological section)*

44 (a) Older age, lower frequency of baseline enuretic events, and greater bladder capacity are associated with better response to DDAVP treatment. However, increased urinary osmolality and

nocturnal polyuria are associated with poor response. *(Ref. 1, Ch. 21, Pharmacological section)*

45 **(d)** Investigation of the physiological explanation of the bell and pad alarm system shows that those who achieve remission have an increased ability to concentrate urine, which appears to be related to an increased level of vasopressin. *(Ref. 1, Ch. 21, Other Treatment section)*

46 **(b)** The approximate prevalence rate of encopresis in children between 7 and 8 years of age is 1.5%. The male to female ratio is 3:1. Similar to enuresis, the prevalence of encopresis tends to decrease over time as the child ages. *(Ref. 1, Ch. 21, Encopresis section)*

47 **(d)** Postprandial pancreatic polypeptide level peaks earlier and remains higher in children with encopresis compared to the control group. Children with encopresis also show lower motilin response. However, the investigators could not rule out that these findings might be secondary to chronic constipation. *(Ref. 3, Ch. 5.12, Encopresis section)*

48 **(c)** Hypercalcaemia can be a medical cause of encopresis along with others such as constipation, medical conditions that produce diarrhea, side effects from certain medications, a painful lesion, thyroid disease, pseudo-obstruction, cerebral palsy, rectal stenosis, anal fissure, anorectal trauma, etc. Frequently associated with retentive encopresis, chronic constipation is the major factor in the evaluation of encopresis. *(Ref. 2, Ch. 11, Encopresis section)*

Matching

49 **(c); 50 (b); 51 (a)** Manualized family-based treatment for AN (FBT-AN) was used in a controlled study by J. Lock et al. 2005. The results show significant weight gain and improvements in psychological symptoms of AN as measured by Eating Disorder Examination (EDE). The FBT-AN needs to follow clearly defined phases: phase 1, restoring the adolescent's weight; phase 2, handing control over eating back to the adolescent; and phase 3, discussion of adolescent development. Family-based treatment for adolescents with BN (FBT-BN) also includes three phases: phase 1, reestablishing healthy eating; phase 2, helping the adolescent eat independently; and phase 3, adolescent developmental issues. In using FBT-BN, the focus is not on weight restoration; instead, it should focus on the regulation of eating patterns and elimination of purging. The FBT-BN approach is more collaborative between parents and the affected youth. Youth with BN are more likely to have psychiatric comorbid conditions that need to also be addressed in the treatment. *(Ref. 1, Ch. 19, Family-based treatment section)*

8

SOMATIC SYMPTOMS AND RELATED DISORDERS AND SLEEP–WAKE DISORDERS

DOI: 10.4324/9781003308805-9

QUESTIONS

Directions: Select the best response for each of the questions 1–30.

1 In the DSM-5 category of somatic symptoms and related disorders, which of the following terms is *not* included to describe a psychiatric condition?

a Somatic symptom disorder

b Hypochondriasis

c Conversion disorder

d Psychological factors affecting other medical conditions

e Factitious disorder

2 Which of the following statements regarding the diagnostic criteria for somatic symptom disorder is *incorrect*?

a Presence of distressing somatic symptom(s) may lead to significant disruption of daily life.

b There are excessive thoughts, feelings, or behaviors related to the somatic symptoms.

c A particular somatic symptom may not be present continuously; the state of being symptomatic has to be persistent, typically longer than six months.

d Upon appropriate investigation, the symptoms cannot be explained by a known general medical condition.

e A specifier "with predominant pain" is included for individuals whose somatic symptoms predominantly involve pain (describes previous "pain disorder" in DSM-IV).

3 All of the following are characteristics of somatic symptom disorder more commonly manifesting in children as compared to adults *except*:

a The most common symptoms are recurrent abdominal pain, headache, fatigue, and nausea.

b Multiple somatic symptoms are usually present.

c Younger children tend to experience more somatic complaints but less concern about "illness" per se compared to adolescents.

d The parents' response to the symptoms may have important effects on the child's level of associated distress.

e The parents may have a strong influence on how to interpret the symptoms.

4 All of the following statements regarding conversion disorder (functional neurological symptom disorder) are correct *except*:

a There is at least one symptom of altered voluntary or sensory function, which is not better explained by another medical or mental disorder.

b Hoover's sign can be potentially used to demonstrate incompatibility.

c The diagnosis of this disorder requires the judgment that the symptoms cannot be intentionally produced as seen in factitious disorder or malingering.

d The prognosis seems to be better in younger children than in adolescents or adults.

e History of childhood abuse and neglect can be a risk factor.

5 All of the following statements regarding factitious disorder are accurate *except*:

a The core feature of this disorder is the falsification of physical or psychological symptoms or manifestations, or induction of injury or disease in self or others.

b The falsification is associated with identified deception.

c When an adult falsifies symptoms in his or her child, both the adult and the child get the diagnosis.

d It is estimated that about 1% of individuals in hospital settings present with symptoms that are consistent with factitious disorder.

e Some aspects of factitious disorder might represent criminal behavior, which is not mutually exclusive of mental illness.

6 Which of the following therapeutic approaches to help children with somatic symptom disorder is *not* appropriate?

a Diminish perceived threats associated with the child's symptoms.

b Modulate affective and physiological reactions to associated environmental or physical precipitating factors.

c Encourage using accommodative coping strategies.

d Encourage avoidance and denial.

e Appropriately balance positive and negative reinforcement.

7 All of the following statements regarding insomnia disorder are correct *except*:

a The core feature of insomnia disorder is dissatisfaction with sleep quantity or quality, which causes clinically significant distress or impairment in important areas of functioning.

b The common complaints are difficulty starting sleep, difficulty maintaining sleep, and early morning awakening with difficulty going back to sleep.

c Children may manifest with difficulty starting sleep or maintaining sleep without caregiver intervention (such as presence of a parent and consistent sleep routines).

d The sleep disturbance occurs at least three nights a week for at least three months.

e The diagnosis should not be given to an individual who has a breathing-related sleep disorder.

8 Which of the following is the *most* common presentation of insomnia?

a Sleep onset insomnia

b Sleep maintenance insomnia

c Late insomnia

d   Nonrestorative sleep

e   Combination of sleep maintenance and sleep initiation

9   The core feature of hypersomnolence disorder is an excessive quantity of sleep, deteriorated quality of wakefulness, and sleep inertia. What is the *minimal* required maintained length of sleep per day to qualify for the diagnostic Criterion A for the disorder?

a   6 hours

b   7 hours

c   8 hours

d   9 hours

e   10 hours

10   All of the following statements regarding narcolepsy are correct *except*:

a   The core feature of narcolepsy is recurrent daytime excessive sleepiness that results in naps or sleep.

b   In individuals with long-standing disease, cataplexy manifests as brief episodes of sudden loss of muscle tone while maintaining consciousness.

c   In children or individuals within six months of onset, cataplexy can manifest as spontaneous grimaces or jaw-opening episodes, or low-grade continuous hypotonia.

d   Low serum hypocretin-1 level is seen in certain individuals with narcolepsy.

e   Rapid eye movement (REM) sleep latency measured by nocturnal sleep polysomnography is shortened in some individuals with narcolepsy.

11   All of the following statements regarding the development and course of narcolepsy are accurate *except*:

a   Onset of narcolepsy is usually in youth and young adults, with two peaks: at ages 15–25 and ages 30–35 years.

b   Onset can be abrupt or progressive, and severity is highest when onset is abrupt in children.

c   Abrupt onset in latency-age children is associated with low body mass index (BMI).

d   Sleep paralysis typically starts around puberty in those with latency-age onset.

e   Youth with narcolepsy may develop aggression along with other behavioral problems due to their sleepiness and/or nighttime sleep disruption.

12   All of the following factors are helpful to distinguish hypersomnolence from narcolepsy *except*:

a   Age at onset

b   Duration of nocturnal sleep

c   Degree of difficulty awakening

d   REM latency

e   Absence of dreaming during daytime naps

13   What is the *minimal* number of obstructive apneas or hypopneas per hour of sleep according to polysomnography required

to meet DSM-5 diagnostic criteria for obstructive sleep apnea hypopnea without accompanying other sleep-related symptoms?

a   5

b   10

c   15

d   20

e   25

14   Which of the following does *not* describe a feature of the sleep of infants as contrasted with that of older children, adolescents, and adults?

a   Shorter sleep cycle

b   Presence of sleep-onset REM sleep

c   Higher proportion of REM sleep

d   Greater variability of NREM-REM proportion across the sleep period

e   Polyphasic circadian cycle (as opposed to diurnal)

15   Among individuals with narcolepsy, which of the following ethnic groups is *more* likely to manifest the disorder without cataplexy or with atypical cataplexy?

a   African Americans

b   American Indians

c   Asian Americans

d   European Americans

e   Latino Americans

16   What is the prevalence of obstructive sleep apnea hypopnea in children?

a   0.5–1%

b   1–2%

c   2–5%

d   5–15%

e   20%

17   All of the following statements regarding the characteristics of obstructive sleep apnea hypopnea in youth are correct *except*:

a   The symptoms and signs of the disorder may be subtler in youth than in adults.

b   Parent-reported snoring episodes are less sensitive.

c   The suspicion of the disorder should be raised if enuresis recurs after a period of continence.

d   The clinical focus of younger children (< 5 years) is more often on observed nighttime symptoms such as apneas and labored breathing.

e   In younger children, obesity is a more common risk factor than in older children.

18   In which of the following ethnic groups is there an increased risk for obstructive sleep apnea hypopnea due to possible craniofacial structural factors?

a   Asians

b   Africans

c American Indians

d Europeans

e Latinos

19 Presence of which of the following conditions indicates the obstructive sleep apnea hypopnea is either very severe or associated with hypoventilation cardiopulmonary comorbidities?

a Diabetes

b Parkinson's disease

c Stroke

d Systemic hypertension

e Pulmonary hypertension

20 Which of the following conditions is *not* associated with "high loop gain"?

a Idiopathic central sleep apnea

b Cheyne-Stokes breathing

c Complex sleep apnea

d Central apnea comorbid with opioid use

e All of the above

21 Which of the following sleep–wake disorders is *most* likely to occur during perinatal periods?

a Idiopathic hypoventilation

b Idiopathic central sleep apnea

c Congenital central alveolar hypoventilation

d Comorbid sleep-related hypoventilation

e Obstructive sleep apnea hypopnea

22 Which of the following conditions is *least* likely seen in children with congenital central alveolar hypoventilation?

a Disorder of autonomic nervous system

b Box-shaped face

c Elongated face

d Hirschsprung's disease

e Neural crest tumors

23 Which of the following is *not* characteristic of circadian rhythm sleep–wake disorder, advanced sleep phase type?

a The main sleep period is advanced more than 3 hours in relation to the desired sleep and wake times.

b Individuals will typically exhibit normal sleep quality and duration when allowed to set their schedule.

c Onset is usually in late adulthood.

d The familial form may occur during childhood.

e The familial form is associated with an autosomal dominant mode of inheritance.

24 What is the prevalence of circadian rhythm sleep–wake disorder, delayed sleep phase type in adolescents?

a 1%

b 2%

c 4%

d 6%

e > 7%

25 Which of the following subtypes of circadian rhythm sleep–wake disorders is *more* prevalent in blind people?

a Delayed sleep phase type

b Advanced sleep phase type

c Irregular sleep–wake type

d Non-24-hour sleep–wake type

e Shift work type

26 All of the following disorders are under the DSM-5 category of parasomnias *except*:

a Non-rapid eye movement sleep arousal disorder

b Sleep terror disorder

c Nightmare disorder

d Rapid eye movement sleep behavior disorder

e Restless legs syndrome (RLS)

27 Which of the following parasomnias is *most* likely to occur in children and diminish in frequency with increasing age?

a Non-rapid eye movement sleep arousal disorders

b Nightmare disorder

c Rapid eye movement sleep behavior disorder

d Restless legs syndrome

e None of the above

28 The symptoms of which of the following conditions are *most* likely to begin in the first third of the night during slow-wave sleep?

a Non-rapid eye movement sleep arousal disorders

b Nightmare disorder

c Rapid eye movement sleep behavior disorder

d Restless legs syndrome

e None of the above

29 All of the following statements regarding differences between nightmare disorder and sleep terror disorder are accurate *except*:

a Only sleep terror disorder involves awakening or partial awakening with fearfulness and autonomic activation.

b Nightmare disorder manifests in the later part of the night during REM sleep.

c Nightmare disorder produces vivid, storylike dreams that are recallable.

d Sleep terror disorder manifests in the first third of the night during stage 3 or 4 NREM sleep.

e Sleep terror disorder does not produce vivid or storylike recallable dreams.

30 Which of the following genes is *not* particularly associated with restless legs syndrome?

a BTBD9

b MAP2K5

c MEIS1

d PER3

e All are associated

Matching

31–40 Match each listed term related to sleep–wake disorders with one of the following descriptions:

a Difficulty falling asleep at bedtime

b Frequent or prolonged awakening throughout the night

c Early morning awakening and difficulty returning to sleep

d Poor sleep quality and feeling unrested despite adequate duration

e Prolonged impaired alertness during the sleep–wake transition

f Vivid perceptual disturbance occurs just after wakening

g Vivid perceptual disturbance occurs before or upon falling asleep

h Reduction in airflow during breathing for at least 10 seconds in adults or two missed breaths in children

i Total absence of airflow during breathing for at least 10 seconds in adults or two missed breaths in children

j A breathing pattern with periodic crescendo–decrescendo variation in tidal volume, which leads to central apneas and hypopneas at a frequency of ≥ 5 events/hour along with frequent arousal

31 Nonrestorative sleep

32 Late insomnia

33 Middle insomnia

34 Initial insomnia

35 Sleep inertia

36 Hypnagogic hallucination

37 Hypnopompic hallucination

38 Cheyne-Stokes breathing

39 Apnea

40 Hypopnea

ANSWERS AND EXPLANATIONS

1 (b) "Hypochondriasis" is not a term used in DSM-5. Under the category of DSM-5 "somatic symptoms and related disorders," all other listed terms are used along with "illness anxiety disorder," "other specified somatic symptoms and related disorder," and "unspecified somatic symptoms and related disorder" to describe different psychiatric conditions. The term "illness anxiety disorder" replaces what was "hypochondriasis" in DSM-IV. *(Ref. 4, pp. 309–327)*

2 (d) "Upon appropriate investigation, the symptoms cannot be explained by a known general medical condition" is not among the diagnostic criteria for somatic symptom disorder. DSM-5 emphasizes that the diagnosis is made based on the *presence* of somatic symptoms and associated distress, abnormal thoughts, feelings, and behaviors in response to the somatic symptoms rather than the *absence* of a medical explanation for the somatic symptoms. In other words, the distinction is not the somatic symptoms per se, but instead how the individual with the disorder manifests and interprets them. *(Ref. 4, pp. 309–311)*

3 (b) A single dominant symptom is a more common presentation in children with somatic symptom disorder than in adults. Young children tend to focus more on the somatic complaints, and do not generally worry too much about "illness" per se until they become adolescents. Parents' response to the symptoms plays an important role in determining how to interpret the symptoms, the level of associated distress, and the associated time off from school and medical help seeking. *(Ref. 4, p. 313)*

4 (c) The diagnosis of conversion disorder (functional neurological symptoms disorder) does *not* require the judgment that the symptoms cannot be intentionally produced as seen in factitious disorder or malingering because there is no reliable way to assess conscious intention. But if there is definite evidence of feigning conversion disorder, factitious disorder (primary goal is to assume sick role) or malingering (primary goal is to obtain a secondary gain) should be considered. The weakness of hip extension that returns to normal strength when the contralateral hip is able to flex against resistance is called Hoover's sign and can be used to assess incompatibility. Evidence of incompatibility between the symptom and recognized neurological or medical conditions through clinical examination is required to diagnose this disorder (Criterion B). *(Ref. 4, pp. 318–321)*

5 (c) When an adult falsifies symptoms in his or her child, only the adult—the perpetrator (not the child—the victim)—gets the diagnosis of "factitious disorder imposed on another"—previously called "factious disorder by proxy"—and the child may be given an abuse diagnosis as a victim. Falsification of symptoms or induction of injury on others may represent criminal behavior that is not mutually exclusive of mental illness. In contrast to factitious disorder that requires the absence of clear rewards, malingering (coded with a V code: V65.2 in DSM-5) requires the presence of intentional reporting of symptoms for clear personal gain, such as money, time off, etc. *(Ref. 4, pp. 324–326)*

6 (d) Using accommodative coping strategies such as acceptance, distractions, self-encouragement, and cognitive reconstructing should be encouraged. However, passive strategies such as avoidance, denial, or wishful thinking should be discouraged. *(Ref. 3, Ch. 5.10, Coping section)*

7 (e) The diagnosis can be given to an individual who has a breathing-related sleep disorder. As a matter of fact, insomnia disorder is commonly comorbid with other medical and mental health conditions. The diagnosis is given regardless of whether it occurs as an independent condition or is comorbid with other conditions (including but not limited to mental disorders, medical comorbidities, and other sleep disorders). However, the insomnia is not better explained by and does not occur exclusively during the course of another condition, and the coexisting condition cannot adequately explain the predominant complaints of insomnia. In DSM-5, there are three specifiers to describe such comorbidities: "with non-sleep disorder mental comorbidity," "with other medical comorbidity," and "with other sleep disorder." *(Ref. 4, pp. 362–363)*

8 (e) The most common presentation of a single symptom of insomnia is difficulty maintaining sleep, followed by difficulty initiating sleep. However, the combination of these symptoms is the most common overall manifestation of insomnia. *(Ref. 4, p. 363)*

9 (b) Based on DSM-5 diagnostic criteria (Criterion A) for *hypersomnolence disorder*, even with sleep of at least seven hours there is still an existence of self-reported excessive sleepiness that is manifested as one of the following: recurrent periods of sleep or lapses into sleep during the same day; a prolonged nonrestorative sleep episode of > 9 hours; or difficulty remaining awake after abrupt awakening. *(Ref. 4, p. 368)*

10 (d) Low cerebrospinal fluid (CSF) hypocretin-1 level is called hypocretin-1 deficiency, which is measured using CSF hypocretin-1 immunoreactivity values, and must be less than or equal to 110/pg/ml. In some individuals with narcolepsy, their rapid eye movement (REM) sleep latency measured by nocturnal sleep polysomnography is shortened ≤ 15 minutes), or a multiple sleep latency test (MSLT) may show a mean sleep latency less than or equal to eight minutes and two or more sleep-onset REM periods. In children or individuals within six months of onset, cataplexy can manifest as spontaneous grimaces or jaw-opening episodes with tongue thrusting ("cataplectic faces"), or low-grade continuous hypotonia, yielding a wobbling walk, which all could occur without obvious emotional triggers. In contrast, typical cataplexy presents with brief episodes of sudden bilateral loss of muscle tone while maintaining consciousness, which is precipitated by laughter or joking. *(Ref. 4, pp. 372–374)*

11 (c) Abrupt onset in latency children can be associated with obesity and premature puberty. In the majority of cases (90%), the initial manifestation of narcolepsy is sleepiness or increased

sleep, followed by cataplexy (50% of the cases within one year, and 85% of the cases within three years). Often accompanied by hypnagogic hallucination, vivid dreaming, and REM sleep behavior disorder, excessive sleep can rapidly progress to an inability to stay awake during the day. *(Ref. 4, p. 375)*

12 (a) Hypersomnolence and narcolepsy are indistinguishable on the degree of daytime sleeping, age at onset, or stable course over time. However, some unique clinical and laboratory features can help to differentiate them. In general, hypersomnolence presents with longer and less disrupted nocturnal sleep, greater difficulty awakening, more persistent daytime sleepiness (no discrete "sleep attacks" that are commonly seen in narcolepsy), longer and less refreshing daytime sleep episodes, and little or no dreaming during daytime naps. Hypersomnolence does not have sleep-related hallucination, sleep paralysis, or shortened REM sleep latency. *(Ref. 4, pp. 368–377)*

13 (c) In the absence of other sleep-related symptoms, the minimal number of obstructive apneas or hypopneas per hour of sleep based on polysomnography is 15 to meet diagnostic criteria for obstructive sleep apnea hypopnea. However, only five obstructive apneas or hypopneas per hour of sleep are needed when present with one of the following two sleep symptoms: nocturnal breathing disturbance or daytime sleepiness, fatigue, or unrefreshing sleep despite sufficient opportunities to sleep. In children, an apnea hypopnea index of 2 is used as the threshold of abnormality. *(Ref. 4, pp. 378–379, 381)*

14 (d) Infants have polyphasic circadian cycles and shorter sleep cycles (approximately 50 minutes) compared to older children, adolescents, and adults (approximately 90–120 minutes). Their sleep cycle includes sleep-onset REM and a greater total proportion of REM sleep. However, the proportions of REM–NREM sleep remain consistent across the sleep period in infants compared to older children and adults, in whom the length of REM periods increases later in the sleep period. *(Ref. 3, Ch. 5.9, Sleep Physiology section)*

15 (a) Among individuals with narcolepsy, African Americans are *more* likely to manifest the disorder without cataplexy or with atypical cataplexy. It can complicate the diagnosis, especially when obesity and obstructive sleep apnea are present. *(Ref. 4, p. 378)*

16 (b) Among breathing-related sleep disorders, obstructive sleep apnea hypopnea disorder is the most common one, which presents in 1–2% in children, 2–15% in middle-aged adults, and > 20% in older adults. It is a highly underdiagnosed disorder in elderly individuals. It is more prevalent in people with obesity and is male predominant (2:1 to 4:1). There is no significant gender difference in latency-aged children and the difference declines in older age, which may indicate increased prevalence in women after menopause. *(Ref. 4, p. 379)*

17 (e) In younger children, obesity is a *less* common risk factor whereas developmental delay, delayed growth, and "failure to thrive" may be present. The diagnosis of the disorder is more difficult to establish in youth because the presentation is subtler and more often manifests as agitated arousals and unusual sleep postures, such as sleeping on the hands and knees. Other common features in children with the disorder may include daytime mouth breathing, difficulty swallowing, and poor speech articulation. Compared to younger children, in children older than 5 years, the disorder is more likely to manifest as sleepiness plus behavioral problems such as ADHD-like symptoms, learning difficulties, and morning headache. *(Ref. 4, p. 380)*

18 (a) Despite a relatively low BMI, people of Asian ancestry may be at a higher risk for obstructive sleep apnea hypopnea because of their relatively narrow nasopharynx. *(Ref. 4, p. 381)*

19 (e) Pulmonary hypertension and right heart failure present either in very severe cases of obstructive sleep apnea hypopnea or when associated with hypoventilation or cardiopulmonary comorbidities. Diabetes, coronary artery disease, stroke, and systemic hypertension are more common in moderate to severe cases. In addition, cerebrovascular disease, Parkinson's disease, and depression are also common comorbidities. *(Ref. 4, p. 383)*

20 (d) High loop gain refers to increased gain of the ventilator control system, which leads to instability in ventilation and $PaCO_2$ levels. The underlying pathogenesis of central sleep apnea comorbid with opioid use is believed to be related to the effects of opioid on the respiratory rhythm generator in the medulla and opioid's differential effects on hypoxic versus hypercapneic respiratory drive. All other listed conditions are associated with high loop gain. Complex sleep apnea refers to central sleep apnea that occurs in association with obstructive sleep apnea. *(Ref. 4, p. 384)*

21 (c) Congenital central alveolar hypoventilation can occur at birth with shallow, erratic, or absent breathing. It can persist into infancy, childhood, and adulthood depending on the severity that is related to variable penetration of the *PHOX2B* mutation. Its core feature is episodic decreased respiration (measured by polysomnography) associated with elevated CO_2 levels or persistent low levels of hemoglobin oxygen saturation unassociated with apneic/hypopneic events. *(Ref. 4, pp. 387–388)*

22 (c) Elongated face is a characteristic facial feature of Fragile X syndrome. On the other hand, box-shaped face (the face is short relative to its width) is the characteristic facial feature of congenital central alveolar hypoventilation. Comorbid with pulmonary disorders, neuromuscular or chest wall disorders, and certain medication use (such as benzodiazepines and opiates), it may also occur in association with autonomic dysfunction and Hirschsprung's disease. *(Ref. 4, pp. 389–390)*

23 (a) Circadian rhythm sleep–wake disorder, advanced sleep phase type, is characterized by the timing of the major sleep period being advanced usually more than 2 hours in relation to the desired sleep and wake times, with symptoms of early morning insomnia and excessive daytime sleepiness. While usual onset is in late adulthood, the familial form can have onset in childhood and is associated with an autosomal dominant mode of inheritance, with mutations in PER2 and CKI. *(Ref. 4. pp. 390–394)*

24 (e) The prevalence of delayed sleep phase type of circadian rhythm sleep–wake disorder is low in the general population (about 0.17%). However, the prevalence in adolescents is higher than 7%, which may be secondary to both behavioral and physiological factors such as hormonal changes from onset of puberty. *(Ref. 4, p. 391)*

25 **(d)** With unclear prevalence in the general population, non-24-hour sleep–wake type occurs among an estimated 50% of people who are blind, and rarely occurs in sighted people. *(Ref. 4, p. 396)*

26 **(b)** Sleep terrors (along with sleepwalking) are classified under the category of non-rapid eye movement sleep arousal disorders, and they are further identified by specifiers as two different types: sleep walking type and sleep terror type. Nightmare disorder is a separate disorder, and restless legs syndrome is another separate disorder. *(Ref. 4, pp. 399–413)*

27 **(a)** Non-rapid eye movement sleep arousal disorders are more likely to start in childhood, and diminish in frequency over time with increasing age. The prevalence of nightmare disorder increases over time with increasing age. More commonly affecting males > 50 years, REM sleep behavior disorder is also seen in females and younger individuals. The prevalence of RLS increases with age. *(Ref. 4, pp. 401, 405, 408, 411)*

28 **(a)** Both sleep walking and sleep terror of non-rapid eye movement arousal disorders usually begin in the first third of the night during slow-wave sleep. They are the repeated occurrence of incomplete arousals or precipitous awakenings from sleep, typically brief, lasting 1–10 minutes, but occasionally lasting longer, especially in children. *(Ref. 4, p. 400)*

29 **(a)** Both sleep terror disorder and nightmare disorder can involve awakening or partial awakening with fearfulness and autonomic activation. Nightmares usually lead to mild autonomic arousal and complete awakenings, whereas sleep terrors lead to partial awakenings and may leave the individual confused, disoriented, minimally responsive, and with significant autonomic arousal. Sleep terrors do not lead to elaborate dreams. *(Ref. 4, p. 406)*

30 **(d)** Genome-wide association studies have confirmed RLS is significantly associated with genetic variants of three genes: MEIS1 (on chromosome 2p), BTBD9 (on chromosome 6p), and MAP2K5 (on chromosome 15p). BTBD9 represents 80% of excessive risk when in the presence of a single allele. Pathophysiologically, RLS is involved with central dopaminergic and iron metabolic disturbances, and the endogenous opiate system may be involved. Response to dopaminergic drugs (such as D_2 and D_3 non-ergot agonists) supports the involvement of the dopaminergic system. Mutations in circadian genes (including PER2, PER3, and CKIe) are associated with delayed sleep phase type and advanced sleep phase type of certain circadian rhythm sleep–wake disorders. *(Ref. 4, pp. 392, 394, 412)*

Matching

31 **(d); 32 (c); 33 (b); 34 (a); 35 (e); 36 (g); 37 (f); 38 (j); 39 (i); 40 (h)** Insomnia can manifest differently at different sleep periods. *Initial insomnia* (*sleep onset insomnia*) refers to difficulty initiating sleep or falling asleep at bedtime. *Middle insomnia* (*sleep maintenance insomnia*) refers to difficulty maintaining sleep and having frequent or prolonged awakenings throughout the night. *Late insomnia* refers to early morning awakening and difficulty returning to sleep. *Nonrestorative sleep* refers to poor-quality, unrefreshed, and unrested sleep despite adequate duration of sleep. *Sleep inertia* (i.e., sleep drunkenness) refers to prolonged, impaired performance and alertness and reduced vigilance during the sleep–wake transition. It commonly occurs in hypersomnolence disorder. Individuals with narcolepsy may experience vivid hallucinations before or upon falling asleep, which are called *hypnagogic*, and the experience can also occur right after awakening, which is called *hypnopompic*. Defined as a breathing pattern with periodic crescendo–decrescendo variation in tidal volume, which leads to central apneas and hypopneas at a frequency of ≥ 5 events/hour along with frequent arousal, *Cheyne-Stokes breathing* is one of the specifiers used to diagnose *central sleep apnea*. Apnea is defined as the total absence of airflow during breathing for at least 10 seconds in adults or two missed breaths in children. Hypopnea is defined as the reduction in airflow during breathing for at least 10 seconds in adults or two missed breaths in children. *(Ref. 4, pp. 363, 369, 374–375, 379, 383)*

9

SUBSTANCE-RELATED AND ADDICTIVE DISORDERS

DOI: 10.4324/9781003308805-10

QUESTIONS

Directions: Select the best response for each of the questions 1–23.

1 Which of the following disorders is formally included under the category of substance-related and addictive disorders in DSM-5?

a Exercise addiction disorder

b Gambling disorder

c Internet gaming disorder

d Sex addiction disorder

e Shopping addiction disorder

2 All of the following substances are known to cause intoxication. Which of the following substances is *least* likely to cause withdrawal?

a Alcohol

b Caffeine

c Cannabis

d Inhalant

e Opioids

3 Which of the following is the *least* likely sign of inhalant intoxication?

a Nystagmus

b Lethargy

c Hypersensitive reflexes

d Euphoria

e Psychomotor retardation

4 Which of the following is the estimated 12-month prevalence rate of alcohol use disorder among American youth between ages 12 and 17 years?

a 1.2%

b 4.6%

c 8.5%

d 12.5%

e 15%

5 Which of the following laboratory tests may have the *highest* sensitivity and specificity in detecting ongoing heavy alcohol drinking?

a Alanine aminotransferase (ALT)

b Alkaline phosphatase

c Carbohydrate-deficient transferrin (CDT)

d Gamma-glutamyltransferase (GGT)

e Combination of CDT and GGT

6 All of the following statements regarding the development and course of cannabis use disorder are accurate *except*:

a The most common age of onset of cannabis disorder is during early adolescence.

b The progression of the disorder is more rapid in adolescents.

c Compared to alcohol intoxication, cannabis intoxication leads to less severe behavioral or cognitive dysfunction.

d Changes in mood stability, energy level, and eating patterns are commonly seen in adolescents who use cannabis.

e Cannabis use prior to age 15 years indicates a higher risk for developing cannabis use disorder.

7 All of the following names commonly refer to the natural cannabis plant *except*:

a Dope

b Gangster

c Grass

d Hashish

e Spice

8 Amotivational syndrome is *most* likely to be associated with which of the following substance use disorders (SUDs)?

a Alcohol use disorder

b Cannabis use disorder

c Phencyclidine use disorder

d Inhalant use disorder

e Stimulant use disorder

9 Which of the following neurological conditions is *least* likely to occur during phencyclidine intoxication?

a Dyskinesia

b Catalepsy

c Hypothermia

d Hypotonia

e Hyperthermia

10 Which of the following hallucinogens has longer duration of effects than the others listed?

a 2, 5-dimethoxy-4-methylamphatamine (DOM)

b Mescaline

c Dimethyltryptamine (DMT)

d Lysergic acid diethylamide (LSD)

e Psilocin

11 Based on updated epidemiologic studies, all of the following descriptions regarding opioid use disorder are accurate *except*:

a Females are more likely to have an opioid use disorder than males.

b Twelve-month prevalence of this disorder among American teens aged 12–17 years (community population) is about 1%.

c The onset of this disorder can occur at any age, but most commonly begins in the late teens or early 20s.

d Whereas 20–30% of individuals with this disorder achieve long-term abstinence, the long-term mortality rate may be as high as 2%.

e Prevalence decreases with increasing age above 29 years because of early mortality and the remission of symptoms after age 40 years.

12 Which of the following opioids is *not* detectable by standard urine drug tests?

a Codeine

b Fentanyl

c Heroin

d Morphine

e Oxycodone

13 Which of the following signs is *least* likely to occur in opioid withdrawal?

a Dysphoric mood

b Lacrimation, rhinorrhea, and sweating

c Muscle aches

d Nausea and vomiting

e Pupillary constriction

14 Which of the following sedative, hypnotic, or anxiolytic drugs *does not* result in sedative, hypnotic, or anxiolytic use disorder?

a Benzodiazepines

b Buspirone

c Glutethimide

d Secobarbital

e Zolpidem

15 Up to how long after the administration of amphetamine-type stimulants can hair samples be used for detecting the substances?

a One week

b One month

c Three months

d Six months

e One year

16 Which of the following conditions is *most* likely to increase the risk of starting and continuing tobacco use and tobacco use disorder in children?

a ADHD

b Anxiety

c Bipolar disorders

d Depression

e Psychotic disorders

17 All of the following statements regarding gambling disorder are accurate *except*:

a A pattern of behavior involving an urgent need to keep gambling to undo a loss or series of losses is often called "chasing one's losses."

b The onset of the disorder can start in adolescence and young adulthood, as well as in older individuals.

c Males are more likely to initiate gambling earlier in life than females.

d Younger individuals are more likely involved with different forms of gambling than older ones.

e Larger amounts of money spent wagering indicate a gambling disorder.

18 All of the following are recommended in the assessment and treatment of children and adolescents with SUDs *except*:

a An appropriate level of confidentiality should be observed during the assessment and treatment.

b More formal evaluation for SUDs should be conducted if the screening raises concerns about substance use.

c Toxicology should be a routine part of formal evaluation and the ongoing assessment during and after treatment.

d Residential treatment should be recommended if SUDs are confirmed by positive toxicology.

e Family involvement should be a component of treatment of SUDs.

19 All of the following are selected instruments for screening of substance use problems in adolescents *except*:

a CRAFFT

b Conners

c Screen to Brief Intervention (S2BI)

d Substance Abuse Subtle Screening Inventory (SASSI)

e Screening, Brief Intervention, and Referral to Treatment (SBIRT)

20 Which of the following regarding nicotine use is *false*?

a In the 2010s, adolescent vaping dramatically increased.

b Nicotine use increases risk of other substance use.

c Nicotine replacement therapy is FDA approved for nicotine dependence in adolescents.

d Bupropion can be used to treat nicotine dependence in adolescents.

e While common in adolescents with SUDs or psychiatric disorders, nicotine dependence is under-diagnosed and under-treated in adolescents.

21 Which of the following conditions is *least* likely to be comorbid with a SUD?

a Depression

b Bipolar disorder

c Anxiety disorder

d ADHD

e Anorexia nervosa, restricting type

22 All of the following stages of change are suggested in motivational interviewing *except*:

a Precontemplation

b Contemplation

c Preparation

d Recognition of higher power

e Action

23 All of the following are general principles that effective substance use prevention programs should follow *except*:

a Protective factors should be enhanced.

b Addressing the most popular drug of choice in the community should be the focus to save limited resources and to enhance efficiency.

c High-risk families and children should not be singled out.

d The program should be long term, with repeated booster programs.

e Multiple programs can be combined to enhance efficacy.

Matching

24–26 Match each SUD with one of the following listed pharmacotherapies:

a Disulfiram

b Bupropion

c Methadone

24 Opioid use disorder

25 Tobacco use disorder

26 Alcohol use disorder

ANSWERS AND EXPLANATIONS

1 (b) Gambling disorder (former "pathological gambling" in DSM-IV-TR under the category of "impulse-control disorders not elsewhere classified") is recategorized under "substance-related and addictive disorder" in DSM-5, which reflects evidence that gambling behaviors activate reward systems similar to those activated by drugs of abuse. The behavioral manifestations elicited are similar to those elicited by the SUDs. However, other addictive, repetitive behaviors such as exercise addiction, Internet gaming addiction, sex addiction, and shopping addiction are not recognized as disorders in DSM-5 because there is a lack of empirical research evidence or peer-reviewed consensus to support their listing. *(Ref. 4, p. 481)*

2 (d) In DSM-5, inhalant-related disorders include inhalant use disorder, inhalant intoxication, other inhalant-induced disorders, and unspecified inhalant-related disorder. Inhalants do not cause typical withdrawal symptoms that are seen in other substances listed in the question. Thus, no diagnosis of "inhalant withdrawal" is included in DSM-5. Common inhalants used include glue, shoe polish, toluene, gasoline, lighter fluid, and spray paints. Approximately one-tenth of 13-year-old American youth report having used inhalants ≥ once. The prevalence rate of inhalant use disorder among Americans aged 12–17 years is approximately 0.4% in the past 12 months and is highest among Native Americans and lowest among African Americans. Withdrawal symptoms or signs with hallucinogens have not been established. Thus, no diagnosis of "hallucinogen withdrawal" is included in DSM-5 either. *(Ref. 4, pp. 523–525, 533–540)*

3 (c) Depressed reflexes can be one of the signs or symptoms of inhalant intoxication among others: dizziness, nystagmus, incoordination, slurred speech, unsteady gait, lethargy, psychomotor retardation, tremor, generalized muscle weakness, blurred vision or diplopia, stupor or coma, and euphoria, which usually develop during or shortly after use of or exposure to the inhalant. Volatile inhalant intoxication can also lead to unconsciousness, anoxia, cardiac arrhythmia or arrest, and "sudden sniffing death." In 2009 and 2010, 0.8% of all Americans > 12 years reported inhalant use in the past year, and the highest age group is among those between 12 and 17 years with a prevalence of 3.6%. The prevalence drops to 1.7% for an older age group between 18 and 25 years. *(Ref. 4, pp. 538–539)*

4 (b) The estimated 12-month prevalence rate of alcohol use disorder among American youth between ages 12 and 17 years is 4.6%, which increases to 8.5% among adults aged 18 years and older in the United States. Among those youth between ages 12 and 17 years, the prevalence rates are highest in Hispanic and Native Americans/Alaska Natives than among whites, and are lowest in African Americans and Asian Americans/Pacific Islanders. The first episode of alcohol intoxication commonly occurs during the mid-teens. *(Ref. 4, p. 493)*

5 (e) The combination of CDT and GGT can provide even higher sensitivity and specificity in detecting ongoing heavy alcohol drinking than either test used alone. People who are drinking heavily show modest elevation or high–normal levels of GGT. GGT is a relatively sensitive test. CDT is another test with even higher sensitivity and specificity. The GGT and CDT tests return to normal a few days after stopping drinking. Thus, they can be used to monitor abstinence and relapses. The combination of GGT and CDT can achieve even higher sensitivity and specificity. Elevated ALT and alkaline phosphatase indicate liver injury, but do not necessarily indicate ongoing heavy drinking. Elevated mean corpuscular volume (MCV) is seen in individuals who drink heavily. However because of the long half-life of red blood cells, it is a less useful test to monitor abstinence. There are some nonspecific laboratory markers for detecting alcohol use, such as elevated lipids and uric acids. *(Ref. 4, p. 495)*

6 (a) The most common age of onset of cannabis disorder is during adolescence and young adulthood, although onset of the disorder at other ages such as in the preteen years or in the late 20s and older can occur. Less severe presentation of cannabis intoxication may explain its more frequent use in more diverse situations than alcohol, which may also contribute to the potential rapid transition from "cannabis use" to "cannabis use disorder." Adolescents with cannabis use disorder may not only present with mood instability and energy level and eating pattern changes, but also demonstrate a dramatic drop in grades, increased truancy, and decreased interest in school activities and performance. Cannabis use prior to age 15 years is a strong predictor of the development of cannabis use disorder along with other SUDs and comorbid mental illnesses during young adulthood, and is associated with concurrent externalized and internalized problems. *(Ref. 4, p. 513)*

7 (e) Spice, K2, JWH-018, and JWH-073 are all synthetic cannabinoid compounds in the form of plant material that has been sprayed with a cannabinoid formulation. The cannabis plant has many names (e.g., weed, pot, herb, grass, reefer, mary jane, dagga, dope, bhang, skunk, boom, gangster, kif, ganja, and hashish). Most commonly smoked via pipes, water pipes, and cigarettes, cannabis is at times ingested orally by mixing it into food and is inhaled via vaporization. *(Ref. 4, pp. 510–511)*

8 (b) Amotivational syndrome refers to a reduction in prosocial goal-directed activity, along with deterioration of school- or job-related performance, which results from cannabis use disorder (either from pervasive intoxication or recovery from the effects of intoxication). *(Ref. 4, p. 514)*

9 (d) Dyskinesia, catalepsy, hypothermia, hyperthermia, dystonia, and seizure are signs of possible neurological toxicity. Other effects may include deficits in memory, speech, and cognition, intracranial hemorrhage, rhabdomyolysis, respiratory problems, and occasionally cardiac arrest. *(Ref. 4, pp. 522, 528)*

10 (d) Lysergic acid diethylamide (LSD) and 3,4-methlenedioxymethamphetamine (MDMA)—also known as ecstasy—have longer duration of effects than other hallucinogens, and it takes a longer time to recover from LSD or MDMA use. MDMA has both hallucinogenic and stimulant properties. In adolescents, MDMA use increases the rate of using other hallucinogens, which is in turn associated with other SUDs and major depressive disorder. Compared to males, female adolescents seem to have increased odds of other hallucinogen use disorder. *(Ref. 4, pp. 524–526)*

11 **(a)** Men have higher rates of opioid used disorder than women. *(Ref. 4, p. 543)*

12 **(b)** Fentanyl is *not* detectable by standard urine drug tests but can be identified by more specialized procedures up to several days after administration. However, most opioids such as codeine, heroin, morphine, oxycodone, and propoxyphene are readily detectable by standard urine tests within 12–36 hours after administration. Methadone, buprenorphine (or buprenorphine/naloxone combination), and L-alpha-acetylmethadol (LAAM) will not cause a positive result on routine tests for opioids, and they can be tested through specialized tests up to one week after administration. *(Ref. 4, p. 544)*

13 **(e)** Pupillary dilation (*not* constriction) is more likely to occur along with other potential signs and symptoms of opioid withdrawal. They are dysphoric mood, nausea, vomiting, muscle aches, lacrimation, rhinorrhea, piloerection, sweating, diarrhea, yawning, fever, and insomnia. They can occur within minutes to several days after cessation or reduction of opioid use that has been heavy and prolonged. Administration of an opioid antagonist after a period of opioid use can trigger withdrawal as well. *(Ref. 4, pp. 547–548)*

14 **(b)** Buspirone is a non-benzodiazepine antianxiety agent, and is not associated with significant misuse or sedative, hypnotic, or anxiolytic use disorder. However, all benzodiazepines and benzodiazepine-like agents (e.g., zolpidem, zaleplon) and all barbiturates (e.g., secobarbital) and barbiturate-like agents (e.g., glutethimide, methaqualone) can be misused and lead to sedative, hypnotic, or anxiolytic use disorder. The 12-month prevalence of this disorder is estimated to be higher among adolescents of ages 12–17 years (0.3%) than among adults (0.2%). It is a more male-predominant disorder in adults, but it is more female predominant in adolescents aged 12–17 years (female to male ratio: 0.4% versus 0.2%). *(Ref. 4, pp. 552–553)*

15 **(c)** The presence of amphetamine-like stimulants is still detectable by testing the hair samples up to 90 days after administration. However, by using urine samples, it is generally only detectable for one to three days, and potentially up to four days depending on dosage and individual metabolism. *(Ref. 4, pp. 565–566)*

16 **(a)** ADHD and conduct disorder can increase the risk of developing tobacco use or tobacco use disorder in children. Adults with bipolar/depressive disorders, personality disorders, psychotic disorders, and other SUDs have a higher risk of developing tobacco use or tobacco use disorder. *(Ref. 4, pp. 573–574)*

17 **(e)** The amount of money spent wagering does not necessarily indicate a gambling disorder and depends on affordability because some individuals can wager a huge amount of money gambling and do not have a gambling disorder, whereas others may suffer a serious gambling disorder while wagering a much smaller amount. In addition to "chasing one's losses," individuals who experience gambling problems may lie to their family members to cover up their illegal activities, such as forgery, fraud, theft, or embezzlement, to obtain money, etc. *(Ref. 4, pp. 585–588)*

18 **(d)** Adolescents with SUDs should receive specific treatment for their substance use, but they should be treated in the least restrictive setting that is safe and effective. The treatment programs should be designed to minimize treatment dropouts and to maximize motivation, compliance, and completion of treatment. Nonuser peer support, family involvement, and comprehensive services involving other domains (e.g., vocational, recreational, medical, and legal) are encouraged. Comorbid psychiatric disorders should be screened, assessed, and appropriately treated. Posttreatment aftercare should be arranged to avoid relapses. *(Ref. 1, Ch. 12, Evaluation section, Treatment section)*

19 **(b)** The Conners rating scale is one of the most commonly used instruments for screening of ADHD, ODD, and conduct disorder in children, but it cannot be used for screening substance use problems. *(Ref. 1, Ch. 12, Screening section)*

20 **(a)** No pharmacologic treatments are FDA approved for nicotine dependence for adolescents under 18 years. For adults, nicotine replacement therapy, bupropion, and varenicline are FDA approved for smoking cessation. The American Academy of Pediatrics recommends offering pharmacologic treatments to youth with nicotine dependence given the risks of nicotine dependence and the effectiveness of these treatments in adults. *(Ref. 1, Ch. 12, Pharmacological Treatments section)*

21 **(e)** A comorbid psychiatric disorder with a SUD is referred to as a "dual diagnosis." Adolescents and adults with SUDs have a higher chance than the general population of having another psychiatric condition, such as depression and other mood disorders, anxiety disorders, oppositional defiant disorder, conduct disorder, antisocial personality disorder, ADHD, schizophrenia, and bulimia. It is often difficult to distinguish whether a SUD is the primary or secondary disorder. Therefore, careful assessment and evaluation for a possible dual diagnosis and appropriate treatments for both disorders are important. *(Ref. 1, Ch. 12, Comorbidity section)*

22 **(d)** Prochaska and DiClemente suggested several stages that people usually go through when trying to stop addictive behaviors. These stages are: precontemplation, contemplation, preparation, action, and maintenance. Recognition of a higher power belongs to the 12-step program (Step 2). Motivational interviewing, a nonconfrontational counseling approach developed by Miller and Rollnick, has been used as a treatment modality in patients with alcohol and SUDs. *(Ref. 5, p. 581, 2218)*

23 **(b)** Addressing all forms of drug abuse, alone or in combination, is an important principle of effective prevention programs. This may include underage use of otherwise legal substances for adults (e.g., alcohol and tobacco, and recently, in certain states, cannabis), inappropriate use of legally obtained substances (e.g., inhalants) and prescribed or over-the-counter medications. *(Ref. 1, Ch. 12, Prevention section)*

Matching

24 **(c)** Methadone can be considered for adolescents (< 18 years) with opioid use disorder who have failed at least two documented drug-free detoxifications, and it has to be prescribed at a certified clinic. A randomized clinical trial shows the effectiveness of using buprenorphine for adolescent detoxification. Naltrexone can be also considered for opioid use disorder. *(Questions 24–26: Ref. 3, Table 5.8.5)*

25 **(b)** Bupropion is an FDA-approved drug for smoking cessation in adults, which can be potentially considered for adolescents with tobacco use disorder.

26 **(a)** Disulfiram as well as acamprosate and naltrexone are FDA-approved drugs for alcohol use disorder ("alcohol dependence" in DSM-IV) in adults. They may be considered for adolescents with serious alcohol use disorder. Topiramate (not FDA approved) shows some effectiveness for alcohol use disorder in adults.

10

SPECIAL ISSUES (DIVERSE POPULATIONS, MEDICALLY ILL CHILDREN, SUICIDE, AND ABUSE)

DOI: 10.4324/9781003308805-11

QUESTIONS

Directions: Select the best response for each of the questions 1–50.

1 Which of the following statements is most accurate regarding cultural concepts of distress as defined in DSM-5?

   a The three categories of cultural concepts are culture-bound syndromes, cultural idioms of distress, and cultural explanations or perceived causes.

   b Cultural idioms of distress are ways of expressing distress that provide shared ways of experiencing and talking about concerns and may not involve specific symptoms or syndromes.

   c Culture-bound syndromes are combinations of psychiatric and somatic symptoms that are recognizable primarily within a specific society or culture.

   d Cultural concepts generally do not correspond one-to-one with specific DSM diagnostic entities.

   e Cultural concepts are defined in part by stability over time and relative imperviousness to global influence.

2 Which of the following is *not* a category assessed in the DSM-5 Outline for Cultural Formulation?

   a Cultural identity of the individual

   b Cultural conceptualizations of distress

   c Psychosocial stressors and cultural features of vulnerability and resilience

   d Cultural features of the relationship between the individual and the clinician

   e All are categories

3 All of the following statements regarding gender dysphoria are accurate *except*:

   a In DSM-5, there are two different sets of diagnostic criteria for either gender dysphoria in children or gender dysphoria in adolescents and adults.

   b The specifier "posttransition" is only available for gender dysphoria in adolescents and adults.

   c Latency-age girls (assigned gender) with gender dysphoria express the wish to be a boy, prefer boys' clothing and hairstyles, and like to participate in contact sports and rough-and-tumble play.

   d Latency-age boys (assigned gender) with gender dysphoria express the wish to be a girl, prefer dressing in girls' clothes, and like to participate in traditionally feminine activities and games.

   e Younger children with this disorder are more likely than older ones to express extreme anatomic dysphoria.

4 All of the following statements regarding the development and course of gender dysphoria are accurate *except*:

   a The onset of cross-gender behaviors occurs usually between ages 2 and 4 years during which time most children start expressing gendered behaviors and interests.

   b Relatively few young children express anatomic dysphoria, but it becomes a more common concern when approaching and anticipating puberty.

   c Most male (assigned gender) children whose gender dysphoria does not persist become sexually attracted to males.

   d Some female (assigned gender) children whose gender dysphoria does not persist become sexually attracted to females.

   e Male (assigned gender) individuals with late-onset gender dysphoria are mostly attracted to males and cohabit with natal males.

5 Which of the following is the most appropriate situation in which to consider initiating a gender-affirming medical intervention?

   a Gender-affirming testosterone treatment for a pre-pubertal trans masculine patient

   b A gender-affirming phalloplasty for a 16-year-old trans masculine patient

   c Pubertal suppression for a 12-year-old trans feminine patient who has entered Tanner stage 2 of puberty

   d Gender-affirming estrogen treatment for a 12-year-old trans feminine patient entering Tanner stage 2 of puberty

   e Gender-affirming testosterone treatment for a 12-year-old trans masculine patient entering Tanner stage 2 of puberty

6 Which of the following are true regarding the "affirmative approach" for treating transgender children?

   a The approach recommends psychotherapeutic interventions to encourage a child to identify with their sex assigned at birth.

   b The approach recommends against a "social transition" prior to the onset of puberty.

   c The approach considers all gender identity outcomes (e.g., transgender, cisgender, non-binary) to be equally desirable.

   d All of the above.

   e Both A and B.

7 All of the following are research findings of the study "Lesbian, Gay, Bisexual, and Transgender Adolescents School Victimization: Implications for Young Adult Health and Adjustment" (S. T. Russell et al. 2011) regarding lesbian, gay, bisexual, and transgender-related school victimization *except*:

   a It is strongly associated with young adult mental health problems.

   b It increases risk for STDs and HIV.

   c It increases risk for depression.

   d It increases risk for suicidal ideation among males.

   e It is strongly associated with substance use or abuse.

8 Which of the following factors is the *strongest* predictor of future suicide?

a History of suicide attempt

b History of suicidality

c History of suicidal ideation

d History of nonsuicidal self-injurious behavior

e None of the above

9 How many folds of increased risk could a loaded gun in the home lead to completed suicide?

a 2-fold

b 10-fold

c 20-fold

d 30-fold

e 50-fold

10 All of the following statements regarding risk factors of completed suicide are accurate *except*:

a Among all the comorbid conditions, major mood disorders are the most strongly associated with completed suicide.

b Other high-risk comorbid conditions may include disruptive, anxiety, and substance use disorders.

c In older adolescents, there is a higher risk of using more lethal means while being influenced by substances.

d Studies find a link between perfectionism and completed suicide.

e Hopelessness seems to be an independent risk factor beyond its association with depression.

11 Which of the following is the most strongly associated with suicide attempts among adolescents?

a Depression

b Anxiety

c Borderline personality disorder

d Nonsuicidal self-injury

e Impulsivity

12 Which of the following is the most common precipitant for adolescent suicide attempts and suicide?

a Interpersonal conflict

b Disciplinary problems

c Financial problems

d Physical abuse

e Sexual abuse

13 Which of the following components should *not* be included during the exploration of suicidal intent?

a Belief about intent

b Preparatory behavior

c Prevention of discovery

d Communication of suicidal intent

e None of the above

14 Which of the following statements regarding assessment of suicidality is *least* correct?

a Suicidal intent, suicide plan, access to means, lethality, precipitants, motivation, and consequences should all be included as components during the assessment.

b Suicidal ideation should be evaluated based on both severity (intent) and pervasiveness (frequency and intensity).

c Nonsuicidal self-injurious behaviors should be separated from suicide attempt because they are involved in separate populations with different lethality and risks.

d Interpersonal conflict or loss, legal disciplinary problems, and chronic and ongoing physical and sexual abuse can all be precipitants.

e Naturally occurring environmental contingencies may reinforce suicidality.

15 Based on the study "Clinical and Psychosocial Predictors of Suicide Attempts and Nonsuicidal Self-Injury in the Adolescent Depression Antidepressant and Psychotherapy Trial" (Wilkinson et al. 2011), all of the following conclusions were reported *except*:

a High suicidality, nonsuicidal self-injury, and poor family functioning at study entry are significant independent predictors of suicide attempts over the 28 weeks of follow-up.

b Nonsuicidal self-injury is an independent predictor of nonsuicidal self-injury over the follow-up period.

c Hopelessness is an independent predictor of suicidal attempts over the follow-up period.

d Anxiety disorder at baseline is an independent predictor of nonsuicidal self-injury over the follow-up period.

e Being younger and female at study entry is an independent predictor of nonsuicidal self-injury over the follow-up period.

16 Which of the following statements regarding clinical management of adolescent suicidal behavior is *not* fully accurate?

a Treatment of depression may not be sufficient to reduce suicide risk.

b Clinical interventions include safety planning, psychosocial treatment package, and hospitalization.

c Safety planning refers to negotiating a detailed written no-harm contract with the adolescent to prevent suicide.

d Removal of guns from the homes of at-risk adolescents is highly recommended.

e Receiving written contact after discharge from hospital reduces reattempt.

17 All of the following statements regarding psychotherapy approaches for treating youth suicidality are accurate based on the updated research *except*:

a In one study (TADS, 2004), the combination of fluoxetine and CBT is associated with decreased suicidal ideation as compared to placebo.

b Dialectical behavior therapy (DBT) focuses on developing mindfulness, emotional regulation, distress tolerance, and interpersonal skills.

c Modified DBT was developed for use with suicidal adolescents to decrease the length of treatment.

d Inpatient treatment with DBT for adolescents hospitalized for suicidal ideation or attempt reduces reattempts and rehospitalization as compared to the inpatient treatment without DBT.

e Multisystemic therapy reduces the rates of reattempt as compared to usual care group.

18 All of the following groups are at increased risk for maltreatment *except*:

a Children under 3 years of age

b Girls

c Mother under 21 years of age

d Living in poverty

e Product of multiple births

19 All of the following reflect accurate epidemiological data available regarding sexual abuse *except*:

a Prior to the age of 18 years, 10–25% of girls are sexually victimized in some fashion.

b The most common age of initial sexual abuse is between 5 and 7 years.

c The most common perpetrators of sexual abuse against girls are male parents or male parent figures.

d 20% of cases are perpetrated by adolescents.

e Unrelated males are the most common perpetrator of sexual abuse against boys.

20 Which of the following behaviors in a child is most suggestive of a sexual abuse history:

a Talking about sexual acts

b Asking others to engage in sexual acts

c Wanting to watch movies that show nudity

d Knowing more about sex than most same-age children

e Hugging adults they do not know well

21 Which of the following is the therapeutic intervention with the strongest evidence for reducing physically abusive parenting behaviors?

a Treatment of parental substance use disorders

b Trauma-focused cognitive-behavior therapy for the parent

c Trauma-focused cognitive-behavior therapy for the child

d Parent–child interaction therapy

e There are no therapeutic interventions with evidence for reducing physical abuse

22 All of the following are parts of a common constellation of clinical findings of whiplash shaken baby syndrome in infants and toddlers *except*:

a Retinal hemorrhage

b Subdural hemorrhage

c Subarachnoid hemorrhage

d Apparent external cranial trauma

e None of the above

23 Which of the following technologies should be considered as the *first-line* choice in assessing children with suspected acute brain or head injury?

a CT scanning

b Bone scans

c MRI

d EEG

e Ultrasound

24 Which of the following is the *least* likely sign of sexual abuse?

a Vague somatic complaints

b Primary enuresis or encopresis

c Anal fissures or blood in the stool

d Anogenital injuries

e Redness or irritation of the vulva

25 Which of the following psychiatric disorders and conditions is *least* commonly associated with childhood physical abuse?

a PTSD

b Attachment dysregulation

c Aggression

d Obsessive-compulsive disorder

e ADHD

26 Which of the following is the *least* likely outcome of sexual abuse in youth?

a Sexual abuse and emotional abuse are independent risk factors for future engagement in sex trade work.

b Long duration, use of force, penetration, and being victimized by perpetrators known to the victims are all associated with worse outcomes.

c Overstimulation of the hypothalamic-pituitary-adrenal (HPA) axis leads to decreased cortisol levels.

d Decreased hippocampus size is detected by MRI and PET scans in patients with PTSD due to severe sexual or physical abuse.

e Dissociation may be temporarily protective and may become maladaptive over time.

27 All of the following statements accurately describe the relationship between childhood maltreatment and substance use/ nonsuicidal self-injury (NSSI) *except*:

a Head banging, self-mutilation, rocking, and other painful stimuli may activate endogenous opiates, which facilitates dissociation.

b Children with a maltreatment history are more likely to develop substance abuse as a way of self-medicating.

c Alcohol activates the mesolimbic reward system in children deprived of true rewards in their lives.

d Both emotional abuse and sexual abuse have the strongest link to NSSI.

e Emotional abuse leads to NSSI, which might be due to the development of self-critical cognitive style.

28 Which of the following is the *most* predictive factor that is linked to resilience or lack of it based on Daigneault et al. (2007)?

a Family violence

b Interpersonal trust

c Maternal conflicts

d Out-of-home placements

e None of the above

29 All of the following statements regarding legal considerations during the evaluation of child maltreatment are correct *except*:

a All 50 states mandate physicians and mental health clinicians to report suspected child abuse to authorities.

b Specific requirements and guidelines vary across different states.

c The most important factor is prompt report and referral to ensure appropriate collection and validation of data.

d The forensic evaluation and data collection should be completed by the treating provider who suspects the abuse.

e Confidentiality issues need to be clarified prior to a forensic evaluation.

30 Which of the following types of child maltreatments may be *most* prevalent?

a Emotional maltreatment (psychological maltreatment)

b Physical abuse

c Neglect

d Sexual abuse

e Sexual assault

31 Based on the "Childhood Trauma and Children's Emerging Psychotic Symptoms: A Genetically Sensitive Longitudinal Cohort Study" (L. Arseneault et al. 2011), which of the following types of maltreatment is *most* associated with reporting psychotic symptoms?

a Maltreatment by siblings

b Sexual abuse by parents

c Neglect by caregivers

d Emotional abuse by parents

e Bullying by peers

32 Based on the "Childhood Trauma and Children's Emerging Psychotic Symptoms: A Genetically Sensitive Longitudinal Cohort Study" (L. Arseneault et al. 2011), which of the following childhood trauma factors is *most* strongly associated with reporting psychotic symptoms?

a Timing of the trauma

b Accumulative effect

c Forms of trauma

d Age of the victim

e Sex of the victim

33 Which of the following statements is *least* accurate regarding the relationship between childhood maltreatment and psychiatric outcomes?

a Childhood maltreatment is associated with earlier age of onset, more severe course, and response to treatment of psychiatric illness.

b More than half of individuals with bipolar disorder report a history of childhood maltreatment.

c Emotional abuse alone is less predictive of suicidal ideation and behavior compared to other forms of abuse.

d Dissociation may be more common in victims of sexual abuse than in victims of physical abuse.

e Polyvictimization in childhood increases the overall likelihood of psychopathology with particularly increased likelihood of mood disorders.

34 All of the following interventions for foster families are used to treat children during middle childhood *except*:

a Attachment and Biobehavioral Catch-up (ABC)

b Fostering Individualized Assistance Program (FIAP)

c Incredible Years (IY)

d Keeping Foster Parents Trained and Supported (KEEP)

e Middle School Success (MSS)

35 Children who have received certain central nervous system (CNS) cancer treatments are at risk for cognitive impairment, including learning problems. Which of the following is (are) common area(s) that can be affected by such medical treatments?

a Attention and concentration

b Handwriting

c Math

d Memory

e All of the above

36 All of the following statements regarding organ transplantation are accurate *except*:

a Current use of tobacco is considered an absolute contraindication to lung transplantation.

b Alcohol use by a liver transplant adolescent patient is extremely dangerous.

c Liver failure can be insidious and unpredictable.

d Most transplant services view occasional experimentation with alcohol by adolescents as an absolute contraindication for future liver transplant.

e Adolescents with end-organ failure other than liver failure are at risk of use or abuse of alcohol or other drugs.

37 Which of the following is the *least* common cause of seizure?

a Hyperthermia

b Hyperglycemia

c Head trauma

d Meningitis

e Tuberous sclerosis

38 A child presents with staring spells and multiple brief episodes of behavioral arrests. Which type of seizure does the child *most* likely have?

a Absence seizure (petit mal)

b Frontal lobe epilepsy

c Juvenile myoclonic epilepsy (JME)

d Parietal/occipital lobe epilepsy

e Rolandic epilepsy

39 Which of the following sets of clinical features commonly occurs in temporal lobe epilepsy?

a Mouth twitching, drooling, nocturnal predisposition

b Gastric or olfactory aura, confusion, automatisms

c Hypermotor activity, change in behavior, nocturnal predisposition

d Myoclonic jerks and staring spells with older age of onset

e Brief myoclonic jerks and generalized tonic-clonic seizures

40 Which of the following psychotropic medications does not seem to lead to clinically significant drug–drug interactions with commonly used antiepileptic drugs?

a Guanfacine

b Risperidone

c Fluoxetine

d Trazodone

e Alprazolam

41 Under the personality disorder section of DSM-5, there are ten specific personality disorders included. Which of the following is *not* one of them?

a Antisocial personality disorder

b Borderline personality disorder

c Histrionic personality disorder

d Passive-aggressive personality disorder

e Schizoid personality disorder

42 According to DSM-5, all of the following personality disorders can be potentially assigned to individuals under the age of 18 years *except*:

a Antisocial personality disorder

b Dependent personality disorder

c Narcissistic personality disorder

d Obsessive personality disorder

e Schizotypal personality disorder

43 What is the *minimal* duration of symptoms of personality disorders that must be present in order to diagnose personality disorders in individuals younger than 18 years?

a Three months

b Six months

c One year

d Two years

e Five years

44 All of the following statements regarding borderline personality disorder are accurate *except*:

a Prevalence of this disorder is higher in older age groups than in the young adult group.

b The risk of suicide is highest in the young adult group.

c Youth and young adults with identity problems may be misperceived temporarily as having a personality disorder.

d This disorder is five times more likely to occur in those who have first-degree biological relatives with the disorder.

e This disorder is female predominant (about 75%).

45 All of the following biological findings based on neuroimaging studies are associated with adolescents with borderline personality disorder *except*:

a Decreased fractional anisotropy in the fornix

b Reduced volume in the left anterior cingulate cortex and right orbitofrontal cortex

c Increased amygdala and hippocampal volume

d Decreased fractional anisotropy in the inferior longitudinal fasciculus

e All are associated with adolescents with borderline personality disorder

46 Which of the following should be *excluded* from the potential psychosocial factors for youth developing borderline personality disorder?

a History of trauma (physical abuse, sexual abuse, and other maltreatment)

b History of neglect

c History of separation from primary caregivers

d Serious parental psychopathology

e None of the above

47 In comparison of the prevalence rates of comorbid conditions between youth with borderline personality disorder and those without, which of the following conditions is significantly *more* prevalent in youth with borderline personality disorder?

a ADHD

b Conduct disorder

c Major depressive disorder

d Oppositional defiant disorder

e Separation anxiety disorder

48 Multimodal treatments of borderline personality disorder usually include all of the following *except*:

a Individual therapy

b Parental/family therapy

c ECT

d Pharmacological interventions

e Partial and inpatient hospitalization and residential programs

49 Which of the following statements is *least* accurate regarding psychiatric disorders in children with epilepsy?

  a Psychopathology appears to be partly, but not entirely, attributable to the effects of having a chronic illness.

  b Rates of suicide attempts are up to 15 times that of the general population.

  c Childhood absence epilepsy is the only epilepsy syndrome not associated with increased rates of depression and anxiety.

  d ADHD in children with epilepsy is more likely to be characterized by inattention than by hyperactivity-impulsivity.

  e All statements are accurate.

50 Based on the DSM-5 diagnostic criteria for pedophilic disorder, what is the *minimum* age difference required between an individual with pedophilic disorder and the potential child victim?

  a 1 year

  b 3 years

  c 5 years

  d 10 years

  e 15 years

Matching

51–55 Choose one from the following descriptions that describes the terms *most* accurately:

  a Self-inflicted destructive conduct with intent to physically harm self without intent to die

  b The person begins to make a suicide attempt but stops themselves prior to experiencing injury

  c Thoughts of death without engaging in the behavior

  d Self-inflicted destructive conduct with explicit or implicit intent to die, but not necessarily leading to injury

  e The person begins to make a suicide attempt but is stopped by another person or circumstance prior to experiencing injury

51 Interrupted attempt
52 Suicide attempt
53 Suicidal ideation
54 Aborted attempt
55 Nonsuicidal self-injurious behavior
56–59 Match each of the following descriptions to the term as it is defined in DSM-5:

  a Gender identity

  b Gender dysphoria

  c Gender assignment

  d Gender identity disorder

56 No longer a term in DSM-5
57 "Natal gender"
58 A diagnostic category in DSM-5
59 An individual's identification as male, female, or another category
60–70 Choose one from the following descriptions that best describes each term as currently commonly used:

  a Refers to the types of individuals toward whom one is romantically and/or sexually attracted

  b Individual's psychological understanding of one's own gender

  c Sexual attraction to males

  d Sexual attraction to females

  e Generally based on physical characteristics

  f Variation from norms in gender role behavior

  g Psychological distress in relationship to one's experienced gender

  h Refers to an individual whose gender identity is incongruent with that of one's gender assigned at birth

  i Attraction to neither males, females, nor another gender

  j Refers to an individual whose experience matches one's gender assigned at birth

  k An individual's psychological understanding of one's own gender in one who has transitioned socially to living as that understood gender

60 Experienced gender
61 Androphilia
62 Sexual orientation
63 Affirmed gender
64 Cisgender
65 Aphilia
66 Transgender
67 Gender dysphoria
68 Gender nonconforming
69 Gender assigned at birth
70 Gynephilia
71–74 Match each antiepileptic drug with the best-fitting description of its neurobehavioral side effect profile:

  a Declines in word fluency and attention

  b Behavioral side effects including irritability, anxiety, and depression

  c Impaired decision making and attention, as well as aggression, irritability, and hyperactivity

  d Little or no cognitive impairment but can have stimulant effects

71 Lamotrigine
72 Valproic acid
73 Levetiracetam
74 Topiramate

ANSWERS AND EXPLANATIONS

1 (d) *Culture-bound syndrome* was a DSM-IV concept that underemphasized the importance of cultural differences in explanations or experience of distress (rather than culturally distinctive combinations of symptoms) and overemphasized the degree to which cultural concepts of distress are localized to limited regions and groups. In DSM-5, this terminology has been replaced by *cultural concepts of distress*, which include cultural syndromes, cultural idioms of distress, and cultural explanations or perceived causes. Cultural concepts generally do not correspond one-to-one with specific DSM diagnostic entities. Cultural concepts may change over time and with local or global influence. *(Ref. 4, pp. 758)*

2 (e) The DSM-5 Outline for Cultural Formulation calls for a systemic assessment of each of these factors, along with an overall cultural formulation. DSM-5 also includes a Cultural Formulation Interview, which is a set of 16 questions to guide the clinician in obtaining information about the impact of culture on an individual's clinical presentation and care. *(Ref. 4, pp. 449–750)*

3 (e) Older children, adolescents, and adults with this disorder are more likely than younger children to express extreme and persistent anatomic dysphoria. The incongruence between experienced gender and somatic sex is a core feature of the disorder among adolescent and adult patients. Such distress can be mediated by environmental support and availability of existing biomedical treatment to reduce such incongruence. *(Ref. 4, pp. 452–455)*

4 (e) Natal males with late-onset gender dysphoria are most likely to engage in transvestic behavior with sexual excitement and are likely to be attracted by females and tend to cohabit with or are married to natal females. *(Ref. 4, pp. 454–456)*

5 (c) Medical intervention may be initiated at the earliest signs of puberty (Tanner stage 2 or 3) with pubertal blockade with GnRHa. Cross-sex hormone therapy with estrogen or testosterone may be initiated around age 16. Gender-affirming surgical interventions are generally considered after the individual reaches the legal age of adulthood. There is some variability among different groups' recommendations, with some guidelines allowing for the consideration of some interventions at earlier ages. *(Ref. 3, Ch. 5.14, Therapeutics section)*

6 (e) This particular study is the longest-running prospective longitudinal study of same-sex parented families. The authors concluded that adolescents of both genders raised by lesbian mothers since conception demonstrated healthy psychological adjustment. They were rated higher by their mothers in social, school, and total competence and lower in social or behavioral problems compared to the control group (age-matched youth in Achenbach's normative sample). *(Gartrell and Bos, 2010)*

7 (e) There is no strong association between lesbian, gay, bisexual, and transgender-related school victimization and substance use or abuse. The authors concluded that reduction of school victimization would probably lead to a significant long-term health gain and reduction of health disparities for this population. *(Russell et al., 2011)*

8 (a) History of suicide attempt is the strongest predictor of future suicide. Suicidality is a generic term that refers to all suicide-related behavior and thoughts. Follow-up studies show 6–15% of adolescent suicide attempters will reattempt. The highest risk period is within three months of the initial attempt and/or following discharge from an inpatient psychiatric facility. Youth suicide attempters who have a history of using more lethal means tend to have a higher risk of eventual completed suicide. Younger children may overestimate the lethality of the means they use. Using relatively low lethal means may not reflect low lethality. *(Ref. 1, Ch. 26, Risk Factors section)*

9 (d) Availability of a firearm at home increases risk of death from suicide significantly, especially when the gun is loaded (more likely to be chosen as a means of suicide). One study shows a loaded gun increases by 30-fold the risk for death from suicide, even among youth with no apparent psychopathology. *(Ref. 1, Ch. 26, Risk Factors section)*

10 (d) Studies failed to find a link between perfectionism and death from suicide even though a perfectionism personality trait, along with the personality trait of neuroticism, seems to be associated with suicide attempts in youth. *(Ref. 1, Ch. 26, Risk Factors section)*

11 (d) Chronic nonsuicidal self-injury is one of the strongest predictors for suicide attempts among adolescents. It has been shown to be stronger than depression, anxiety, borderline personality disorder, and impulsivity. Nonsuicidal self-injury in adolescents is also associated with family dysfunction, poor parental mental health, insecure attachment, as well as poor emotion regulation, self-confidence, and problem-solving skills *(Ref. 3, Ch. 5.4.3, Risk Factors for Suicidal Ideation and Acts section)*

12 (a) Interpersonal conflicts and loss are the most common precipitants for adolescent suicide attempts, whereas adults, compared to adolescents, are more likely to have financial and medical problems and less likely to have relationship problems as precipitants. *(Ref. 1, Ch. 26, Assessment section)*

13 (e) Belief about intent, preparatory behavior, prevention of discovery, and communication of suicidal intent are four components that should be explored during the evaluation of suicidal intent. Belief about intent refers to the extent to which the person wishes to die. Preparatory behavior may include giving away prized possessions, writing suicidal notes, etc. Prevention of discovery refers to planning the attempt in a way that rescue is unlikely. Expressing a wish to die, planning the attempt ahead of time, timing the attempt to avoid detection, and confiding suicide plans are all indications of high intent, which are all associated with recurrent suicide attempts and completed suicide. *(Ref. 1, Ch. 26, Assessment section)*

14 (c) Nonsuicidal self-injurious behavior should be differentiated from a suicide attempt. However, the risk factors often overlap, and it is not uncommon for youth to engage in both behaviors, and either behavior can potentially lead to high lethality and poor outcomes (even accidental suicide). Thus, a thorough assessment is warranted for both behaviors. *(Ref. 1, Ch. 26, Risk Factors section)*

15 **(c)** Hopelessness, anxiety disorder, and being younger and female are all independent predictors of nonsuicidal injury over the follow-up period, but not predictors of suicide attempts. *(Wilkinson et al., 2011)*

16 **(c)** Safety plans are the most critical components of clinical management of adolescent suicidality, which involve collaborative efforts among the clinician, patient, and family. Written no-harm contracts alone are not sufficient to prevent suicidality. The plans should include assessment and determination of the appropriate level of care (i.e., outpatient or inpatient), elimination of lethal means, implementation of coping skills, strategies for identifying warning signs, and potential ways of stepping up level of services, etc. Depression is a risk factor for suicidality. However, treatment of depression alone may not necessarily reduce suicidal risk. Specific interventions targeting suicidality per se are often required. The highest risk period for suicide and reattempt happens after discharge from the hospital; studies show that sending out written contact postcards to the patients reduces the risk of reattempt. Aftercare arrangements, such as scheduling the initial outpatient appointment, may be helpful. *(Ref. 1, Ch. 26, Clinical Management section)*

17 **(d)** Inpatient treatment *with* and *without* DBT for adolescents hospitalized for suicidal ideation or attempt both reduce self-reported depression, suicidal ideation, and hopelessness in similar fashions, but there are no differences in reattempts, compliance with outpatient treatment, or rehospitalization. In one study (Huey et al. 2004), at one-year follow-up, the MST group shows significant reduction in reattempts as compared to the usual care group whereas there are higher rates of hospitalization in the MST group. The other potential psychosocial interventions include home-based family therapy, youth-nominated support teams, developmental group therapy, skills-based therapy, and school-based prevention, all of which have variable levels of empirical support. *(Ref. 1, Ch. 26, Clinical Management section)*

18 **(b)** Being a boy (not girl), under the age of 3 years, having a mother under the age of 21, being the product of a multiple birth, and living in poverty are all risk factors for maltreatment. Death from homicide during the first week of life is almost always perpetrated by mothers, whereas death occurring between ages 1 week and 13 years are equally caused by mothers and fathers. However, in older age groups, fathers are more likely to be responsible for the majority of parent-perpetrated homicides: 63% among 13- to 15-year-olds, and 80% among 16- to 19-year-olds. *(Ref. 1, Ch. 24, Epidemiology section)*

19 **(b)** The most common age of initial sexual abuse is 8–11 years. Boys are less willing to disclose sexual abuse and are more likely to be victimized by unrelated males. Sexual abuse of boys has been less well studied than sexual abuse of girls, and sexual abuse of boys may be underreported. *(Ref. 1, Ch. 24, Epidemiology section)*

20 **(b)** Asking others to engage in sexual acts is moderately prevalent in sexually abused children and rare in both psychiatric and normal controls, along with putting mouth on sex parts, masturbating with an object, and inserting object into vagina or anus. Asking others to engage in sexual acts, wanting to watch movies that show nudity, knowing more about sex than most same-age children, and hugging adults they do not know well are all moderately prevalent in both sexually abused children and psychiatric controls and uncommon in normal controls. *(Ref. 3, Ch. 5.15.1, Sequelae section)*

22 **(d)** Parent–child interaction therapy (PCIT) is a play-based model of therapy originally developed for young children with externalizing behavior problems that uses live coaching to help caregivers interact more effectively with their children. PCIT has evidence of effectiveness for improving child behavior as well as reducing parental stress, harsh parenting behaviors, child welfare referrals, and recurrence of physical abuse. *(Ref 3, Ch. 15.1.1, Child and Birth Parent Clinical Interventions)*

23 **(a)** CT scanning has high sensitivity to hemorrhage (intraparenchymal, subarachnoid, subdural, and epidural) and mass effect. Thus, CT scanning should be considered as the first-line choice over MRI or other technologies. *(Ref. 1, Ch. 24, Clinical Presentation section)*

24 **(b)** Secondary (*not* primary) enuresis or encopresis could be a sign of sexual abuse in children among other signs such as vague somatic complaints (headaches, abdominal pain), redness or irritation of the vulva, anogenital injuries (lacerations, scarring, or bruising of genitalia), anal dilation or scarring, repeated urinary tract infections, hematuria, anal fissure, and blood in the stool. *(Ref. 1, Ch. 24, Clinical Presentation section)*

25 **(d)** Obsessive-compulsive disorder is not commonly associated with physical abuse. Other characteristics of abused children include anxiety disorders and PTSD, cognitive and neurological impairments, dissociative disorders, ADHD, depression and suicide, self-destructive behavior, impaired impulse control and aggression, and impaired social relations. *(Ref. 1, Ch. 24, Diagnostic Considerations and Comorbidity section)*

26 **(c)** Overstimulation of the hypothalamic-pituitary-adrenal (HPA) axis leads to increased cortisol levels. *(Ref. 1, Ch. 24, Impact of Abuse section)*

27 **(c)** Stimulants (*not* alcohol) activate the mesolimbic dopaminergic reward system in children deprived of true rewards in their lives. Alcohol usually reduces anxiety, and opiates trigger soothing dissociation, which all can lead to higher rates of use of such substances by youth with a maltreatment history. *(Ref. 1, Ch. 24, Impact of Abuse section)*

28 **(b)** All of the factors listed are predictive of resilience studied by Daigneault et al. (2007), among which interpersonal trust is the most predictive of resilience. Thus, development of a trusting relationship and promotion of a sense of empowerment and self-efficacy in treating youth with traumas are critically important. Other positive factors that can enhance resilience include the child's above-average intelligence, high self-esteem, internal locus of control, external attribution of blame, presence of spirituality, and high ego control. Family cohesiveness, competent foster care, and positive school experiences can also promote resilience. *(Ref. 1, Ch. 24, Resilience section; Daigneault, Hébert, and Tourigny, 2007)*

29 **(d)** The forensic evaluation should be completed by a forensic-trained clinician separate from the treating provider who suspects the abuse in the first place. From a legal standpoint, the

initial clinician who suspects the abuse is only obligated to report to appropriate authorities according to the local state laws and regulations, but is not responsible for performing a forensic evaluation on the case. The treating clinician should try to document direct statements of disclosure (e.g., quotations) in the medical record. The confidential issues should be addressed and clarified prior to a forensic evaluation because such an evaluation is done for the purpose of court proceedings. *(Ref. 1, Ch. 24, Resilience section)*

30 **(a)** Emotional maltreatment (psychological maltreatment) may be the most prevalent form of child maltreatment, and may be the most likely to be underreported. Unfortunately, there is no universally agreed upon definition of such maltreatment. Six types of psychopathologically abusive behaviors by caregivers are proposed to indicate possible emotional or psychological maltreatment including: spurning, terrorizing, isolating, exploiting/corrupting, denying emotional responsiveness, and mental health/medical/educational neglect. *(Hibbard et al., 2012)*

31 **(e)** Both bullying by peers and maltreatment by an adult with intent to harm are strongly associated with self-reported psychotic symptoms, which suggests that intention to harm and perceived threat could be factors regardless of the forms of maltreatments per se. *(Arseneault et al., 2011)*

32 **(b)** The accumulative effect of abuse or trauma confers the highest risk for developing psychotic symptoms. (*Arseneault et al., 2011*)

33 **(c)** Childhood emotional abuse is independently associated with adolescent suicidal ideation and behavior. Sexual abuse and emotional abuse may be more significant in explaining suicidal behavior than physical abuse and neglect). *(Ref. 1, Ch. 24, Diagnostic Considerations and Comorbidity section)*

34 **(a)** As one of the interventions for foster families during early childhood, Attachment and Biobehavioral Catch-up (ABC) is designed to help caregivers to be highly responsive to the child's emotional needs and to promote the caregiver in providing nurturing care and attachment security. *(Ref. 1, Ch. 24, Parent and Child Treatment section)*

35 **(e)** All listed are common areas of learning that can be affected by cancer treatment to the CNS. In addition, organizing or sequencing of tasks can be affected. *(Ref. 3, Ch. 7.2.1, School section)*

36 **(d)** Most transplant services do not view occasional experimentation with alcohol by adolescents as an absolute contraindication for a future liver transplant. In adults, a liver transplantation program requires at least six months to one year of sobriety before liver transplantation can be considered because alcohol or addictive drug use is usually a contraindication to liver transplant. Lecturing to youth about the serious negative consequences of alcohol use is less productive than having developmentally appropriate discussions with them about alcohol use. *(Ref. 3, Ch. 7.7.2, The Pretransplantation Psychiatric section)*

37 **(b)** Hypoglycemia can induce seizure. Other common causes of seizure include: systemic infection-induced high fever, cerebral palsy, phenylketonuria, encephalitis, intracranial bleed, lesions, and neoplasm, electrolyte disturbance, carbon monoxide poisoning, lead toxicity, cocaine, certain medications, lupus, and multiple sclerosis. *(Ref. 3, Table 7.2.4.1)*

38 **(a)** Absence seizure (petit mal) often manifests as staring spells and multiple brief episodes of behavioral arrests in younger children. In older children, it may also present with myoclonic jerks along with staring spells. Absence seizure should be considered in the differential diagnosis of ADHD. Mouth twitching, drooling, and nocturnal predisposition are clinical features of Rolandic epilepsy. Temporal lobe epilepsy may present with gastric aura, automatisms, and tonic posturing. Frontal lobe epilepsy manifests as hypermotor activity (e.g., repetitive motor activities) with a change in behavior. Parietal/occipital lobe epilepsy may induce somatosensory/visual phenomena. Juvenile myoclonic epilepsy (JME) may present with brief myoclonic jerks, which can be repetitive and lead to generalized seizure. *(Ref. 3, Table 7.2.4.5)*

39 **(b)** Gastric or olfactory aura, confusion, and automatisms commonly occur with temporal lobe epilepsy. Mouth twitching, drooling, and nocturnal predisposition are features commonly associated with benign Rolandic epilepsy with centrotemporal spikes. Hypermotor activity, change in behavior, and nocturnal predisposition can occur in frontal lobe epilepsy. Myoclonic jerks and staring spells with older age of onset are characteristic of juvenile absence epilepsy. Brief myoclonic jerks and generalized tonic-clonic seizures are often associated with juvenile myoclonic epilepsy. *(Ref 3, Ch. 7.2.4, Table 7.2.4.5)*

40 **(a)** Alpha agonists do not appear to have clinically significant interactions with antiepileptic drugs (AEDs). Risperdidone, trazodone, and alprazolam levels may be reduced by some AEDs through cytochrome P450 3A4 induction. Fluoxetine may increase some AED levels through 3A4 inhibition. *(Ref. 3, Ch. 7.2.4, Table 7.2.4.8)*

41 **(d)** Passive-aggressive personality is not listed as a formal personality disorder in DSM-5. However, it can be considered under "other specified personality disorder and unspecified personality disorder" if the individual meets the general criteria for a personality disorder, but cannot be categorized into one of the former personality disorders. In addition to the personality disorders listed in the question, the other six are: paranoid personality disorder, schizotypal personality disorder, narcissistic personality disorder, avoidant personality disorder, obsessive-compulsive personality disorder, and dependent personality disorder. *(Ref. 4, pp. 645–646)*

42 **(a)** Antisocial personality disorder is the only personality disorder that has an age diagnostic requirement in DSM-5 (at least age 18 years). However, there must be a history of symptoms of conduct disorder before age 15 years, manifested as a repetitive and pervasive pattern of disregard for and violation of the rights of others or age-appropriate societal norms/rules. *(Ref. 4, pp. 659–660)*

43 **(c)** Personality disorder diagnoses can be given in individuals younger than 18 years (except for antisocial personality disorder). However, the symptoms must be present for more than one year. In these cases, the maladaptive personality traits must be pervasive, persistent, and unlikely to be limited to a particular developmental stage or be related to another mental disorder. In general, personality traits observed in childhood often end up changing over time into adulthood. *(Ref. 4, p. 647)*

44 **(a)** The prevalence of borderline personality disorder decreases as people age and is lower in the older age groups. The overall

impairment and suicide risk associated with this disorder gradually decreases when people age. Studies show half of the individuals no longer meet the criteria at ten-year follow-up. In primary care settings, the prevalence rate is about 6%, about 10% in outpatient mental health clinics, and about 20% in psychiatric hospital settings. *(Ref. 4, pp. 665–666)*

45 **(c)** Decreased amygdala and hippocampal volume is found in adults with borderline personality disorder by structural MRI. The other findings have all been seen in studies of adolescents with borderline personality disorder. *(Ref. 3, Ch. 5.13, Etiology section)*

46 **(e)** None of the listed factors should be excluded as psychosocial risk factors for developing borderline personality disorder. Among them, sexual abuse is more discriminatory between borderline personality disorder and other personality disorders, although such a correlation does not imply causality, and studies show most abused children do not grow into adults with borderline personality disorder. *(Ref. 3, Ch. 5.13, Etiology section)*

47 **(b)** All of the listed conditions are commonly comorbid conditions with borderline personality disorder and are quite prevalent in youth without borderline personality disorder. However, only conduct disorder is statistically significant in being more prevalent among youth with borderline personality disorder than those without the disorder. *(Ref. 3, Ch. 5.13, Diagnosis and Clinical Features section)*

48 **(c)** Many different interventions have been used for treating borderline disorder in children and adolescents without any published, well-controlled studies indicating the best therapeutic modality. Because of the complex nature of the disorder, multimodal treatment approaches are proposed, relying on no single approach but rather combining them when clinically indicated. ECT, however, has not been considered as one of the recommended approaches. *(Ref. 3, Ch. 5.13, Treatment section)*

49 **(c)** Children with childhood absence epilepsy have been found to have, relative to healthy controls, more depression and anxiety symptoms as well as general psychosocial difficulties such as isolation and low self-esteem. *(Ref. 3, Ch. 7.2.4, Psychiatric Disorders in Children with Epilepsy section)*

50 **(c)** The core feature of pedophilic disorder is recurrent, intense sexually arousing fantasies, sexual urges, or sexual acting-out behaviors with a prepubescent child or children lasting more than six months, which causes marked distress or interpersonal difficulty. The individual with the disorder has to be at least 16 years old and five years older than the victim(s). *(Ref. 4, pp. 697–698)*

Matching

51 **(e); 52. (d); 53. (c); 54. (b); 55. (a)** Suicide refers to fatal, self-inflicted, destructive conduct with explicit or implicit intent to die. Suicide attempts are nonfatal, self-inflicted, destructive conduct with explicit or implicit intent to die, which may not necessarily lead to injury. Aborted attempts are stopped by the individual prior to injury. Interrupted attempts are stopped by another person or circumstance prior to injury. Suicidal ideation refers to thoughts of harming or killing self. Nonsuicidal self-injurious behavior refers to any self-inflicted, destructive conduct with full intent to inflict self-harm without intent to die. *(Ref. 1, Ch. 26, Definitions section)*

56 **(d); 57. (c); 58 (b); 59. (a)** The assigned gender at birth is sometimes referred to as the "natal gender." Gender identity refers to an individual's identification as male, female, or another category. Gender identity disorder was a diagnosis in DSM-IV that was replaced in DSM-5 with gender dysphoria, which focuses on dysphoria as the clinical problem, not the gender identity itself. *(Ref. 4, pp. 451)*

60 **(b); 61 (c); 62 (a); 63 (k); 64 (j); 65 (i); 66 (h); 67 (g); 68 (f); 69 (e); 70 (d)** Experienced gender is also referred to as gender identity. Terms describing sexual orientation such as androphilia (attraction to males), gynephilia (attraction to females), biphilia (attraction to males and females), and aphilia (attraction to neither males nor females) correspond to older terms such as heterosexual, bisexual, homosexual, and asexual. Gender nonconforming and gender variant are terms that encompass a range of variations from developmental norms in gender role behavior, which may include incongruency between experienced gender and gender assigned at birth. *(Ref. 3, Ch. 5.14, Terminology and Definitions section)*

71 **(d)** Lamotrigine is associated with little or no cognitive impairment or effect on attention, psychomotor speed, or memory. It can cause tremulousness, irritability, aggressive behavior, and insomnia.

72 **(c)** Valproic acid can be effective in the treatment of mania, but in some children can cause dose-dependent aggression, irritability, and hyperactivity.

73 **(b)** The behavioral side effects of levetiracetam are common and are more likely in children with developmental delays.

74 **(a)** Topiramate carries significant concern about adverse effects on cognition, most notably declines in word fluency and attention. It is advisable to monitor school performance in children taking topiramate. *(Ref. 3, Ch. 7.2.4, Neuropsychiatric Effects of Antiepileptic Drugs section)*

References

Arseneault, L., Cannon, M., Fisher, H. L., Polanczyk, G., Moffitt, T. E., & Caspi, A. (2011). Childhood trauma and children's emerging psychotic symptoms: A genetically sensitive longitudinal cohort study. *The American Journal of Psychiatry, 168*(1), 65–72. https://doi.org/10.1176/appi.ajp.2010.10040567

Daigneault, I., Hébert, M., and Tourigny M. (2007). Personal and interpersonal characteristics related to resilient developmental pathways of sexually abused adolescents. *Child Adolesc Psychiatr Clin N Am, 16*(2), 415–434.

Gartrell, N. and Bos, H. (2010). US National Longitudinal Lesbian Family Study: Psychological Adjustment of 17-year-old Adolescents. *Pediatrics, 126*, 28–36.

Hibbard, R. et al.(2012). Psychological maltreatment. *Pediatrics, 130*(2), 372–378.

Russell, S.T. et al. (2011). Lesbian, Gay, Bisexual, and Transgender Adolescents School Victimization: Implications for Young Adult Health and Adjustment. *Journal of School Health, 81*, 223–230.

Wilkinson, P. et al. (2011). Clinical and Psychosocial Predictors of Suicide Attempts and Nonsuicidal Self-Injury in the Adolescent Depression Antidepressant and Psychotherapy Trial/ADAPT. *Am J Psychiatry, 168*, 495–501.

11

PSYCHOLOGICAL TESTING AND RATING SCALES

DOI: 10.4324/9781003308805-12

QUESTIONS

Directions: Select the best response for each of the questions 1–20.

1. All of the following statements regarding referral questions for psychological testing describe good practice *except*:
   a. Referral for assessment of a child's developmental process.
   b. Referral for assessment of a child's intellectual capacity and academic achievement.
   c. Referral for clarification of a child's diagnoses and assistance with therapeutic interventions.
   d. Referral questions should be explained to the parents.
   e. Referral questions should be formulated by the testing clinician after evaluation.

2. Which of the following is the *best* definition of construct validity on a testing instrument?
   a. The test's capacity to measure what it is supposed to measure (such as underlying theoretical, intangible qualities or traits in which individuals differ)
   b. The test's effectiveness in predicting an individual's performance in specific areas
   c. The fact that the test's content covers a representative sample for the property being measured
   d. The degree to which the test results can be reproduced
   e. Pretesting of the test on a large, demographically representative group of individuals

3. All of the following intelligence tests can be used in younger children (< 4 years) *except*:
   a. Differential Ability Scales, Second Edition (DAS-II)
   b. Kaufman Assessment Battery for Children, Second Edition (KABC-2)
   c. Stanford-Binet Intelligence Scale, Fifth Edition (SB-5)
   d. Wechsler Abbreviated Scale of Intelligence (WASI)
   e. Wechsler Preschool and Primary Scale of Intelligence, Third Edition (WPPSI-III)

4. All of the following statements regarding the Vineland Adaptive Behavior Scales, Second Edition are accurate *except*:
   a. It is an excellent measurement of adaptive behavior.
   b. It assesses psychosocial functioning.
   c. It can be used in individuals with cognitive delay.
   d. It can be completed by the child's teacher.
   e. It measures academic achievement.

5. The Rorschach inkblots can be used for children as young as:
   a. 2 years
   b. 5 years
   c. 9 years
   d. 12 years
   e. 16 years

6. All of the following are projective assessment procedures that can be used in children *except*:
   a. Rorschach Inkblot Test
   b. Children's Apperception Test (CAT)
   c. Personality Inventory for Children (PIC-2)
   d. Sentence and Story Completion Tasks
   e. Draw-A-Person Test

7. All of the following instruments can be used during early infancy *except*:
   a. Bayley Scales of Infant Development-II
   b. Gesell's Developmental Schedules (GDS)
   c. Denver Developmental Screening Test-II
   d. Brazelton Neonatal Behavioral Assessment Scale-2
   e. Draw-A-Person Test (DAP)

8. Which of the following rating scales has the *best* performance data and the *greatest* usage in measuring childhood behavior problems?
   a. Child and Adolescent Psychiatric Assessment (CAPA)
   b. Child Behavior Checklist (CBCL) (Achenbach)
   c. Child Schedule for Affective Disorders and Schizophrenia (K-SADS)
   d. Diagnostic Interview for Children and Adolescents (DICA)
   e. Diagnostic Interview Schedule for Children (DISC)

9. Neuropsychological evaluation is useful in the assessment of all of the following areas *except*:
   a. Sensory perception
   b. Motor function and visuomotor integrity
   c. Executive functions
   d. Specific brain damage site
   e. Language, memory, and concept formation

10. All of the following areas can be reliably assessed in children and adolescents using psychological tests *except*:
    a. Intellectual ability
    b. Personality functioning
    c. Life expectancy
    d. Educational accomplishment
    e. Adaptive behaviors

11 Which of the following statements regarding intelligence tests is *inaccurate*?

   a Intelligence tests measure both a global/overall capacity and separate/subscale abilities.

   b IQ score is not used to determine severity of intellectual disability in DSM-5.

   c The most widely used tests to assess intelligence and cognitive functioning are the Wechsler scales.

   d Individuals' IQ scores demonstrate wide variability after the age of 5 years.

   e IQ testing can be used to assist making diagnoses of specific learning disabilities.

12 Which of the following is *not* a nonverbal and language-free test?

   a Comprehensive Test of Nonverbal Intelligence (CTONI-2)

   b Mullen Scales of Early Learning (MSEL)

   c Leiter International Performance Scale, 3rd ed. (Leiter-3)

   d Raven's Progressive Matrices

   e Wechsler Nonverbal Scale of Ability (WNV)

13 All of the following are achievement tests *except*:

   a Kaufman Test of Educational Achievement, Second Edition (KTEA-II)

   b Kaufman Assessment Battery for Children, Second Edition (KABC-II)

   c Peabody Individual Achievement Test, Revised (PIAT-R)

   d Wide Range Achievement Test, Fourth Edition (WRAT4)

   e Woodcock-Johnson, Third Edition Test of Achievement (WJ-III ACH)

14 Which of the following tests can be used for assessing receptive language but *not* expressive language?

   a Clinical Evaluation of Language Fundamentals (CLEF)

   b Developmental Neuropsychological Assessment-Second Edition (NEPSY-II)

   c Peabody Picture Vocabulary Test (PPVT)

   d Test of Language Competence (TOLC)

   e Woodcock-Johnson-III (WJ-III)

15 Which of the following tests is *not* a commonly used projective test for clinical hypothesis generation?

   a Thematic apperception test

   b Wisconsin card sorting test

   c Draw-A-Person test

   d Kinetic family drawing

   e Sentence completion test

16 Which of the following objective personality measures can be administered to children as young as five years old?

   a Millon Adolescent Personality Inventory (MAPI)

   b Millon Adolescent Clinical Inventory (MACI)

   c Millon Pre-Adolescent Clinical Inventory (M-PACI)

   d Minnesota Multiphasic Personality Inventory, Adolescent (MMPI-A)

   e Personality Inventory for Children, Second Edition (PIC-2)

17 Which of the following is *not* an instrument based on interviewing the parents and the parents' reports for assessment of communication?

   a Autism Diagnostic Interview, Revised

   b Children's Communication Checklist-2

   c Woodcock Language Proficiency Battery–Revised

   d Language Development Survey

   e MacArthur-Bates Communication Development Inventory

18 All of the following are considered as interrelated and interdependent domains of executive function *except*:

   a Inhibition

   b Set shifting

   c Planning

   d Working memory

   e None of the above

19 Which of the following reliability concepts is measured by the consistency obtained by the same person who takes the same test on two different occasions?

   a Alternate-form reliability

   b Interitem reliability

   c Interrater reliability

   d Split-half reliability

   e Test-retest reliability

20 Which of the following T-scores is equivalent to a typical mean score of 100?

   a 20

   b 30

   c 40

   d 50

   e 60

Matching

21–25 Select from the following descriptions the one that *best* matches each psychological test or rating scale:

   a Preschool intelligence test

   b Modified Beck Inventory

   c Comprehensive symptom rate scale

   d Attention-deficit/hyperactivity disorder (ADHD)

   e Internalizers-externalizers

21 Behavior Assessment System for Children (BASC-3)

22 Wechsler Preschool and Primary Scale of Intelligence, Third Edition (WPPSI-III)

23 Conners' Rating Scale, Revised (CRS-R)
24 Child Behavior Checklist (CBCL)
25 Children's Depression Inventory (CDI)
26–30 Select from the following descriptions the one that *best* matches each of the following terms related to psychological testing:

a Continued rise in IQ test performance

b Lack of enough easy items

c Lack of enough hard items

d Effects of level of language, memory, and speed of processing on the overall IQ scores

e Improvement of the score due to the familiarity of the test

26 Practice effects
27 Item content differences
28 Ceiling effects
29 Floor effects
30 The Flynn effect

ANSWERS AND EXPLANATIONS

1 **(e)** To ensure the efficiency and efficacy of the assessment, it is critical to develop a list of referral questions to be answered by the psychological evaluations. The specific relevant referral questions should be formulated by the referring clinician and explained to the parents of the child being assessed. Several areas referral questions commonly address are: assessments of developmental process, intellectual capacity, academic achievement, learning disabilities, diagnoses, treatments, and prediction of course of treatment. *(Ref. 3, Ch. 4.4, The Assessment Process section)*

2 **(a)** Answer (b) defines criterion-related validity, answer (c) defines content validity, answer (d) defines reliability, and answer (e) defines standardization. It is important to know the reliability and validity of a particular test in interpreting the results. *(Ref. 3, Table 4.4.3)*

3 **(d)** The Wechsler Abbreviated Scale of Intelligence (WASI) is designed to be used for individuals 6:0 to 89:0 years of age. The DAS-II is designed for children 2:6 to 17:11 years, the KABC-2 for children age 3:0 to 18:11 years, the SB-5 for children age 2:0 to adults age 89:11 years, and the WPPSI for those age 2:6 to 7:3. *(Ref. 3, Table 4.4.8)*

4 **(e)** The Vineland does not measure academic achievement, as does the Woodcock-Johnson Psychoeducational Battery or the Wide Range Achievement Test. Many factors can influence the assessment of adaptive functioning, and there is some reported fluctuation in means and standard deviations across age groups with the Vineland. It does come with a teacher form. *(Ref. 2, Table 2-7)*

5 **(b)** Besides the Thematic Apperception Test, the Rorschach is also a projective test. It is used to assess personality organization and provides data regarding the child's developmental capacities for reality testing, integration of affect, and maturational level of object relations in children as young as five years. It can be used to evaluate personality development and help to reveal children's hidden emotions or internal conflicts. *(Ref. 3, Table 4.4.9)*

6 **(c)** The Personality Inventory for Children (PIC-2) is one of the objective personality measures for children among others including: High School Personality Questionnaire (HSPQ), Millon Adolescent Personality Inventory (MAPI), Millon Adolescent Clinical Inventory (MACI), Millon Pre-Adolescent Clinical Inventory (M-PACI), Minnesota Multiphasic Personality Inventory, Adolescent (MMPI-A), and Personality Inventory for Youth, Second Edition (PIY). Besides all the listed projective measures, other such measures may include Projective Drawings, Roberts Apperception Test for Children, Second Edition (Roberts-2), Thematic Apperception Test (TAT), and Tell-Me-A-Story (TEMAS). *(Ref. 3, Table 4.4.9)*

7 **(e)** The Draw-A-Person Test (DAP) can be used as a projective test in subjects 5–17 years. The other tests listed are measures of neonate, infant, and toddler development, and can all be used during early infancy. *(Ref. 3, Table 4.4.9)*

8 **(b)** The CBCL has been considered a gold standard among behavioral rating scales. It is validated and is the most widely used instrument in research and clinical settings to measure a range of internalizing and externalizing behaviors. The K-SADS, CAPA, DISC, and DICA are diagnostic interviews, not behavior rating scales. *(Ref. 3, Table 4.4.8; Ref. 5, p. 1072)*

9 **(d)** Variability in cerebral organization makes it impossible to determine that one specific brain region is involved or damaged, especially using one particular test. Neuropsychological testing is rarely used to find the "site of lesion," and brain regions are interrelated in a manner that makes it very unlikely that only one particular brain region is involved. All other areas listed are commonly assessed through neuropsychological testing. *(Ref. 3, Ch. 4.4, Neuropsychological Assessment section)*

10 **(c)** Psychological testing cannot assess life expectancy. All other listed areas can be reliably assessed by psychological testing. Psychological testing can also provide concrete, standardized data about language skills, visual-motor coordination, developmental level, neurocognitive functioning, and occupational interest and aptitude. *(Ref. 3, Ch. 4.4, Psychological Assessment section)*

11 **(d)** Individual IQ scores are relatively stable after about age five, although there may be individual differences. The Wechsler scales are most widely used for testing intellectual functioning. IQ score per se is no longer used as a diagnostic criterion for intellectual disability in DSM-5 (in contrast to DSM-IV). The severity of the intellectual disability is based on adaptive functioning, but not IQ scores. Deficits of intellectual functioning must be confirmed by both clinical assessment and individualized, standardized intelligence testing. *(Ref. 3, Ch. 4.4, Psychological Assessment section; Ref. 4, pp. 33–37)*

12 **(b)** Mullen Scales of Early Learning (MSEL) is a measure of cognitive development consisting of five scales: gross motor, visual reception, fine motor, expressive language, and receptive language. It is a good assessment tool for measuring general strength and weakness in young children. The other listed instruments are all considered as nonverbal and language free or culture free. Some of them depend more on abstract pattern recognition and make fewer demands on language systems, which are considered as less biased by cultural differences. *(Ref. 5, p. 3417)*

13 **(b)** The Kaufman Assessment Battery for Children, Second Edition (KABC-II) is not an achievement test. Instead, it is an intelligence test that consists of subtests including measures of sequential and simultaneous processing, fluid reasoning and crystallized ability, and long-term retrieval. Most of the intellectual, achievement, and processing tests are structured in a similar way using 100 as the mean score and 15 as the standard deviation in order to be compared across instruments. *(Ref. 5, p. 3417)*

14 **(c)** The Peabody Picture Vocabulary Test (PPVT) can be used only to assess receptive language. The rest of the tests listed can be used to assess both receptive and expressive language. *(Ref. 5, p. 3418)*

15 **(b)** The Wisconsin card sorting test (not a projective test) is used to measure executive functioning and attention capacity. All of the other tests listed are projective tests useful for generating clinical hypotheses regarding children's feelings about themselves and their families. The information generated needs to be integrated into the clinical evaluation and cannot be used alone. *(Ref. 3, Table 4.4.9; Ref. 5, p. 3434)*

16 **(e)** The Personality Inventory for Children, Second Edition (PIC-2) can be administered for youth between the ages of 5 and 19 years. The PIY is for older children (between the ages of 9 and 19 years. The rest of the listed tests are all for adolescents. *(Ref. 3, Table 4.4.9; Ref. 5, p. 3404)*

17 **(c)** The Woodcock Language Proficiency Battery–Revised is administered by the examiner and is not based on the parents' report. The rest of the listed instruments are used for assessing communication based on interviewing the parents and the parents' report. *(Ref. 3, Table 4.5.2)*

18 **(e)** Inhibition, set shifting, planning, working memory, and self-monitoring are all domains of executive function in children and adolescents. *(Ref. 3, Ch. 4.4, Neuropsychological Assessment)*

19 **(e)** Test-retest reliability is measured and obtained by the same person taking the same test on two different occasions. On the other hand, the interrater reliability is obtained by getting the same results when the same test is administered by different examiners. *(Ref. 3, Table 4.4.3)*

20 **(d)** A T-score of 50 is equivalent to a typical standard mean score of 100. Standard scores are very useful for making comparisons across tests. Thus, most cognitive and achievement tests use standard mean scores of 100 with a standard deviation of 15. However, many behavioral checklists use T-scores that have a mean of 50 with a standard deviation of 10. *(Ref. 3, Table 4.4.5)*

Matching

21 **(c)** The BASC is a comprehensive symptom rating scale with parent, teacher, and youth forms. *(Ref. 5, p. 3399)*

22 **(a)** The WPPSI-III is intended for use in children age 2:6–7:7 years. *(Ref. 3, Table 4.4.8)*

23 **(d)** The Conners' Rating Scale-Revised is a measure of externalizing behaviors and is best known for use in the assessment of ADHD. *(Ref. 3, Table 4.4.9)*

24 **(e)** The CBCL uses factor-derived scores to classify behaviors as externalizing or internalizing. It has been the gold standard for research and clinical work among broad-band behavior rating scales. *(Ref. 5, p. 1072)*

25 **(b)** The CDI is derived from the adult Beck Depression Inventory, written at first grade level and used in both young children and teenagers. *(Ref. 5, p. 3399)*

26 **(e); 27. (d); 28. (c); 29. (b); 30. (a)** Practice effects refer to improved scores due to familiarity with or prior exposure to the test items. Item content differences refer to the differences in the measures of the content. Ceiling effects occur when there are not enough hard items. Floor effects occur when there are not enough easy items. The Flynn effect refers to the continuous increase in IQ performance over years. *(Ref. 3, Table 4.4.7)*

12

PSYCHOPHARMACOLOGY AND MEDICATION-INDUCED MOVEMENT DISORDERS AND OTHER ADVERSE EFFECTS OF MEDICATION

DOI: 10.4324/9781003308805-13

QUESTIONS

Directions: Select the best response for each of the questions 1–50.

1 Which of the following statements regarding developmental changes in neurochemical systems that can influence both therapeutic and side effects of psychotropic medications is *not* accurate?

   a Adolescents have a higher risk of dystonic reactions to conventional antipsychotics in comparison to adults.

   b Younger children have a higher risk of activating side effects to the SSRIs.

   c Developmental differences in the maturation of the noradrenergic neurotransmission system may in part explain the lack of effectiveness of tricyclic antidepressants in children.

   d Major neurochemical systems that are altered by psychotropic medications are subject to age-related effects.

   e None of the above.

2 Which of the following is *not* one of four functionally distinct phases of pharmacokinetics?

   a Absorption

   b Distribution

   c Excretion

   d Metabolism

   e Neurotransmission and receptor binding

3 All of the following statements regarding the effect of age on the absorption of psychotropic medications are correct *except*:

   a The pH-dependent diffusion has a major influence on gastrointestinal absorption.

   b During the first week of infancy, the gastric pH is nearly neutral.

   c The gastric pH reaches adult level by age 3 years.

   d In toddlers, weakly acidic drugs tend to be more likely ionized in the stomach because of less acidic stomach content.

   e In young children, intestinal transit time is decreased and the intestinal absorptive surface area is increased.

4 Relatively lower plasma concentration of lithium in the pediatric population compared to adults is *most* likely to be due to which of the following factors?

   a The first pass effect

   b Fat distribution

   c Body weight

   d Volume of distribution

   e Cytochrome enzymes (CYPs)

5 What percentage of Caucasians have a genetic deficiency of CYP 2D6, which causes less efficiency at metabolizing CYP 2D6 substrates?

   a 0.5–1%

   b 3–5%

   c 7–10%

   d 12–15%

   e 16–20%

6 Which one of the following syndromes is associated with a reduced activity of UDP-glucuronylsyltransferase 1A1 (UGT-1A1)?

   a Down syndrome

   b Fragile X syndrome

   c Gilbert's syndrome

   d Prader-Willi syndrome

   e Williams syndrome

7 All of the following statements regarding unique developmental characteristics of CYPs and Phase II enzymes are correct *except*:

   a CYP 3A4 are higher in youth than in adults.

   b CYP 2D6 matures to adult level by age 10 years.

   c CYP 2C19 are highly variable from 5 months to 10 years.

   d UGT1A1 is immature in premature infants.

   e UGT 1A19 only develops after the second year of life.

8 Which one of the following statements can clearly explain the reason(s) why children under 10 years require larger, weight-adjusted doses of most hepatically metabolized medications than adults to achieve comparable blood levels and therapeutic responses?

   a Children have greater liver to body mass ratio compared to adults.

   b Children have more efficient CYP enzymes than adults.

   c Children have uniformly increased phase II conjugates.

   d All of the above.

   e None of the above.

9 An adolescent who develops Steven-Johnson syndrome because of an elevated level of lamotrigine after combining lamotrigine with valproate is *most* likely the result of which of the following mechanisms?

   a Valproate as an inhibitor of CYP 2C19

   b Valproate as an inhibitor of 2D6

   c Valproate as an inhibitor of UGT2B7

   d Lamotrigine as a self-inducer of UGT 1A4

   e Lamotrigine as an inhibitor of CYP3A4

10 Paroxetine is both substrate and inhibitor of which of the following CYPs?

   a CYP1A2

   b CYP2B6

c CYP2C9

d CYP2C19

e CYP2D6

11 All of the following general principles of psychopharmacological treatment are appropriate *except*:

a A thorough psychiatric assessment is the first step prior to starting the treatment.

b An appropriate biopsychosocial formulation and treatment planning improves treatment compliance and outcomes.

c Target symptoms should be the key focus regardless of diagnoses or disorders.

d Unique pharmacokinetic and pharmacodynamics difference in youth should be considered.

e Start medications with relatively low doses and titrate slowly.

12 Clomipramine (Anafranil) potentially benefits all of the following disorders *except*:

a OCD

b ADHD

c Trichotillomania (hair-pulling disorder)

d OCD-like symptoms in children with autism

e Self-injury and stereotypic behaviors

13 Based on our current knowledge, all of the following statements regarding the use of amphetamine and methylphenidate in the treatment of ADHD are correct *except*:

a Amphetamine is FDA approved for children as young as 3 years of age.

b They both invariably worsen tics when used in children with ADHD comorbid with tic disorders.

c In general, an effective dose of amphetamine is lower than that of methylphenidate.

d Methylphenidate blocks the reuptake of dopamine and facilitates the release of stored dopamine.

e Amphetamine more specifically facilitates the release of newly synthesized dopamine in addition to blocking its reuptake.

14 All of the following statements regarding long-acting stimulants are true *except*:

a They do not cause insomnia.

b The peak levels come later than those of immediate-release agents.

c They help overcome tachyphylaxis.

d Usually, children do not need to take a dose in school, which can minimize missed doses.

e They may minimize the rebound phenomenon commonly seen in immediate-release formulations.

15 All of the following statements regarding atomoxetine (Strattera) reflect the current state of our knowledge *except*:

a It has both noradrenergic reuptake and dopaminergic properties.

b The FDA approved it for treatment of ADHD in both children and adults.

c It can increase diastolic blood pressure and heart rate.

d It can have drug–drug interactions with MAOIs and CYP 2D6 inhibitors.

e It can rarely cause serious hepatotoxicity.

16 Which of the following is *not* a required baseline medical test prior to initiating treatment with lithium?

a Urinalysis

b Blood urea nitrogen (BUN)

c Thyroid function test

d Liver function test

e Electrolytes test

17 Which of the following SSRIs is the *most* potent serotonin reuptake inhibitor?

a Citalopram

b Escitalopram

c Fluoxetine

d Fluvoxamine

e Paroxetine

18 Which of the following SSRIs follows linear (first-order) kinetics?

a Fluoxetine

b Fluvoxamine

c Paroxetine

d Sertraline

e None of the above

19 Which of the following SSRIs has the *lowest* incidence of sexual side effects?

a Citalopram

b Fluoxetine

c Fluvoxamine

d Paroxetine

e Sertraline

20 Which of the following SSRIs shows a significant increase in plasma levels when administered with food?

a Citalopram

b Fluoxetine

c Fluvoxamine

d Paroxetine

e Sertraline

21 Small studies show which of the following properties of bupropion (Wellbutrin) explains its effectiveness in the treatment of ADHD?

a Norepinephrine-dopamine reuptake inhibition

b Selective serotonin-norepinephrine reuptake inhibition

c   Noradrenergic and specific serotonergic

d   Serotonin agonist and serotonin reuptake inhibition

e   Selective serotonin reuptake inhibition

22 All of the following antidepressants have almost no sexual side effects *except*:

a   Bupropion (Wellbutrin)

b   Duloxetine (Cymbalta)

c   Mirtazapine (Remeron)

d   Trazodone (Desyrel)

e   Venlafaxine (Effexor)

23 All of the listed antidepressants follow linear kinetics *except*:

a   Bupropion (Wellbutrin)

b   Duloxetine (Cymbalta)

c   Mirtazapine (Remeron)

d   Trazodone (Desyrel)

e   Venlafaxine (Effexor)

24 Lithium has all of the following effects on the central nervous systems (CNS) at the second messenger level *except*:

a   Block the activity of inositol polyphosphatase 1-phosphatase

b   Inhibit adenyl cyclase by competing with magnesium

c   Up-regulate hippocampal serotonin (5-HT$_{1A}$) receptors

d   Increase the proportion of low-affinity beta receptors

e   Induce sensitivity of alpha 2 receptors

25 Which of the following agents demonstrated the highest response rate in the initial treatment of childhood mania in the Treatment of Early Age Mania (TEAM) study?

a   Carbamazepine

b   Lamotrigine

c   Valproate

d   Risperidone

e   Lithium

26 A genetic variant inherited by patients of Chinese ancestry, strongly associated with Stevens-Johnson syndrome induced by carbamazepine, is present on which of the following human leukocyte antigen (HLA) genes?

a   HLA-A

b   HLA-B

c   HLA-C

d   HLA-DR

e   HLA-DQ

27 Which of the following agents or types of agents is *least* likely to have an increased drug level when co-administered with carbamazepine?

a   Atypical antipsychotics

b   Lamotrigine

c   Oral contraceptives

d   Phenobarbital

e   Tricyclic antidepressants

28 Which of the following numbers reflects the approximate elevated risk of developing serious rashes in youth taking lamotrigine younger than 16 years compared to older individuals?

a   Three times greater

b   Five times greater

c   Eight times greater

d   Ten times greater

e   Twenty times greater

29 Which of the following agents is *not* metabolized or protein bound and does *not* alter hepatic enzymes or interact with other anticonvulsants?

a   Gabapentin

b   Lamotrigine

c   Oxcarbazepine

d   Topiramate

e   Valproate

30 Which of the following agents is *most* likely to be associated with nephrolithiasis?

a   Gabapentin

b   Lamotrigine

c   Oxcarbazepine

d   Topiramate

e   Valproate

31 Blocking which of the following receptors can *best* explain certain antipsychotics' less frequent association with extrapyramidal symptoms (EPS)?

a   Dopamine D$_2$

b   Alpha-1 adrenergic

c   Alpha-2 adrenergic

d   Muscarinic M$_{2-4}$ (peripheral)

e   Serotonin 5-HT$_{2A}$

32 Compared to most of the other antipsychotics, which of the following antipsychotics requires a higher level of occupancy of the D2 receptor to achieve an equivalent level of blockade and therapeutic effect?

a   Aripiprazole

b   Clozapine

c   Paliperidone

d   Risperidone

e   Ziprasidone

33 The pharmacokinetic rebound effect experienced during switching of antipsychotics is *least* likely to be seen in which of the following situations?

a   When a patient is nonadherent to the new antipsychotic or the dose of the new antipsychotic is too low.

b When there is a lack of adequate overlap during the switching.

c When the dose of the new agent is titrated up rapidly.

d When there is a low bioavailability because of taking it without food (e.g., ziprasidone).

e When it is less ready to cross the blood–brain barrier.

34 All of the following antipsychotic-induced side effects are more prevalent in children and adolescents *except*:

a Sedation

b Akathisia

c Withdrawal dyskinesia

d Weight gain and metabolic abnormalities

e Prolactin abnormalities

35 Based on updated research data, all of the following statements regarding antipsychotic-induced weight gain in youth are accurate *except*:

a Longer exposure to antipsychotics increases risk of weight gain or obesity.

b Associated with a relatively lower risk of gaining weight, aripiprazole and ziprasidone are not weight neutral, especially in subgroups of pediatric patients.

c Combination of an antipsychotic with a stimulant medication can attenuate the antipsychotic-induced weight gain.

d Combination of an antipsychotic with a mood stabilizer is associated with more weight gain than with mood stabilizer monotherapy or treatment with combined mood stabilizers.

e Olanzapine carries a higher risk for weight gain, whereas risperidone and quetiapine carry intermediate risk.

36 A 16-year-old boy who has been treated with risperidone for his psychotic symptoms develops gynecomastia. Which of the following antipsychotics should be considered *first* as an alternative?

a Aripiprazole

b Clozapine

c Paliperidone

d Quetiapine

e Ziprasidone

37 Which of the following antipsychotics is associated with myocarditis, especially early in treatment?

a Aripiprazole

b Clozapine

c Paliperidone

d Risperidone

e Ziprasidone

38 Which of the following ethnic groups is associated with benign ethnic (or cyclic) neutropenia?

a African descent

b Asian descent

c Latinos

d American Indians

e Europeans

39 Which of the following symptoms is a cardinal feature of neuroleptic malignant syndrome (NMS)?

a Akinesia

b Dysphagia

c Generalized rigidity ("lead pipe")

d Sialorrhea

e Tremor

40 Which of the following SSRIs is *most* likely to be associated with antidepressant discontinuation syndrome?

a Citalopram

b Fluoxetine

c Fluvoxamine

d Paroxetine

e Sertraline

41 All of the following statements regarding the study "ADHD Drugs and Serious Cardiovascular Events in Children and Young Adults" (W. O. Cooper et al. 2011) are accurate *except*:

a This is a retrospective study of data collected from about 1.2 million children and young adults who use ADHD drugs.

b Serious cardiovascular events (sudden cardiac death, acute myocardial infarction, and stroke) are identified.

c The incidence of serious events is 3.1 per 100,000 person-years.

d Use of ADHD drugs is not associated with an increased risk of serious cardiovascular events in children and young adults.

e Because of the upper limit of the 95% confidence interval, a doubling in the risk has been ruled out.

42 All of the following statements regarding the study "A Double-Blind Randomized Controlled Trial of N-Acetylcysteine in Cannabis-Dependent Adolescents" (Gray et al. 2012) are correct *except*:

a As an over-the-counter supplement, N-acetylcysteine (NAC) down-regulates the cysteine-glutamate exchanger in the nucleus accumbens.

b This eight-week trial enrolled 116 youth (ages 15–21) who have cannabis dependence.

c Either 1200 mg NAC or placebo twice daily was provided to the subjects (two groups of 58 patients each).

d The primary outcome measure is the odds of negative weekly urine tests comparing the two groups.

e Via an intent-to-treat analysis, the drug group has more than twice the odds of having negative urine tests compared to the placebo group.

43 Which atypical antipsychotic appears to be associated with the fewest adverse effects in children and adolescents?

   a Aripiprazole

   b Risperidone

   c Quetiapine

   d Ziprasidone

   e Lurasidone

44 All of the following are the conclusions made by authors Scahill et al. (2012) in the study "Effects of Risperidone and Parent Training on Adaptive Functioning in Children with Pervasive Developmental Disorder and Serious Behavioral Problems" *except*:

   a Both medication only (MED) and combination (COMB) groups show improvement over the 24-week trial on all Vineland domains.

   b The COMB group shows greater improvement than the MED group in the Vineland Socialization and Adaptive Composite Standard Scores.

   c The COMB group shows a greater improvement than the MED group on age-equivalent scores in the Socialization and Communication domains.

   d The COMB group shows a significantly greater gain in the Vineland Daily Living Skills domain than the MED group.

   e There is evidence to show additive benefits of parent training to medication management in school-aged children with PDDs and serious behavioral problems.

45 Based on the American Academy of Child and Adolescent Psychiatry "practice parameter for the use of atypical antipsychotic medications in children and adolescents," all of the following recommendations are considered as "clinical standards" *except*:

   a Clinicians should follow the most current available evidence in the scientific literature when selecting any atypical antipsychotic agent (AAA).

   b Clinicians should obtain baseline BMI and monitor it throughout treatment course.

   c Clinicians should monitor the risk of developing diabetes, and baseline blood glucose and other parameters should be obtained and monitored at regular intervals.

   d Clinicians should obtain baseline measurements of movement disorders using structured measures and continue to monitor at regular intervals and during the tapering of the AAAs.

   e Clinicians should obtain baseline EKG and again when a stable dose is achieved when prescribing ziprasidone.

46 Weight gain on atypical antipsychotics has been shown to be greatest in which of the following groups?

   a Children with disruptive behavior disorders

   b Children with early-onset schizophrenia

   c Children with tic disorders

   d Children with autism spectrum disorders

   e Children with bipolar disorder

47 All of the following statements regarding desmopressin (DDAVP) are correct *except*:

   a Desmopressin is an analog of the hormone arginine vasopressin (AVP) that is naturally secreted by the neurohypophysis.

   b The primary role of AVP is to concentrate urine.

   c AVP decreases urine output by increasing urine reuptake in the renal tubules.

   d AVP has a more potent antidiuretic effect than DDAVP.

   e AVP also has a vasopressor effect and can play a role in regulating blood pressure.

48 Which of the following is the *most* likely mechanism of the action of buspirone?

   a Binding to a GABA receptor

   b Binding to a histamine receptor

   c Binding to a noradrenergic receptor

   d Binding to a serotonin receptor

   e Binding to a muscarinic receptor

49 Which of the following agents is approved by the FDA for the treatment of pediatric insomnia?

   a Clonidine

   b Eszopiclone (Lunesta)

   c Melatonin

   d Zaleplon (Sonata)

   e Zolpidem (Ambien)

50 Among all of the following sedative-hypnotics, which one has a totally different mechanism of action compared to others?

   a Eszopiclone (Lunesta)

   b Ramelteon

   c Zaleplon (Sonata)

   d Zolpidem (Ambien)

   e Zolpidem CR (Ambien CR)

Matching

51–54 For each of the following medications, select the relative neurotransmitter effect that provides the *best* description of its action. Use each effect profile only once.

   a Primarily noradrenergic

   b Serotonergic and noradrenergic

   c Primarily serotonergic

   d Dopaminergic and noradrenergic

51 Venlafaxine

52 Clomipramine

53 Atomoxetine

54 Bupropion

55–58 For each of the following neuroleptics, select the profile that *best* describes its side effects. Use each side-effect profile only once.

   a Relatively high risk of extrapyramidal symptoms

   b Blood disorder and seizure

    c   Relatively low risk of EPS

    d   QTc prolongation

55 Quetiapine (Seroquel)

56 Ziprasidone (Geodon)

57 Risperidone (Risperdal)

58 Clozapine (Clozaril)

59–70 Select from the following the description that *best* matches each of the pharmacological terms:

    a   Conversion of drugs to forms more suitable for elimination

    b   Drug concentration is reduced before reaching target tissues

    c   Availability of unbound drugs reaching target tissues

    d   Measurement of medication through concentration level in blood

    e   Lowest concentration of a drug in serum required to produce a desired effect

    f   An equilibrium between the amount of drug ingested and the amount of drug eliminated

    g   The concentration of drug decreases by one-half

    h   Fixed amount of drug being eliminated per unit of time

    i   Amount of drug eliminated being proportional to its amount circulating in the bloodstream

    j   Biochemical and physiological effects of drugs at the effect sites

    k   Handling and disposition of drugs within the body

    l   Conjugation of drug metabolites

59 Pharmacokinetics

60 Pharmacodynamics

61 First-order kinetics

62 Zero-order kinetics

63 Elimination half-life

64 Steady-state concentration (Css)

65 Minimal effective concentration (MEC)

66 Therapeutic drug monitoring (TDM)

67 Bioavailability

68 First pass effect

69 Phase I metabolic reactions

70 Phase II metabolic reactions

ANSWERS AND EXPLANATIONS

1 (e) All of the statements correctly reflect how developmental changes in neurochemical systems influence both therapeutic and side effects of psychotropic medications. *(Ref. 3, Ch. 6.1.2, Pharmacokinetics and Pharmacodynamics section)*

2 (e) Neurotransmission and receptor binding are a part of pharmacodynamics, which refers to what a drug does to the body. In contrast, pharmacokinetics refers to what the body does to a drug, which involves four functionally distinct phases: absorption, distribution, metabolism, and excretion. The speed of onset of drug effect is determined by the first two phases, whereas metabolism and excretion are responsible for terminating the action of the drugs by removing the active form of the agent from the body. Overall, the four phases determine the duration of drug activity. *(Ref. 3, Ch. 6.1.2, Basic Principles section)*

3 (e) In young children, intestinal transit time is increased and the intestinal absorptive surface area is reduced, which can potentially lead to incomplete absorption of sustained-release drugs and certain drugs with long phases of absorption (e.g., carbamazepine). Weakly acidic drugs may be absorbed more slowly in young children because they are more likely to be ionized. *(Ref. 3, Ch. 6.1.2, Factors Affecting Drug Disposition section)*

4 (d) The volume of distribution is higher in youth than in adults. There is increased body water in children. Because lithium is primarily distributed in body water, the levels can be relatively lower in youth than in adults. Plasma concentration (Cp) = drug absorbed (D)/volume distribution (Vd). Lithium is a drug that is renally excreted unmetabolized, bypassing phase I metabolic reactions (hydroxylation, reduction, and hydrolysis) and phase II reactions (conjugation). *(Ref. 3, Ch. 6.1.2, Factors Affecting Drug Disposition section)*

5 (c) About 7–10% of Caucasians have a genetic deficiency of CYP 2D6, which causes less efficiency at metabolizing CYP 2D6 substrates (such as a lot of psychotropic medications). Some Asians also have a 2D6 genetic variant that leads to their being "somewhat slow" in metabolizing the substrates. Some African Americans also have an allelic variant of 2D6, which can cause slow or poor metabolism. People with variants in 2D6, in general, require lower dosages of relevant medications to achieve therapeutic levels. There are some other ethnic genetic differences in CYPs, which are also relevant in considering dosing psychotropic medications. *(Ref. 3, Ch. 6.1.2, Hepatic Influx and Efflux Transporters and Metabolism section)*

6 (c) With a reduction of UGT1A1 activity (about 70%), Gilbert's syndrome manifests with fluctuating bilirubinemia and can lead to toxic levels of certain drugs that are metabolized through UGT1A1 during the phase II metabolic reactions. Genetic polymorphisms of individual UGTs have been linked to clinical outcomes of certain psychotropic medications. The psychiatric field is becoming more aware of the increasing clinical relevance of UGTs in regard to psychotropic

medication metabolism. The FDA has approved a genetic test for UGT1A1. *(Ref. 3, Ch. 6.1.2, Hepatic Influx and Efflux Transporters and Metabolism section)*

7 (a) CYP 3A4 are lower in youth than in adults. A lot of medications are metabolized through this system. Jaundice in premature births is associated with immature hepatic UGT1A1, which leads to bilirubinemia. Most UGTs reach adult levels by 3–6 months, although both UGT1A9 and UGT2B4 do not start to develop until after the second year of life. *(Ref. 3, Ch. 6.1.2, Hepatic Influx and Efflux Transporters and Metabolism section)*

8 (e) Clinical observation and experience confirm that children under 10 years require larger, weight-adjusted doses of most hepatically metabolized medications than adults to achieve comparable blood levels and therapeutic responses. However, the reason behind the phenomenon is not obvious or clear. None of the reasons listed in the question can sufficiently or clearly explain the phenomenon based on recent studies. The phase II conjugates do not show uniform increases in young children. *(Ref. 3, Ch. 6.1.2, Hepatic Influx and Efflux Transporters and Metabolism section)*

9 (c) Valproate is an inhibitor of UGT2B7 that is likely the phase II conjugate besides UGT 1A4, which are both responsible for metabolizing lamotrigine. Combining valproate with lamotrigine can inhibit such enzymes, which leads to an elevation of the lamotrigine blood level that can result in severe rashes, such as Steven-Johnson syndrome. *(Ref. 3, Ch. 6.1.2, Hepatic Influx and Efflux Transporters and Metabolism section)*

10 (e) Paroxetine is both substrate and inhibitor of CYP2D6. This can explain the nonlinear kinetic nature of paroxetine (e.g., a dose of 10 mg being changed to 20 mg can potentially increase plasma concentration more than sixfold rather than twofold). *(Ref. 3, Ch. 6.1.2, Linear and Nonlinear Pharmacokinetics section)*

11 (c) Target symptoms should not be the key focus of psychotropic medications. Instead, treating psychiatric disorders/syndromes should be the primary focus. *(Ref. 1, Ch. 33, General Principles of Psychopharmacological Assessment, Diagnosis, and Treatment Planning section)*

12 (b) Clomipramine has its greatest effect on the serotonergic system, which is abnormal in obsessive-compulsive disorder (FDA approved) and trichotillomania (hair-pulling disorder). It also shows beneficial effects on OCD-like symptoms and repetitive behaviors in children with autism. It has not been effective in the treatment of ADHD. However, desipramine (a stronger noradrenergic agent) shows efficacy in treating ADHD. *(Ref. 1, Ch. 35, Tricyclic Antidepressants section)*

13 (b) Studies show that children with ADHD comorbid with tic disorders do not necessarily experience tic exacerbation during treatment with stimulants. Even though more research data support the efficacy of methylphenidate agents in treating ADHD in children younger than 6, only amphetamine agents (such as Dexedrine and Adderall) have been approved by the

FDA for use in children ages 3 and up. Although the exact mechanisms of stimulants are not fully understood, amphetamine agents seem to have a different mechanism of action than that of methylphenidate agents. *(Ref. 1, Ch. 24, Stimulants section)*

14 (a) Long-acting preparation stimulant agents can cause insomnia depending on the length of duration of different preparations, the time of administration, and metabolism of the drug. In general, long-acting preparations are considered as effective as immediate-release agents, needing no additional dose during school time, minimizing missed doses and behavioral rebound. *(Ref. 3, Ch. 6.1.4.1, Stimulants section)*

15 (a) Atomoxetine is mostly a noradrenergic reuptake inhibitor without dopaminergic properties, and is not a controlled substance. It may cause mild appetite suppression, but no data indicate long-term growth suppression. Having a better side-effect profile compared to TCAs, it can still cause increased blood pressure and heart rate. Potential drug–drug interactions should be considered. There are case reports of serious hepatotoxicity. *(Ref. 1, Ch. 34, Noradrenergic Reuptake Inhibitors section; Ref. 3, Ch. 6.1.4.1, Nonstimulant Treatments of ADHD section)*

16 (d) Liver function tests are not mandatory. The rest of the listed tests are needed prior to initiation of lithium treatment. Because preexisting cardiac conduction problems can be exacerbated by lithium, many recommend a baseline EKG even though some scholars believe this should not be a mandatory test. These tests along with a lithium level should be repeated and monitored with each dose change and every three to six months. *(Ref. 1, Ch. 26, Lithium section; Ref. 3, Ch. 6.1.4.4, Lithium section)*

17 (b) Escitalopram is the S-enantiomer of citalopram, and is twice as potent as citalopram in regard to serotonin reuptake inhibition. They are the most serotonin selective of all SSRIs. The S-enantiomer of citalopram is the active compound of serotonin reuptake inhibitor, and the R-enantiomer of citalopram is inactive. *(Ref. 1, Ch. 35, Selective Serotonin Reuptake Inhibitors section)*

18 (d) Only sertraline along with citalopram and escitalopram are the SSRIs that follow first-order (linear) kinetics. The rest of SSRIs all follow zero-order (nonlinear) kinetics. In children and adolescents, dose titration of these SSRIs with nonlinear kinetics should be more careful because doubling the dose of such a drug may lead to many folds increase of plasma drug level. *(Ref. 3, Ch. 6.1.4.2, Selective Serotonin Reuptake Inhibitors section)*

19 (c) Fluvoxamine has the lowest incidence of sexual side effects among all the SSRIs. The peak plasma concentration is significantly higher in female children than male children, but no such difference is observed in adolescents. This indicates female children may need lower doses than males. With multiple CYPs involvements, drug–drug interactions should be monitored. Fluvoxamine is FDA approved for the treatment of pediatric OCD. *(Ref. 1, Ch. 35, Selective Serotonin Reuptake Inhibitors section)*

20 (e) The maximum plasma drug level increases about 25% and time to the peak plasma concentration is reduced when sertraline is taken along with food. Studies show that in lower dose ranges sertraline has decreased half-lives in youth. Thus, instead of once-a-day dosing, twice-daily dosing may be considered when using the lower dose range. Sertraline is FDA approved for the treatment of pediatric OCD. *(Ref. 1, Ch. 35, Selective Serotonin Reuptake Inhibitors section)*

21 (a) Bupropion (Wellbutrin) is a norepinephrine-dopamine reuptake inhibitor, with FDA-approved indications for depression and smoking cessation in adults. A small study shows its effectiveness in treating both depression and ADHD symptoms in youth, although more rigorous random controlled trials are needed to verify the finding. The effectiveness is likely due to its norepinephrine-dopamine reuptake inhibition property. *(Ref. 1, Ch. 35, Atypical Antidepressants section)*

22 (d) Among all the listed antidepressants, only trazodone seems to show significant potential sexual side effect (priapism). Bupropion is a norepinephrine-dopamine reuptake inhibitor. Duloxetine and venlafaxine are both selective serotonin/norepinephrine reuptake inhibitors. Mirtazapine is a noradrenergic and specific serotonergic antidepressant. Trazodone is a serotonin agonist and serotonin reuptake inhibitor. They should not be taken together with any monoamine oxidase inhibitors (MAOIs), or within two weeks of beginning or discontinuing MAOIs to avoid potential serious side effects such as confusion, hypertension, tremor, hyperactivity, and death. Only duloxetine has a current FDA-approved indication for children or adolescents (for generalized anxiety disorder). *(Ref. 1, Ch. 35, Atypical Antidepressants section)*

23 (d) Among all the listed antidepressants, only trazodone (Desyrel) follows nonlinear kinetics. It is associated with priapism, and unfortunately one-third of such cases need surgery, which can potentially comprise erectile functioning permanently. *(Ref. 1, Ch. 35, Atypical Antidepressants section)*

24 (c) The CNS effects caused by lithium include down-regulating hippocampal serotonin ($5-HT_{1A}$) receptors along with increasing dopamine levels in tuberoinfundibular pathway along with the others listed. In addition, based on recent data, lithium along with valproate may have neurotrophic effects through regulating a number of factors involved in cell survival pathways indirectly. These factors may include cAMP response element-binding protein, brain-derived neurotrophic factor, bcl-2, and mitogen-activated protein kinases. *(Ref. 1, Ch. 36, Lithium section)*

25 (d) In the Treatment of Early Age Mania (TEAM) trial, risperidone was superior both to lithium and divalproex sodium for initial treatment of childhood mania both in likelihood of response and in overall symptoms of mania. The response rate for acute mania was 65% for risperidone, 36% for lithium, and 24% for valproic acid. *(Ref. 3, Ch. 6.1.4.4, Mood Stabilizers section)*

26 (b) HLA-B*1502 is an inherited variant present in some individuals of Asian ancestry, and is strongly associated with the risk of developing Stevens-Johnson syndrome and toxic epidermal necrolysis (TEN) during treatment with carbamazepine. Testing for HLA-B*1502 is recommended prior to starting carbamazepine in patients of Asian ancestry and a positive result is considered as a contraindication for carbamazepine. Interestingly, this variant is largely absent in individuals of non-Asian origin. *(Ref. 1, Ch. 36, Carbamazepine section)*

27 **(a)** Serum levels of many atypical antipsychotics can be decreased when co-administered with carbamazepine. Drug–drug interactions of carbamazepine can be extensive; they can also increase the lithium level. Some medications such as erythromycin, cimetidine, fluoxetine, verapamil, and valproate can also increase the carbamazepine level. *(Ref. 1, Ch. 36, Carbamazepine section)*

28 **(a)** There is about three times greater risk of developing serious rashes in youth (younger than 16 years) who are taking lamotrigine than in adults. The frequency of serious rashes associated with lamotrigine is about 1% in youth younger than 16 years versus about 0.3% in adults. *(Ref. 1, Ch. 36, Lamotrigine section)*

29 **(a)** Eliminated from systemic circulation by renal excretion, gabapentin is not appreciably metabolized in humans. It is an FDA-approved anti-seizure medication for the treatment of partial seizure in individuals older than 12 years. Adult studies show it plays a role as an adjunct agent to lithium or valproate, or other mood stabilizing agents, but show no benefit as a monotherapy agent. *(Ref. 1, Ch. 36, Gabapentin section)*

30 **(d)** Because of carbonic anhydrase inhibition, nephrolithiasis occurs in about 1–2% of patients taking topiramate. Several adult trials failed to demonstrate the efficacy of this drug in treating bipolar disorder, which led to an early termination of a double-blind, placebo controlled clinical trial in children in 2005. Even though a weak inducer of CYPs, it is potentially associated with failure of oral contraceptives. It can also lower the serum levels of risperidone and valproate. *(Ref. 1, Ch. 36, Topiramate section)*

31 **(e)** Tighter binding of certain non-dopaminergic receptors (such as Histamine H_1, Muscarinic M_1-central, 5-HT_{1A}, and 5-HT_{2A}) by certain antipsychotics seems to be associated with less propensity for EPS. Blocking D_2 is the primary cause of EPS. Blocking alpha-1 may cause postural hypertension, dizziness, and syncope. Blocking alpha-2 may cause increased alertness and hypertension. Blocking H_1 can cause sedation, weight gain, and anxiolytic effects. Blockade of central M_1 may interfere with memory and cognition. Dry mouth, constipation, and urinary retention are associated with the blockade of peripheral M_{2-4}. *(Ref. 1, Ch. 36, Pharmacology section)*

32 **(a)** Aripiprazole is a partial agonist and requires a higher degree of D_2 occupancy (80–85%) to achieve the equivalent level of blockade and therapeutic effect. In general, most other antipsychotics only need 60–70% dopamine receptor occupancy to achieve therapeutic efficacy. *(Ref. 1, Ch. 36, Pharmacology section)*

33 **(c)** When the new agent requires a slower titration, pharmacokinetic rebound is more likely to occur, which may be avoided by using an overlapping or "plateau" cross-titration. *(Ref. 1, Ch. 36, Pharmacology section)*

34 **(b)** Compared to adults, children and adolescents are more sensitive to most antipsychotic-induced side effects, including EPS, but not akathisia. The risk of akathisia is less known in youth and seems to be comparable to that experienced by adults. Relatively higher rates of akathisia in placebo groups in pediatric schizophrenia trials may reflect a carryover effect from prior antipsychotic treatment or withdrawal after the brief washout period. *(Ref. 1, Ch. 36, Adverse Effects section)*

35 **(c)** Combination of an antipsychotic with a stimulant medication does not seem to attenuate the antipsychotic-induced weight gain. *(Ref. 1, Ch. 36, Adverse Effects section)*

36 **(a)** Because of its partial D_2 agonistic property, aripiprazole does not cause an increased level of prolactin. Instead, it may decrease the prolactin level. The likelihood of prolactinemia increases with increased potency of antipsychotics and follows the pattern: paliperidone ≥ risperidone > haloperidol > olanzapine > ziprasidone > quetiapine ≥ clozapine > aripiprazole. Prolactinemia is associated with amenorrhea or oligomenorrhea, erectile dysfunction, decreased libido, hirsutism, gynecomastia/breast engorgement/pain, and galactorrhea. *(Ref. 1, Ch. 36, Adverse Effects section)*

37 **(b)** Clozapine seems to be the only second-generation antipsychotic that is associated with myocarditis risk that is highest early in treatment. The associated signs and symptoms may include palpitation, chest pain, shortness of breath, syncope, and EKG changes such as ectopic beats, atrioventricular block, atrial fibrillation or flutter, intraventricular conduction disturbance, ventricular tachycardia or fibrillation, and low QRS voltage. Among antipsychotics, thioridazine and ziprasidone are associated with higher risks of QTc prolongation. EKGs may be needed if there is a family history of early sudden death, prolonged QT syndrome, or a personal history of irregular heartbeat, tachycardia at rest, shortness of breath, dizziness on exertion, or syncope. *(Ref. 1, Ch. 36, Adverse Effects section)*

38 **(a)** A subgroup (about 25–50%) of individuals of African descent and some people of Middle Eastern origin have low white blood cell (WBC) counts without signs of any infection. The phenomenon is called benign ethnic (or cyclic) neutropenia. Males have lower WBCs than females independent of ethnicity. Monitoring WBCs during treatment with clozapine among certain ethnic groups can be adjusted accordingly. *(Ref. 1, Ch. 36, Adverse Effect Assessment and Monitoring section)*

39 **(c)** Generalized rigidity ("lead pipe") is a cardinal feature of NMS, and it does not usually respond to anti-Parkinsonian agents. Another distinguishing feature is hyperthermia (> 100.4° F) with profuse diaphoresis. Other associated symptoms and signs are elevated creatine kinase, changes in mental status, autonomic activation and instability, and other neurological symptoms such as sialorrhea, tremor, akinesia, dystonia, trismus, myoclonus, dysphagia, dysarthria, and rhabdomyolysis. Epidemiological data suggest incidence rates of 0.01 to 0.02% among individuals treated with antipsychotics, with fatality rates of 10–20% when the disorder is not recognized, even though total resolution of the symptoms can be obtained in most cases. *(Ref. 4, pp. 709–710)*

40 **(d)** The short-acting SSRI paroxetine is most likely associated with antidepressant discontinuation syndrome because of its relatively short half-life. The symptoms can be nonspecific such as dizziness, ringing in the ears, "electric shocks in the head," insomnia, and increased anxiety, etc. The severity of the syndrome also depends on the dosage of medication used and the length of time it takes to taper off. Abrupt discontinuation is associated with a higher risk. *(Ref. 4, p. 713)*

41 **(e)** Because of the upper limit of the 95% confidence interval, a doubling in the risk cannot be ruled out at this time, although the absolute magnitude of any increased risk should be low. *(Cooper et al. 2011)*

42 **(a)** As an over-the-counter supplement, N-acetylcysteine (NAC) up-regulates the cysteine-glutamate exchanger in the nucleus accumbens. Animal studies have shown that chronic self-administration of the drug down-regulates the cysteine-glutamate exchanger in the nucleus accumbens, and NAC's role is to reverse the process via glutamate modulation and other mechanisms. *(Gray et al. 2012)*

43 **(c)** In a pooled analysis across eight second-generation antipsychotics with data in children and adolescents (risperidone, quetiapine, aripiprazole, lurasidone, paliperidone, ziprasidone, olanzapine, and asenapine) (Solmi et al. 2020), lurasidone appeared to have the fewest adverse effects that were significantly more frequent compared to placebo. *(Ref 1., Ch. 37, Adverse Effects section)*

44 **(d)** Based on the results of the study, the COMB group did not show a significantly greater gain in the Vineland Daily Living Skills domain than did the MED group. *(Scahill et al. 2012)*

45 **(e)** EKG monitoring and related recommendations are under the category of "clinical guideline," not "clinical standard," based on strong empirical evidence and/or overwhelming clinical consensus but lack of rigorous empirical evidence. *(Findling et al. 2011)*

46 (d) Children with autism spectrum disorders have greater observed weight gain on atypical antipsychotics compared to children in other diagnostic groups. This effect is thought to be related to their being younger and more antipsychotic-naïve. *(Ref. 1, Ch. 37, Adverse Effects section)*

47 **(d)** DDAVP has a more potent antidiuretic effect than that of AVP, but it is less potent as a vasopressor. *(Ref. 1, p. 21, Enuresis section)*

48 **(d)** Acting as a partial agonist, buspirone selectively binds to the 5-HT_{1A} receptor, and has a weak dopamine antagonist effect. It is not an additive drug because it does not bind to benzodiazepine receptors or enhance GABA. Thus, it cannot be used for benzodiazepine withdrawal. It is FDA approved for the treatment of GAD only in adults, and there is no strong empirical evidence to support its use in children and adolescents. However, some case reports and open-label trials indicate that it can be considered for the treatment of mild anxiety or as an adjunctive agent to SSRIs in the pediatric population. *(Ref. 1, Ch. 15, Treatment section)*

49 **(c)** The FDA has not approved any medications for the treatment of pediatric insomnia. Medications for insomnia can mask or exacerbate other sleep disorders (such as obstructive sleep apnea and restless legs syndrome), which should be ruled out. Commonly used medications for pediatric insomnia include melatonin, alpha-2 agonists such as clonidine and guanfacine, and antihistamines. Side effects, limited efficacy, and tolerance are limiting factors in the use of many medications for insomnia, and benefits and risks should be considered carefully. *(Ref. 3, Ch. 5.9, Insomnia section)*

50 **(b)** Ramelteon is an FDA-approved medication for the treatment of initial insomnia in adults and has potent agonistic effects on melatonin receptors (MT_1 and MT_2). It has major drug–drug interactions with fluvoxamine, and its common side effects may include nausea, dizziness, somnolence, fatigue, and depression. *(Ref. 1, Ch. 22, Insomnia Disorder section)*

Matching

51 **(b); 52 (c); 53 (a); 54 (d)** In addition to the antidepressants listed: desipramine—primarily noradrenergic; trazodone and nefazodone—both serotonin reuptake blockers and 5-HT_{2A} antagonists. *(Ref. 1, Ch. 35, Atypical Antidepressants section; Ref. 1, Ch. 34, Noradrenergic Reuptake Inhibitors section)*

55 **(c)** Seroquel has a relatively lower risk of EPS. *(Ref. 1, Ch. 37, Adverse Effects section)*

56 **(d)** QTc prolongation has been associated with Geodon based on premarketing data. An EKG may be needed. *(Ref. 1, Ch. 37, Adverse Effects section)*

57 **(a)** Among atypical antipsychotics, risperidone is more like a high-potency typical agent, with a relatively high risk for EPS. *(Ref. 1, Ch. 37, Adverse Effects section)*

58 **(b)** The prominent side effects of clozapine, used for treatment-refractory psychosis, include lowered seizure threshold, as well as granulocytopenia and agranulocytosis. *(Ref. 1, Ch. 37, Adverse Effects section)*

59 **(k); 60 (j)** Pharmacokinetics refers to how the body handles and disposes of drugs within the body through biological processes: absorption, distribution, metabolism, and excretion. Pharmacodynamics refers to how a drug has biomedical and physiological effects on the body. *(Ref. 3, Ch. 6.1.2, Pharmacokinetics and Pharmacodynamics section)*

61 **(i); 62 (h)** First-order kinetics refers to the amount of drug eliminated, which is proportional to the amount of drug circulating in the bloodstream. Zero-order kinetics refers to only a fixed amount of drug that can be eliminated per unit of time because of the saturation of the eliminating mechanisms. *(Ref. 3, Ch. 6.1.2, Pharmacokinetics and Pharmacodynamics section)*

63 **(g); 64 (f)** Elimination half-life refers to the time required for the plasma concentration of a drug to be decreased by one-half. Steady-state concentration (Css) refers to a stable and steady plasma concentration level reached because of the establishment of an equilibrium between the amount of drug ingested and the amount of drug eliminated. *(Ref. 3, Ch. 6.1.2, Pharmacokinetics and Pharmacodynamics section)*

65 **(e); 66 (d)** The minimal effective concentration refers to the lowest plasma concentration of drug required to produce clinical effects. Therapeutic drug monitoring refers to measuring and monitoring the medication concentration level in the blood, which should be checked at "trough" level (just prior to the next dose). TDM is an important tool to use for those drugs that have narrow therapeutic windows, significant consequences associated with drug toxicity, and a wide range of inter-patient variability. It can help reveal individuals with unusual metabolism, uncover noncompliance, and confirm toxicity. *(Ref. 3, Ch. 6.1.2, Therapeutic Drug Monitoring section)*

67 **(c); 68 (b)** Bioavailability refers to the availability of unbound drugs in the systemic circulation that can exert biological effects on the target tissues. The first pass effect (also called pre-systemic clearance) refers to drugs being metabolized through the liver before they reach their target

tissues in the systemic circulation. Different drugs have very different first pass effects, which lead to different bioavailability. *(Ref. 3, Ch. 6.1.2, Factors Affecting Drug Disposition section)*

69 (a); **70** (l) The phase I metabolic reactions refer to the process of converting drugs to forms more suitable for elimination through hydroxylation, reduction, and hydrolysis. The phase II metabolic reactions refer to the process of conjugating of metabolites generated by the phase I metabolic reactions by phase II enzymes in order to be excreted in urine or through other body fluids. However, some drugs can be processed directly through the phase II metabolic reactions without going through any phase I metabolic reaction. *(Ref. 3, Ch. 6.1.2, Hepatic Influx and Efflux Transporters and Metabolism section)*

References

Cooper, W. O. et al. (2011). ADHD Drugs and Serious Cardiovascular Events in Children and Young Adults. *N Engl J Med, 365,* 1896–1904.

Findling, R. L. et al. (2011). Practice Parameter for the Use of Atypical Antipsychotic Medications in Children and Adolescents. AACAP, www.aacap.org.

Gray, K. M. et al. (2012). A Double-Blind Randomized Controlled Trial of N-Acetylcysteine in Cannabis-Dependent Adolescents. *Am J Psychiatry, 169,* 805–812.

Scahill, L. et al. (2012). Effects of Risperidone and Parent Training on Adaptive Functioning in Children with Pervasive Developmental Disorder and Serious Behavioral Problems. *JAACAP, 51,* 136–146.

13

PSYCHOTHERAPIES

DOI: 10.4324/9781003308805-14

QUESTIONS

Directions: Select the best response for each of the questions 1–27.

1 Which of the following is (are) the reason(s) that delay(s) the conduct of the kind of research that might enable nonmanualized individual psychotherapy to reach the current criteria for being "evidence based"?

a Difficulty in following control subjects as long as some individual cases actually take in therapy

b Difficulty in locating proper comparison groups

c Challenge of "double blinding"

d Difficulty in getting funding and institutional approval

e All of the above

2 All of the following tactics for working with parents in parent counseling should be recommended *except*:

a Model appropriate parent–child interactions for the parents to follow.

b Guide parents to understand the purposes of consequences and to find an appropriate consequence that works for the child.

c Eliminate using any punishment and replace it with rewards.

d Refer parents to receive other needed services that you cannot provide.

e Encourage parents to receive therapy for themselves.

3 All of the following are advantages that multifamily psychoeducation groups have in comparison to individual family psychoeducation *except*:

a Cost-effective and delivered in a large clinic

b Chance to discuss and share with both professionals and other families

c Establishment of support network

d Identification with other families and learning from others' success

e Privacy

4 All of the following are appropriate age adjustments needed for psychoeducation targeting children and adolescents with mental illness compared to those programs targeting adults *except*:

a Emphasizing social skills training

b Assisting adjusting environmental expectations

c Emphasizing the important aspects of the home environment

d Higher intensity of service and longer follow-up

e None of the above

5 All of the following are psychoeducation core concepts *except*:

a Behavioral inhibition

b Cognitive restructuring

c Daily routines

d Relapse prevention

e Social functioning

6 All of the following are examples of techniques used in psychoeducation *except*:

a Bibliotherapy

b Daily routine tracking

c Mood chart

d Naming the friend

e Thinking, feeling, doing

7 It is not uncommon for the leaders of a parent group or support group to face some challenges and difficult situations. Which of the responses by the group leaders should be *excluded* if one parent dominates the discussion?

a Setting limits

b Setting amount of time for people to take turns

c Reminding the group of time and schedule

d Thanking the parent who is sharing and asking if others would like to talk

e None of the above

8 Setting treatment goals is an important step of behavioral parent training (BPT). All of the following are appropriate for establishing initial treatment goals between the therapist and the parent *except*:

a Eliciting the parent's goal (commonly involves modifying child's behavior)

b Explicitly identifying the parent's behavior that causes the child's problems

c Finding a goal that is the best fit between parenting practices and the child's personality

d Setting the initial goal at a level where both child and parent can experience success

e Consider usage of shaping process

9 Which of the following descriptions *best* explains the concept of coercive process in regards to BPT?

a Parents overly control their children

b Children's behavior controls the parents' reactions

c External factors influence both children's and parents' behavior

d Parents and children with behavioral problems control each other through negative reinforcement

e None of the above

10 All of the following statements regarding the effectiveness and efficacy of BPT are accurate based on updated research *except*:

a BPT is effective in treating disruptive behavior disorders during preschool and elementary school.

b Family-centered behavioral interventions are effective for adolescents.

c BPT improves parenting skills; improvements of child behavior are associated with the degree of changes in parenting.

d BPT effectiveness does not extend to untreated siblings.

e BPT can alleviate marital stress.

11 All of the following statements regarding the factors that can influence the outcomes of BPT are accurate *except*:

a Lower level of socioeconomic status (SES) predicts poorer overall outcome.

b Lower level of SES predicts differentially more drop-outs for behavior therapy versus other psychosocial interventions.

c Involvement of both parents in treatment may not affect outcome but may increase the maintenance of treatment gains.

d Parental psychopathology, parental involvement with illicit drugs, and severe marital discord all predict reduced efficacy.

e Severity and nature of the child's symptoms strongly influence outcome.

12 Which of the following family therapies emphasizes boundaries?

a Bowen family systems therapy

b Structural family therapy

c Multisystemic therapy (MST)

d Strategic family therapy

e Functional Family Therapy (FFT)

13 Which of the following concepts is *most* closely associated with Winnicott's theory?

a Circular causality

b Constraints

c Holding environment

d Narratives

e Negative affective reciprocity

14 Among all of the following models of family therapy, which is the *newest* one?

a Bowen family systems therapy

b Experiential family therapy

c Integrative module-based family therapy

d Strategic family therapy

e Structural family therapy

15 Interpersonal psychotherapy for depressed adolescents (IPT-A) is *not* recommended for adolescents with all of the following conditions *except*:

a Actively abusing substances

b Actively psychotic

c Actively suicidal or homicidal

d Significantly intellectually disabled

e Very anxious

16 All of the following statements regarding IPT-A are accurate *except*:

a IPT-A, a time-limited and manualized psychotherapy, was originally adapted from IPT for adults.

b IPT is based on interpersonal theories and attachment theory.

c Parental participation is mandatory.

d IPT-A includes three phases: initial, middle, and termination.

e Assigning the adolescent with a "limited sick role" is recommended during psychoeducation.

17 During the initial phase of IPT-A, the therapist helps the client identify interpersonal problem areas. If an adolescent's depression coincides with a relationship conflict, which of the following problem areas should be *primarily* identified?

a Grief due to the death of a loved one

b Interpersonal deficits

c Interpersonal role disputes

d Interpersonal role transitions

e None of the above

18 Which of the following techniques is *not* commonly used in the middle phase of IPT-A?

a Communication analysis

b Decision analysis

c Encouragement of affect and linkage with interpersonal events

d Role playing

e Transference interpretation

19 Which of the following therapy modalities has the best evidence for treatment of depression in youth?

a Behavioral parent training

b Individual psychodynamic psychotherapy

c IPT-A

d Psychoeducation

e Structured family therapy

20 During a session involving cognitive-behavioral therapy (CBT) for anxiety disorder, the therapist suggests the patient remain in contact with the feared stimulus until physiological response and subjective distress dissipate. Which of the following techniques *best* fits this description?

a Between-session habituation

b Graduated exposure

c Implosion

d Relaxation training

e Within-session habitation

21 Which of the following specific intervention(s) is (are) commonly used in CBT for depression?

a Activity scheduling

b Affect regulation

c Assertiveness

d Mood monitoring

e All of the above

22 All of the following factors clearly predict poor outcomes of CBT in the treatment of depression among adolescents *except*:

a Lower functioning

b Greater severity of depression

c Higher chronicity of depression

d Maternal depression

e Presence of comorbidity

23 All of the following are applied behavior analysis (ABA) techniques used as interventions for children with autism spectrum disorders *except*:

a Fading

b Forward chaining

c Prompting

d Shaping

e Task analysis

24 Which of the following stages should be *excluded* from systematic desensitization commonly used in the treatment of anxiety?

a Relaxation training

b Constructing the anxiety hierarchy

c Desensitization in imagination

d In vivo desensitization

e None of the above

25 All of the following are motivational interviewing (MI) processes *except*:

a Engaging

b Focusing

c Exposing

d Evoking

e Planning

26 Which is a core focus of dialectical behavior therapy (DBT) for adolescents?

a Interpersonal effectiveness

b Distress tolerance

c Incorporating family

d Emotion regulation

e All of the above

27 Which is *not* one of the techniques taught in the second, parent-directed stage of parent–child interaction therapy (PCIT)?

a Attending

b Giving effective commands

c Labeled praise

d Selective attention (ignoring)

e Time-out

Matching

28–31 Match the treatment name with the *best* treatment description. Use each description only once.

a Emphasizing the establishment of boundaries within the family

b Addressing the function of symptoms in family interaction, enhancing supportive interactions, and reducing defensive interactions

c Focusing on the "unconscious" life of the family members, disentangling interlocking alliance

d Interrupting rigid feedback, maintaining the family homeostasis, and strengthening the parental alliance using paradoxical instructions

28 Functional family therapy

29 Psychodynamic family therapy

30 Strategic family therapy

31 Structural family therapy

32–37 Match each of the parent training topics with the *best* description or example of such a topic.

a Utilizing more desirable activities as reinforcers for the purpose of completing less desirable ones

b Removing the tokens, points, or privileges the child previously earned because of current negative behaviors

c Removing the child from positive reinforcement or enjoyable activity for a period of time as a consequence of specific target negative behaviors

d Assigning tokens, points, or privileges to each positive behavior and cashing them out for rewards

e Finding salient positive behavior to praise and to reward through reinforcement

f Parent actively attending child-directed activities and paying no attention to mild negative behaviors

32 Attending and ignoring

33 Praise/positive reinforcement

34 Token economy/point system

35 Time-out

36 Response-cost procedures

37 When-Then/If-Then/"Grandma's Rule"

38–41 Cognitive restructuring is a CBT technique involving identifying and challenging cognitive errors. Match each of the cognitive errors with the *best* description.

a Blaming self for events that are outside one's control

b Assuming the worst-case scenario will result

c Placing too much or too little importance on thoughts or events

d Focusing on one detail and ignoring other relevant information

38 Catastrophizing

39 Magnifying/minimizing

40 Personalization

41 Selective abstraction/mental filter

ANSWERS AND EXPLANATIONS

1 **(e)** All of the listed reasons along with difficulty in getting parental and child consents have led to only a few clinical case series and a handful of controlled research projects in this field over many years. *(Ref. 1, Ch. 38, Introduction section)*

2 **(c)** Appropriate punishment should not be eliminated, but the importance of counterbalancing punishment with rewards should be emphasized to the parents. Other tactics may include: assisting parents to reframe the problems in a way that seems manageable and does not place responsibility solely on them; providing parents with supplemental materials for them to review outside of the sessions; and reminding parents to be patient with gradual small incremental progress made without a quick cure. *(Ref. 1, Ch 39, Parent Counseling section)*

3 **(e)** Along with privacy, ease of being implemented by a private practitioner, scheduling flexibility, and flexibility in tailoring topics to meet individual special needs are the advantages that individual family psychoeducation has over the multifamily psychoeducation groups. *(Ref. 1, Ch. 39, Table Relative advantages)*

4 **(e)** All listed are appropriate age adjustments needed for psychoeducation targeting children and adolescents with mental illness compared to those programs for adults. In addition, because children may not have developed a healthy identity separate from the psychiatric symptoms that they suffer, it is important to clarify with the child and family what the disorder is and what the child's traits are. With variable levels of development, developmentally appropriate contents should be used in different age groups. *(Ref. 1, Ch. 39, Table Age adjustments)*

5 **(a)** Behavioral activation (not inhibition) is one of the core concepts of psychoeducation along with others such as types of disorders and symptoms, medication and side effects, problem-solving skills, treatment and services, and communication skills. *(Ref. 1, Ch. 39, Table Core psychoeducation)*

6 **(d)** Naming the enemy (not friend) is one of the techniques used in psychoeducation to help the child and parents distinguish the difference between the child's symptoms and his/her own personality. Bibliotherapy refers to the use of written information, video, and resources from media and the Internet to further educate families. Daily routine tracking and mood charts can help tracking daily routine activities such as sleep–wake cycles, eating, changes in mood, and how different activities or circumstances influence mood. "Thinking, feeling, doing" helps in gaining the insight of parents and child into the connections among their thoughts, feelings, and behaviors. Another technique called "tool kit" refers to the development of a series of pleasure and relaxing activities for the child to use in helping affective regulation. *(Ref. 1, Ch. 39, Table Examples of techniques)*

7 **(e)** All of the listed responses are appropriate in this situation. There are many other frequent challenges and situations group leaders may face, such as arguing among members, crying, discussion of inappropriate topics, discussion shifts away from the scheduled topic, incomplete homework, late arrival, non-participation, lack of time to cover the topic, only one attendee, and silence (please see the referenced section for details). *(Ref. 1, Ch. 39, Table Complications frequently faced)*

8 **(b)** While modifying the parent's behavior is a goal of parent training, this goal may not need to be explicitly stated because the therapist needs to communicate in a way to avoid the parent feeling that she or he is to blame for the child's behavior. *(Ref. 1, Ch. 40, Setting Treatment Goals section)*

9 **(d)** The theory behind behavioral parent training programs is based on the belief that dysfunctional parent–child relationship and interaction patterns are possible driving forces of the child's behavior problems. As a learned process, "coercive process" describes those families with a child having behavioral issues that have a tendency to control one another through negative reinforcement. *(Ref. 1, Ch. 40, Rationale section)*

10 **(d)** Research supports that BPT effectiveness can be extended to the untreated siblings. BPT does have positive effects on parent functioning, which leads to lower parenting stress, marital conflicts, depression; unifying childrearing approaches; gaining parental confidence in managing their child's behavior; and extending benefits to untreated siblings. Parents are more likely to report high levels of satisfaction with this approach. *(Ref. 1, Ch. 40, Research Evidence section)*

11 **(b)** Lower level of SES predicts early termination from the treatment, but it does not differentially predict more dropouts for behavior therapy in comparison to other psychosocial interventions. *(Ref. 1, Ch. 40, Factors Affecting Outcome section)*

12 **(b)** Represented by Salvadore Minuchin, structural family therapy emphasizes shifting from enmeshed or disengaged boundaries to clear and flexible boundaries as seen in functional families. *(Ref. 3, Table 6.2.7.1)*

13 **(c)** Holding environment is a critical component of D. W. Winnicott's theory. This refers to the caregivers providing a safe and nurturing environment to fulfill the child's needs and to facilitate the child's normal growth and development. *(Ref. 1, Ch. 41, Social Environment section)*

14 **(c)** Several newer models of family therapy have been developed to meet the clinical challenges we are facing today. Integrative module-based family therapy is one such model among two others including multisystemic therapy (MST) and metaframeworks. *(Ref. 1, Ch. 41, Integrative Module-Based section; Ref. 3, Table 6.2.7.1)*

15 **(e)** Research shows adolescents with depression can respond to IPT-A even when the depression is comorbid with anxiety disorder, ADHD, and ODD. However, the treatment is most effective when the primary diagnosis is depression with limited comorbidities, and it is not recommended for some of the conditions listed in answers (a) through (d). *(Ref. 1, Ch. 42, Introduction section)*

16 (c) Parental participation is highly encouraged, but not mandatory or required. Parental participation can be helpful at different phases of the treatment (e.g., education about depression and IPT-A treatment itself during the initial phase, providing opportunities to practice during the middle phase, and education about warning signs of depression recurrence in the termination phase). *(Ref. 1, Ch. 42, Course section)*

17 (c) Interpersonal role disputes should be identified in this case because the depression coincides with a relationship conflict, and resolving such a conflict is the goal of the treatment. In general, only one of the four listed areas needs to be identified, but it is also possible to identify a secondary problem area. Adolescents with interpersonal role dispute may fall into one of the following stages: renegotiation stage, impasse stage, and dissolution stage. During the first two stages, the therapist should assist the adolescent to define and to resolve the dispute. However, the treatment strategy will be focused on mourning the loss of the relationship if the adolescent is in the dissolution stage. *(Ref. 1, Ch. 42, Initial Phase section)*

18 (e) Transference interpretation is *not* commonly used in the middle phase of IPT-A. Instead, all of the other techniques listed can be appropriately used in the middle phase of IPT-A. *(Ref. 1, Ch. 42, Middle Phase section)*

19 (c) Among all the listed therapy modalities, IPT-A is the only one that meets the Society of Clinical Child and Adolescent Psychology criteria for a "well-established" psychotherapy for depression in youth. *(Ref. 1, Empirical Support)*

20 (e) Exposure is the key element of CBT for anxiety. Graduated exposure involves introducing the situation that elicits a low level of fear, followed by gradually introducing situations that elicit more intense fear; eventually, the fearful behaviors or responses are eliminated (extinction). In a session when the fear-producing situation remains until the individual's fear response extinguishes, the process is called within-session habituation. If the individual is exposed to the situation that elicits the highest fear (not graduated), this process is called flooding. Flooding is not recommended given the levels of distress it provokes and less durable treatment response. Usually, as an adjunctive approach, relaxation training involves either muscle tension–relaxation sequences or cognitive meditation to decrease patients' physiological fear response and subjective arousal. *(Ref. 3, Ch. 6.2.2, Exposure Techniques section)*

21 (e) All are specific interventions commonly used in CBT among others including introduction and treatment rationale, goal setting, rational problem solving, rationally disputing automatic thoughts and replacing them with adaptive self-statements, correction of cognitive distortions, social skills training, communication and compromise, relaxation, parent training, and relapse prevention. *(Ref. 1, Ch. 43, General Characteristics section)*

22 (e) There are conflicting data regarding whether comorbidity predicts a poor outcome. In addition, lower level of suicidal ideation, higher overall baseline functioning, consistency in completing homework, therapeutic warmth, responsiveness, and cultural sensitivity all predict positive response and outcome. *(Ref. 1, Ch. 43, Factors section)*

23 (b) Backward chaining is an ABA technique, which refers to a complex behavior that is taught by starting with reinforcing the successful performance of the final step, and working backward one step after another to the initial step of the behavior. The goal is to eventually reinforce the child being able to perform the whole behavior. *(Ref. 3, Table 6.2.2.4)*

24 (e) The choices comprise the four stages of systemic desensitization and none of them should be excluded. *(Ref. 3, Ch. 6.2.2, Systematic Desensitization section)*

25 (c) The four processes of MI are engaging (establish therapeutic alliance), focusing (collaborative agenda setting), evoking (elicit and strengthen client motivation for change), and planning (develop a commitment to and process for change). *(Ref. 1, Ch. 44, The Four Processes section)*

26 (e) Core elements of dialectical behavior therapy (DBT) include interpersonal effectiveness, emotion regulation, distress tolerance, and mindfulness. DBT for adolescents additionally incorporates family with caregiver skills training and an additional family-based module, Walking the Middle Path, which helps teens and parents more effectively interact. *(Ref. 3, Ch. 6.2.2, Dialectical Behavior Therapy section)*

27 (a) PCIT is an evidence-based behavioral program developed for preschool and early elementary school ages which uses a "bug-in-the-ear" device to provide in-the-moment parent coaching. The first stage is child directed and involves parents fostering a secure relationship with their child through techniques such as attending. The other techniques listed are taught during the second parent-directed stage *(Ref. 1, Ch. 40, Developmental Issues section; Ref. 5, p. 3711)*

Matching

28 (b) Functional family therapy is an intensive home-based approach and is designed to address the function of symptoms in family interaction. The goals are to enhance supportive interactions and to reduce defensive interactions.

29 (c) Psychodynamic family therapy focuses on the "unconscious" life of family members and encourages them to share their unconscious conflicts and defenses, and intra-familial transference reactions in the therapy. Psychodynamic family psychotherapy is good for families with long-standing but subtle symptoms, and it can be combined with individual therapies. Object relations theory is applied in psychodynamic therapy. To enhance the therapeutic process, attachment theory can be used as well to differentiate between "defensive" and "attachment" affects.

30 (d) Strategic family therapy sees families in terms of process and maladaptive problem-solving efforts. In the therapy, strategies should be developed to identify the family rules, interrupt rigid feedback, strengthen the parental alliance, and maintain the family's homeostasis. Paradoxical intervention, circular questioning, extended family intervention, and narrative therapy techniques can be used.

31 (a) Structural family therapy focuses on adaptive and maladaptive structure, particularly in relation to power, boundaries, and preferred transactional patterns. Reestablishing and realigning

boundaries are emphasized in the therapy. *(Questions 28–31: Ref. 3, Table 6.2.7.1)*

32 **(f); 33 (e); 34 (d); 35 (c); 36 (b); 37 (a)** In addition to those listed in the questions, there are other core topics in parent training, such as psychoeducation/background information, giving effective instruction, developing a plan for homework, homeschool report cards, managing behavior in public places, and planning ahead/anticipating future behavior problems (please review the referenced section for the detailed key elements of each topic). *(Ref. 1, Ch. 40, Core Session Topics section)*

38 **(b); 39 (c); 40 (a); 41 (d)** Other cognitive errors include absolutism, arbitrary inference, ignoring evidence, overgeneralization, and attending to negative features of events. *(Ref. 3, Table 6.2.2.1)*

14

TREATMENT SETTINGS

DOI: 10.4324/9781003308805-15

QUESTIONS

Directions: Select the best response for each of the questions 1–20.

1 All of the following statements regarding wraparound services are accurate *except*:

   a Wraparound services are child and family centered.

   b Wraparound services are community based.

   c Value is placed on cultural competency.

   d A problem is identified based on a deficit model and ameliorating the problem is the treatment focus.

   e The family determines the mix of services.

2 Research shows which of the following groups of youth is *most* likely to respond to multisystemic therapy?

   a Youth with anxiety disorders

   b Youth who are juvenile offenders

   c Youth with depression

   d Youth who are psychotic

   e Youth with bipolar disorders

3 The federal government established the Child and Adolescent Service System Program (CASSP) in 1984. All of the following are major principles of the CASSP *except*:

   a To individualize care that recognizes strengths in the child, family, and community

   b To include the family at every level of the clinical process and system organization

   c To coordinate and collaborate among different agencies and to integrate services across agencies

   d To serve youth in more restrictive and structured environments or settings to meet their clinical needs

   e To provide culturally competent services

4 All of the following are common differences between residential treatment facilities (RTFs) and residential treatment centers (RTCs) *except*:

   a RTFs are typically licensed by state departments of mental health.

   b RTCs typically fall under the purview of state departments of social service.

   c The RTC population is typically more psychiatrically impaired than the RTF population.

   d Some RTFs may be located as cottages within RTCs with different staffing and capabilities.

   e RTCs in many states require that parents relinquish custody of their children.

5 All of the following statements accurately describe the Intensive In-Home Child and Adolescent Psychiatric Service (IICAPS) developed at Yale in 1997 *except*:

   a The IICAPS serves children and adolescents with serious emotional and behavioral problems in home/family settings.

   b The IICAPS believes that the family has the capacity and is essential to make sustainable changes in a child's life.

   c The families have to be partners in the treatment process and co-lead the treatment planning.

   d A psychologist is required to serve as the director to co-lead the interdisciplinary team meetings.

   e The IICAPS provides 24/7 mobile crisis services.

6 All of the following statements regarding milieu treatment (MT) are accurate *except*:

   a Therapeutic milieu is central to inpatient hospital units (IU), partial hospital (PH), day treatment (DT), and residential treatment centers (RTCs).

   b IU, PH, DT, and RTCs are considered as restrictive or intensive services, but federal reports combine IU and RTCs into statistical analysis, and PH and DT are now grouped into outpatient treatments.

   c Managed care involvement has not lessened the difficulty of accessing and appropriately using IU care across the nation.

   d Most outcome studies have used "change analysis" (i.e., the differences between before and after service delivery).

   e Conclusive evidence has demonstrated the effectiveness of MT.

7 All of the following critical factors should be determined prior to admission to MT *except*:

   a Child and family functioning

   b Consistency of discipline within the family

   c Family perceived stress

   d Contact with delinquent peers for those with disruptive disorders

   e None of the above

8 If a child is at high risk of danger to self or others, which of the following MT programs is *not* appropriate?

   a Acute inpatient

   b Day treatment

   c Partial hospital

   d Residential treatment center

   e All of the above

9 Based on the most recent research findings, all of the following statements regarding aggressive behaviors, seclusion, and restraint in MT settings are correct *except*:

   a All MT programs are expected to be able to manage youth with highly aggressive, violent, and destructive behaviors.

b Stricter federal policy on seclusion and restraint is associated with the highly publicized concerns of the adverse effects of mechanical and other forms of restraint.

c Multiple attempts have been made to reduce seclusion and restraint.

d Some case studies have shown how leadership serves to decrease seclusion and restraint through organizational and cultural change.

e A recent study shows hospitalized youth prefer time-out to medication (e.g., chemical restraint and prn medication).

10 Which of the following is the *best* way to prevent elopement from MT programs?

a Effective communication among staff and between staff and patients

b Onsite schooling

c Negative consequences such as time-out, seclusion, and restraint

d Sufficient dosage of psychotropic medications

e Use of video surveillance system

11 Which of the following is (are) the risk factor(s) warranting an admission to an appropriate MT program?

a A suicide attempter with clear abnormal mental state, or an individual with suicidal ideation

b An individual with persistent wish to die

c Lack of adequate supervision or support outside of therapeutic milieu

d Unsafe to return home because of unresolved biopsychosocial risk factors that are unlikely to change

e All of the above

12 All of the following safety factors should be considered prior to discharging youth from an MT program to a lower level of care *except*:

a Crisis issue resolved to acceptable level

b Suicidal potential is minimal

c Home environment is sanitized (e.g., no firearms and medication secured)

d Family-related issues addressed

e None of the above

13 All of the following are recommended to assure effective milieu treatment *except*:

a Optimize safety for patients, peers, and staff members

b Require onsite school education

c Actively involve the family

d Actively address the factors identified in the formulation and treatment plan

e Discharge only when a lower level of care can provide sufficient services

14 All of the following correctly describe the differences between residential treatment centers (RTCs) and inpatient hospital units (IU) *except*:

a RTCs provide more comprehensive services than inpatient hospital units.

b Only IU provides 24-hour nursing and medical care.

c Youth with psychosis are generally served in IUs rather than RTCs because of the complexity of their needs.

d RTCs expect greater independent functioning than IUs.

e Youth view themselves as "residents" in RTCs in contrast to "sick persons" in IUs.

15 All of the following factors predict poor treatment outcome for RTCs *except*:

a Presence of psychosis

b Below-average level of intelligence

c Presence of antisocial and bizarre behavior

d Longer length of stay

e Inadequate aftercare services

16 All of the following are risk factors for readmission to an RTC *except*:

a Suicidal thoughts and behaviors

b Older age

c Harsh parenting

d Permissive parenting

e Caregiver–child conflict

17 All of the following are considered common functions of an acute inpatient psychiatric unit (IU) *except*:

a Minimizing potential for harm (e.g., separation from family and community and monitoring behavior)

b Psychological testing

c Case formulation and diagnosis

d Developing a treatment plan and rapidly implementing it

e Stabilizing symptoms and crisis

18 Which of the following is associated with higher readmission rates after discharge from an IU?

a Severe conduct problems

b Disengaged parent–child relations

c Harsh parental discipline

d All of the above

e None of the above

19 All of the following statements regarding partial hospitalization (PH) and day treatment (DT) are accurate *except*:

a Both PH and DT are less than 24-hour hospital-level daily care to prevent relapses and rehospitalizations.

b Both PH and DT must be part of a hospital clinic or an IU.

c   Youth in the programs are expected to have sufficient self-control to avert dangerous behavior.

d   Chemical or manual restraints are not commonly used in DT.

e   The PH model can be employed in specialized milieu treatments for substance-related disorders, eating disorders, victims of abuse, and those with medical and psychiatric comorbidities.

20   All of the following are considered as routine laboratory tests for a patient undergoing medical clearance prior to admission to a psychiatric facility *except*:

a   Chemistries including glucose and electrolytes

b   Liver functioning tests

c   Electroencephalography (EEG)

d   Thyroid function tests

e   Urine drug screen

ANSWERS AND EXPLANATIONS

1 **(d)** In contrast to the traditional mental health treatment that uses a deficit model, wraparound services use strength-based approaches that uncover positive coping mechanisms and resiliency factors in the family. Wraparound services are especially beneficial to the children and families that have significant emotional and behavioral difficulties and previously experienced treatment failure. They are child and family centered, community and strength based, and contain culturally competent services that integrate the family as an active participant in building the treatment plan. *(Ref. 1, Ch. 45, Wraparound Services section)*

2 **(b)** Youth who are juvenile offenders and youth who are abusing substances and are at risk for out-of-home placement respond to the MST more robustly. Short-term data support the efficacy of reducing inpatient psychiatric hospitalization and out-of-home placements, improving externalizing symptoms and family relationships, and increasing school attendance. *(Ref. 1, Ch. 45, Home-Based Services and Mental Health section)*

3 **(d)** One of the five principles of CASSP is to serve youth in the communities or in the least restrictive environment or setting to meet their clinical needs. *(Ref. 1, Ch. 45, Historical Roots: Emergence of Systems of Care and Wraparound Services section)*

4 **(c)** The residential treatment center (RTC) population is typically less psychiatrically impaired than the residential treatment facility (RTF) population. Many of the youth in RTCs could probably be treated in outpatient settings except for psychosocial circumstances that impair the feasibility of living in the community. *(Ref. 3., Ch. 6.3.2, Overview of Types of Milieu Settings and their Purpose in a System of Care section)*

5 **(d)** IICAPS requires a child and adolescent psychiatrist to serve as the medical director to co-lead the interdisciplinary treatment rounds. Programmatically, IICAPS is designed as the following: six to eight cases per team, four teams to a rounds group, one to four rounds groups to a program, and 15 programs to a network. *(Ref. 1, Ch. 45, Home-Based Services and Mental Health section)*

6 **(e)** Because of the significant difficulties in study design and implementation, even though some studies have shown positive outcomes of RTCs and IU services, conclusive evidence demonstrating MT's effectiveness is still largely lacking. *(Ref. 1, Ch. 46, Parent or Sponsoring Body, Structure, and Administrative Issues section)*

7 **(e)** None of the listed factors should be excluded as critical factors that should be determined prior to admission, and another factor is extent of drug and/or alcohol use or abuse. *(Ref. 1, Ch. 46, Clinical Issues section)*

8 **(d)** A residential treatment center would not be sufficient to provide care for youth at high risk of danger to self or others. Acute inpatient is the most appropriate setting, and partial hospital and day treatment can potentially provide the needed acute services. For those with low risk of danger to self or others, acute inpatient is the least appropriate, but PH, DT, and

RTCs all can provide the appropriate level of care. *(Ref. 1, Ch. 46, Clinical Issues section)*

9 **(e)** A recent study shows hospitalized youth prefer medication to time-out or seclusion in contrast to earlier studies advocating for time-out. *(Ref. 1, Ch. 46, Clinical Issues section)*

10 **(a)** Effective communication among staff and between staff and patients is the best way to prevent elopement and other risky behaviors in the MT programs. *(Ref. 1, Ch. 46, Clinical Issues section)*

11 **(e)** All listed are the risk factors that warrant an admission to an appropriate MT program. *(Ref. 1, Ch. 46, Clinical Issues section)*

12 **(e)** None of the listed safety factors should be excluded when considering discharging youth from an MT program to a lower level of care. Other safety factors may include aftercare planning such as providing appropriate psychoeducation to the family and patient and setting up realistic transition plans (ongoing psychosocial interventions and medication follow-ups). *(Ref. 1, Ch. 46, Clinical Issues section)*

13 **(b)** Onsite school education may not be available to all the MT programs and is a key factor for assuring effective milieu treatment. Providing financial support for duration of needed treatment is also recommended. *(Ref. 1, Ch. 46, Role in a System of Care section)*

14 **(c)** Many residential treatment centers serve youth with psychotic illnesses, and some states even require psychosis as a condition for publicly funded residential treatment. *(Ref. 1, Ch. 46, Residential Treatment Centers section)*

15 **(d)** Shorter or longer stays may be associated with poorer outcomes of residential care, with some studies showing the range of 6–10 months being optimal. Another negative outcome factor is a dysfunctional family. *(Ref. 1, Ch. 46, Residential Treatment Centers section)*

16 **(b)** Younger age, not older age, is associated with increased risk of readmission to RTC *(Ref. 1, Ch. 46, Clinical Issues section)*

17 **(b)** Psychological testing is not a common function of an acute psychiatric inpatient unit. Disposition planning and transition to less restrictive care are other common functions of an IU. *(Ref. 1, Ch. 46, Inpatient Hospitalization section)*

18 **(d)** A 2004 study by J. C. Blader indicates that predictors for the readmission of 109 school-aged children who were previously hospitalized in a psychiatric facility are severe conduct problems, disengaged parent–child relations, and harsh parental discipline. *(Ref. 1, Ch. 46, Inpatient Hospitalization section)*

19 **(b)** Unlike PH, DT can be freestanding or a part of an IU, a hospital clinic, a school, or an RTC. DTs are structured and attend to patients' educational needs and provide multimodal treatments. The restrictive practice (i.e., seclusion and restraints) in DTs is limited to those methods acceptable and available in most school or home environments, whereas the restrictive practice in PH depends on the hospital configuration. Chemical or physical restraints are not used in DT programs, but personal ("therapeutic") holding of young children and quiet rooms are sometimes used in certain DT programs. *(Ref. 1, Ch. 46, Partial Hospital and Day Treatment section)*

20 (**c**) Electroencephalography (EEG) is not a routine test but can be potentially useful in cases of suspected seizure disorders such as Landau-Kleffner syndrome (manifesting as declination of language skills). Neuroimaging studies are not considered as routine laboratory tests but at times can be useful to rule out an alternative etiology of psychosis (such as tumors, hemorrhage, and other brain lesions, etc.). Blood levels of certain psychotropic medications may be useful, and toxicological analysis of urine is a common routine admission test. *(Ref. 3, Ch. 6.3.1, Evaluating and Addressing Medical and Psychosocial Causes of Behavioral Disturbance section)*

15

SPECIAL TOPICS (CONSULTATION, FORENSICS, AND PUBLIC HEALTH)

DOI: 10.4324/9781003308805-16

QUESTIONS

Directions: Select the best response for each of the questions 1–24.

1 All of the following are areas of focus for a school consultant working in a systems consultation model *except*:

a Addressing individual students' needs

b Creating a positive school environment

c Developing and coordinating mental health programs

d Improving attendance

e Valuing diversity in the school

2 During the past 50–60 years, mental health consultation services to schools have undergone five major periods of significant changes triggered by major sociocultural movements. All of the following accurately describe such periods *except*:

a Since World War II, it is believed that schools are appropriate community-based sites to deliver mental health services.

b Educational rights legislation prohibiting discrimination against students with mental disabilities resulted from the civil rights movement in the 1960s.

c Reduction of risky behavior in youth between the 1960s and the 1980s decreased school involvement in providing mental health services.

d In the 1990s, decreases in psychiatric hospitals and residential programs led to the subsequent increased need for mental health services and an increase in school-based mental health treatment.

e Most recently, there has been increased evidence for the benefits of universal social-emotional learning on both academic and social-emotional functioning of students.

3 All of the following are the characteristics of mental health services delivered in school settings compared to those provided in conventional settings *except*:

a Enhancement of access

b Reduction of stigma

c Reduction of generalization and maintenance of treatment effects

d Opportunity for earlier intervention

e More ecologically grounded roles played by mental health clinicians

4 Child abuse is a serious public health concern. Which of the following is an example of a tertiary prevention strategy for childhood maltreatment?

a Trauma-focused cognitive-behavioral therapy

b Educating children about "bad touch"

c Parent education programs

d Parenting hotlines

e Home-visit service for high-risk families

5 A school-based program designed to support social-emotional learning and positive social behavior in all elementary school students is an example of:

a Indicated preventive intervention

b Selective preventive intervention

c Universal preventive intervention

d Secondary prevention

e Tertiary prevention

6 Based on Section 504 of the Rehabilitation Act of 1973, schools need to develop a 504 plan to provide appropriate accommodations to students with physical or mental impairments. A behavioral intervention plan (BIP) should be written in the 504 plan for students with disruptive behaviors, and it is derived from a functional assessment of behavior. Which of the following is a key component of the functional behavioral assessment?

a Define behavior (such as aggression)

b Describe behavior (e.g., Tommy hits the peer who sits next to him, especially when the teacher is not watching)

c Describe antecedents (when bored, when provoked, and when unsupervised)

d Describe consequences (getting attention, suspension, being picked up by mother and going home early)

e All of the above

7 Which of the following processes or procedures is designed to clarify whether a behavior resulting in school suspension is related to the child's disability?

a Functional behavioral assessment

b Behavioral intervention plan (BIP)

c Manifestation determination review (MRD)

d 504 plan

e IEP annual review

8 A student with a disability cannot be expelled or transferred to a temporary alternative placement unless which of the following(s) is (are) present?

a If the student carries a weapon to school or a school function

b If the student possesses, uses, or sells illegal drugs or controlled substances at school or a school function

c If the student causes serious injury to another person at the school

d Both parent and school agree to the change in placement

e All of the above

9 Under the Individuals with Disabilities Education Act (IDEA), a student is eligible for special education services as long as the student meets the criteria for one or more categories of disability. A student diagnosed with ADHD should be categorized into which of the following?

a Emotional disturbance

b Intellectual disabilities

c Multiple disabilities

d Other health impairment

e Specific learning disability

10 Because of the shortage of child psychiatrists, primary care physicians (PCPs), pediatricians, or family physicians are required to provide mental health services in their offices. All of the following are needed for them to feel comfortable to treat mental health problems in primary care settings *except*:

a Ability to recognize signs and symptoms

b Ability to perform psychiatric assessment

c Knowledge to appropriately prescribe psychotropic medications

d Completion of post-residency formal psychiatric training

e Knowledge of when and how to refer for psychotherapy and other treatment options

11 All of the following are core principles of collaborative care in the primary care setting *except*:

a Employ the clinic's own mental health professionals (e.g., psychiatrists) to provide direct mental health services

b Establish clear and regular communication with emergency rooms, psychiatrists, and psychologists, ideally via electronic medical records

c Establish the availability of mental health professionals in the clinic to provide triage, crisis assessment, and patient/family education

d Establish screening protocols, mechanisms, and assessment/intervention pathways in order to provide standard care

e Encourage continuing education via lectures, case discussion, etc., to bring connections among psychiatrists, psychologists, other mental professionals, and the PCPs

12 The level of collaborative care is determined by the acuity of the mental disorders. A child with depression does not respond to SSRIs along with cognitive-behavioral therapy (CBT) provided by an individual therapist. The PCP refers him to a child and adolescent psychiatrist for an emergency consultation, but then participates in the ongoing care of the patient with other providers. Under which of the following levels of collaborative care is this categorized?

a Primarily primary care

b Primarily primary care with consultation

c Shared care

d Shared care and higher levels of care

e Primarily mental health care

13 Which of the following does *not* correlate with more resilience?

a Community social cohesion

b Responsive caregiving

c Secure attachment to an adult

d External locus of control

e Above-average intelligence

14 Studies have found that which of the following aged youth and younger have significantly less understanding and appreciation of the significance of the Miranda warning?

a 8 years

b 10 years

c 15 years

d 17 years

e 18 years

15 Younger children acquire less knowledge about the legal system. During the arrest and interrogation process, all of the following accurately describe the differences in younger children compared to older youth and adults *except*:

a They are more suggestible.

b They are more likely to confess.

c They have less capacity to understand the nature of the charges and the potential consequences.

d They are more likely to cooperate with counsel.

e They are less capable of understanding the nature and process of the proceeding.

16 Execution of juveniles was legally permissible in the United States until which of the following Supreme Court rulings?

a In *Roper v. Simmons*

b In *Kent v. United States*

c In *Santosky v. Krammer*

d In *re Gault*

e In *Rennie v. Klein*

17 What is the standard of proof used in juvenile court?

a Probable cause

b Preponderance of evidence

c Clear and convincing evidence

d Beyond a reasonable doubt

e Within a reasonable degree of medical certainty

18 A consultation child psychiatrist working in a children's hospital is asked to see a child with an acute medical illness and the child says his illness is caused by his bad behavior. Which one of the following cognitive developmental stages according to Piaget's theory is the child in?

a Sensory motor stage

b Preoperational stage

c Concrete operational stage

d Formal operational stage

e None of the above

19 During a court proceeding, the party who calls a witness to testify first questions the witness. Which of the following legal terms *best* fits this description?

a Cross-examination

b Direct examination

c Expert witness

d Fact witness

e Redirect examination

20 Which of the following legal terms explains the process that a court uses to determine or verify a child psychiatrist's credentials, training, and experiences?

a Expert witness

b Fact witness

c Subpoena

d Subpoena duces tecum

e Voir dire

21 All of the following statements regarding a child psychiatrist participating in a testimony as a fact witness are accurate *except*:

a The child psychiatrist cannot bill the patient/family or an insurance company for the time spent for the testimony.

b All the responses have to be verbal because the testimony is recorded or transcribed.

c Only factual information should be given, and speculations or personal opinions should be avoided.

d The child psychiatrist has to answer each question asked.

e When objection is made, the child psychiatrist should not answer the questions or should stop speaking in the middle of the answering.

22 All of the following statements regarding court-ordered evaluations or expert witness testimony are accurate *except*:

a A child psychiatrist should not serve as both therapy and expert witness for any of his or her clients.

b It is important to clarify the specific requests for the expert testimony from the start.

c A child psychiatrist should not feel pressured into taking cases when inadequate time is given to complete a thorough evaluation.

d The expert should seek contingent reimbursement based on the outcome of the trial.

e The expert may be requested to present his or her updated curriculum vitae.

23 All of the following statements regarding impacts on youth from families with separated or divorced parents are accurate *except*:

a Divorce increases overall risk for adjustment problems in youth.

b Preschoolers are more likely to present with regression, intense anxiety, and fear.

c Middle school-aged children are more likely to experience loneliness and a sense of powerlessness.

d Adolescents are more likely to experience acute depression and concern about their own future relationships.

e Girls are more vulnerable than boys in both short-term and long-term consequences.

24 To substantiate malpractice, the plaintiff must establish all of the following points (known as 4Ds) by a preponderance of the evidence *except*:

a Duty of reasonable care

b Deception in treatment

c Dereliction of duty

d Damage, a compensable injury, or harm

e Direct result

Matching

25–36 Match the following titles of school personnel to each description that correctly defines their roles:

a In charge of fiscal responsibilities of the school

b Managing and coordinating activities in all schools within a school district

c Managing all services within a school building

d Facilitating skills of daily living and dealing with sensory integration issues

e Addressing communication and social problems

f Maintaining students' health records and addressing acute health needs

g Helping students with college and vocational planning

h Participating in special education assessments and implementation planning and addressing social problems in social skills groups

i Assessing students for special education eligibility and developing individual education plans (IEP)

j Assisting classroom teachers and/or individual students

k Having received training and being credentialed to provide alternative instruction to students with disabilities

l Having the most extensive involvement with students and providing direct instructions to students

25 Schoolteachers

26 Special education teachers

27 Teacher aides

28 School psychologists

29 School social workers

30 Guidance counselors

31 School nurses

32 Speech therapists

33 Occupational therapists

34 School principals

35 Superintendents

36 School boards

ANSWERS AND EXPLANATIONS

1 (a) Addressing individual students' needs is not a focus of a systems consultation model but is the focus of a direct provider model. Using the principles of organizational psychology, the systems consultation model may also focus on building school connectedness among students and parents, enhancing teacher and staff morale, and planning for crisis situations. *(Ref. 1, Ch. 47, Roles section)*

2 (c) Increased risky behavior in youth between the 1960s and 1980s due to the dramatic changes in social mores led to increased school involvement in providing preventive mental health services in schools. *(Ref. 3, Ch. 7.3, Emergence section)*

3 (c) Enhanced generalization and maintenance of treatment effects is one of the advantages of mental health services being delivered in school settings among the others listed. *(Ref. 3, Ch. 7.3, Mental Health Services section)*

4 (a) Primary prevention decreases the number of new occurrences of a disorder, secondary prevention decreases the rates of an established disorder such as through early detection, and tertiary prevention lowers the level of disability associated with an existing illness through treatment. Trauma-focused cognitive-behavioral therapy is an example of tertiary prevention as it improves PTSD symptoms and behavior problems due to child abuse. The other interventions listed are all examples of primary prevention as they attempt to prevent child abuse before it occurs. *(Ref. 1, Ch. 24, Prevention section; Ref. 3, Ch. 3.2.2, History of Prevention section)*

5 (c) This type of program is an example of a universal preventive intervention. In 1994, the Institute of Medicine's report on Reducing Risk for Mental Disorders divided primary prevention into universal, selective, and indicated interventions. Universal preventive interventions target the entire population, selective preventive interventions target high-risk populations, and indicated preventive interventions target individuals with early symptoms. *(Ref. 3, Ch. 3.2.2, History of Prevention section)*

6 (e) All of the listed are the key components of a functional behavioral assessment. There are two additional key components: to hypothesize function of the identified behavior (attention seeking, anger expression, releasing impulsivity, and an incentive of going home early) and to gather related information (poor academic performance, limited social skills, and dysfunctional family dynamics). *(Ref. 3, Table 7.3.4)*

7 (c) Manifestation determination review (MRD) should be conducted if the number of consecutive days of suspensions exceeds ten days in a given school year to determine whether the behavior associated with the suspensions is secondary to the child's disability. If yes, the child cannot be suspended for more than ten days, and then the IEP and BIP should be reviewed and revised to address this specific behavior problem. If no, the child can be suspended as other students are. However, parents who do not agree with the MRD can appeal. *(Ref. 1, Ch. 47, Response to Intervention section)*

8 (e) Any of the listed situations can trigger the student with disabilities being expelled or transferred to a temporary placement. *(Ref. 1, Ch. 47, Response to Intervention section)*

9 (d) Other health impairment captures both ADHD and sensory processing difficulties. In addition to those listed, other categories include: autism, deaf-blindness, deaf, hearing impairment, orthopedic impairment, speech-language impairment, traumatic brain injury, and visual impairment. *(Ref. 3, Ch. 7.3, The Individual with Disabilities section)*

10 (d) Completion of post-residency formal psychiatric training is not required. However, PCPs should seek additional education that would improve their skill and confidence, and should also actively seek consultation from and work collaboratively with psychiatrists and other mental health professionals. PCPs are expected to be a part of a multidisciplinary team that provides an integrated approach to mental health care for children. The primary care clinic should be both a medical home and a mental health home for youth, where services involving a variety of mental health and medical specialties can be coordinated. *(Ref. 3, Ch. 7.1.1, Primary Care section)*

11 (a) Most primary care clinics do not employ their own mental health professionals to provide direct mental health services. Instead, they establish local or regional connections with mental health professionals who can play roles as team members in the patient's care. *(Ref. 1, Ch. 48, Strategies section)*

12 (c) In this case, it is considered "shared care." As acuity and severity of the cases increase the levels of care will increase on the continuum in the following sequence: primarily primary care, primarily primary care with consultation, shared care, shared care and higher levels of care, and primarily mental health care. *(Ref. 5, Ch. 58.2, The Collaborative Primary Behavioral section)*

13 (d) Resilience is the ability to do well despite experiencing significant adversity and is an important part of understanding prevention of development of psychopathology. Internal locus of control, not external locus of control, is associated with resilience, along with the other factors listed. *(Ref. 1, Ch. 24, Resilience section)*

14 (c) Research has found that youth under the age of 15 years have significantly less understanding and appreciation of the significance of the Miranda warning. They have difficulty understanding an adversarial nature of the interrogation. They are more likely to waive their rights. *(Ref. 3, Ch. 7.4.1, Specialized Forensic Evaluation section)*

15 (d) To cooperate with counsel, children must be able to communicate effectively with their attorney and to able to evaluate the advice provided by the attorney. Younger children, in general, are less capable of doing that. *(Ref. 1, Ch. 31, Children as Witnesses section)*

16 (a) The Supreme Court recognized the developmental differences between adults and adolescents being significant and made juvenile offenders ineligible for execution during the ruling in *Roper v. Simmons* in March 2005. *(Ref. 5, Ch. 60.1, Criminal Competencies section)*

17 (d) Standard of proof is the level of certainty required to make a judgment depending on the type of legal proceeding. Juvenile court as well as criminal proceedings require the highest standard, "beyond a reasonable doubt." The intermediate standard is "clear and convincing evidence," which is required for termination of parent rights. Least strict is preponderance of evidence which is used in most civil proceedings. "Within a reasonable degree of medical certainty" is comparable to the level of certainty physicians use for diagnosis and treatment and is standard for physician testimonies in court. *(Ref. 1, Ch. 31, Overview section)*

18 (c) During the concrete operational stage, children's capacity for linking cause and effect increases. However, their thinking and reason are concrete, and education should be provided to them to dispel their belief that they have brought about their own illness through their behaviors or thoughts. *(Ref. 2, Ch. 16, Physically Ill Children section; Ref. 3, Ch. 2.3.1, Cognitive Development section)*

19 (b) Direct examination refers to the initial questioning of a witness by the party that called the witness to testify in a trial or other court proceeding to elicit evidence to support a claim or defense. Cross-examination refers to the questioning and interrogation of a witness called by the opponent's party to discredit the witness, which occurs after the direct examination. Redirect examination occurs after the cross-examination, which gives a chance for the witness to explain, but the scope is usually limited to the areas brought out on the cross-examination. *(Ref. 3, Table 7.4.1.1)*

20 (e) Voir dire refers to the process of determining the qualification of a witness and questioning of prospective jurors to determine whether they are biased or not. Functioning either as an expert witness or a fact witness, a child psychiatrist can be questioned about his or her credentials, training, and experiences during a court procedure. In this case, the process is also called voir dire. *(Ref. 3, Table 7.4.1.1)*

21 (d) The child psychiatrist does not have to answer each question asked. The psychiatrist should let the attorney or judge know if a question is posed in a way that it cannot be answered or is misleading. The psychiatrist should be allowed to ask for repeating or rephrasing the questions or inform the court that he or she simply does not know the answer. *(Ref. 3, Ch. 7.4.1, Fact Witness section)*

22 (d) It is unethical for a child psychiatrist/expert witness to negotiate a contingency fee based on the potential outcome or settlement of a trial because this could potentially undermine the objective position expressed by the witness. *(Ref. 3, Ch. 7.4.1, Expert Witness section)*

23 (e) Some studies show that boys are more vulnerable than girls in both short-term and long-term consequences. However, the data on the effects of gender differences regarding the outcomes of divorce is not very clear. The most important predictors of a child's adjustment to divorce are inter-parental conflicts, psychological health of the parents, and the quality of the parent–child relationships. *(Ref. 3, Ch. 7.4.2, Divorce—An Update section)*

24 (b) Deception of treatment is not one of the 4Ds. To substantiate a malpractice case, the plaintiff has to establish that the clinician had a Duty of reasonable care to the patient; presence of a Dereliction of that duty that was judged by the standard of the average, prudent practitioner; Damage (a compensable injury or harm) was sustained by the patient; and the damage was a Direct result of the clinician's failure to exercise a reasonable standard of care. *(Ref. 3, Ch. 7.4.4, The Law of Malpractice section)*

Matching

25 (l); **26** (k); **27** (j); **28** (i); **29** (h); **30** (g); **31** (f); **32** (e); **33** (d); **34** (c); **35** (b); **36** (a) School teachers are involved with students most extensively, providing instruction many hours a day to a relatively large group of students. Special education teachers are specially trained and credentialed to provide alternative instruction to smaller group of students with disabilities. Requiring no advanced education or training, teacher aides assist teachers and/or individual students in the classroom. The primary role of school psychologists is to assess students for special education eligibility and develop the IEP. They play a role in consulting with teachers regarding classroom management strategies and providing individual and/or group therapy to students. School social workers are a part of special education assessments and program planning, and may also provide limited therapies to students and their families. Guidance counselors primarily assist students in college preparation and vocational planning, and also occasionally provide therapy to students. School nurses are responsible for addressing acute health needs of students and maintaining their health records. Speech therapists are responsible for assessing and addressing speech, language, and communication difficulties as well as social problems. Occupational therapists help with daily living skills training and address sensory integration problems. School principals are fully responsible for managing all services within their schools. Superintendents manage and coordinate activities in all schools within the same school district. School boards are in charge of fiscal responsibilities and exert tremendous influence over the allocation of funds and resources for external consultants and programs. School administrators report to a school board and may have competing agendas with special education administrators (who are responsible for determining the special education needs of students) because of the concerns about finding resources to meet special education needs. *(Ref. 5, Ch. 55.8, Roles of School Personnel section)*

16

RESEARCH DESIGN, STATISTICS, AND TECHNOLOGIES

DOI: 10.4324/9781003308805-17

QUESTIONS

Directions: Select the best response for each of the questions 1–25.

1 All of the following statements regarding reliability and validity are accurate *except*:

  a The validity of an instrument refers to the extent to which it measures what it was intended to measure.

  b Reliability refers to the extent to which results obtained with an instrument can be reproduced.

  c Validity ensures reliability.

  d Test-retest reliability is a strenuous test of interrater reliability.

  e Validity includes predictive validity, factorial validity, and construct validity.

2 Randomized experimental research designs are usually preferred over quasi-experimental designs because they:

  a Are easier to execute

  b Eliminate bias

  c Are less expensive to carry out

  d Have one active independent variable

  e Require little training to perform

3 Variable refers to a characteristic of the participants or situations that has different values in the study. The predictors, antecedents, or presumed causes under investigation in the study should be considered as which of the following variables?

  a Dependent variable

  b Demographic variable

  c Extraneous variable

  d Independent variable

  e Operational variable

4 On a normal curve measuring the IQs of a large group of youth, how many of them will fall within the one standard deviation range from either side of the mean?

  a 68%

  b 78%

  c 88%

  d 95%

  e 99%

5 All of the following are broad types of evidence that support validity *except*:

  a Content

  b Responses

  c External structure

  d Relations to other variables

  e The consequence of testing

6 Effect size can be measured by the strength of the relationship in applied behavioral sciences, using the r value. Which of the following r values implies an acceptable level of support?

  a $r \geq 0.1$

  b $r \geq 0.2$

  c $r \geq 0.3$

  d $r \geq 0.5$

  e $r \geq 0.8$

7 In the *ex post facto* research method, there are usually a few levels or categories for the independent variable, and between-group comparisons are made. Which of the research approaches does this method belong to?

  a Associational research approach

  b Comparative research approach

  c Description research approach

  d Quasi-experimental research approach

  e Randomized experimental research approach

8 Which of the following statements regarding associational research designs and data analysis is *incorrect*?

  a They are designed to examine the relationship between two continuous variables.

  b Variables are both independent and dependent.

  c Coefficient r expresses the Pearson product moment correlation.

  d A strong positive relationship is found if $r > 0.5$.

  e The r can be expressed with degrees of freedom and significance level.

9 Which of the following is used to measure statistical significance?

  a The *p* value

  b The *r* value

  c The κ value

  d The *d* score

  e The $x2$ value

10 All of the following statements regarding logistic regression analysis and discriminant analysis are correct *except*:

  a Logistic regression requires fewer assumptions than discriminant analysis and performs better.

  b Logistic regression estimates the probability an event will occur.

  c The coefficient is expressed as an odds score in logistic regression.

  d An odds ratio (the ratio of two odds, OR) is essential to logistic regression.

  e OR = 0 means random association.

11 Which of the following neuroimaging techniques is most broadly suited to study developmental brain abnormalities in children?

a Computed tomography (CT)

b Magnetic resonance imaging (MRI)

c Positron emission tomography (PET)

d Magnetic resonance spectroscopy (MRS)

e Single-photon emission computed tomography (SPECT)

12 Magnetic resonance spectroscopy (MRS) can be used to measure all of the following *except*:

a Energy metabolism

b Amino acids

c Neuronal structural integrity

d Cerebral blood flow

e Neurotransmitters

13 All of the following statements regarding SPECT are accurate *except*:

a It is capable of monitoring brain activity.

b It provides clear spatial resolution of white matter changes.

c It is capable of measuring neurotransmitter activity.

d It is useful for identifying focal epileptogenic brain regions.

e Radiation exposure is a potential limitation.

14 Which of the following statements regarding the type II error is correct?

a Null hypothesis is not rejected when it is true.

b Null hypothesis is rejected when it is false.

c Null hypothesis is not rejected when it is false.

d Null hypothesis is rejected when it is true.

e The alternative hypothesis is rejected when it is false.

15 Which of the following statements regarding sensitivity and specificity is *incorrect*?

a Sensitivity is the percentage of negative results among individuals who do not have the disease for which they are being tested.

b Sensitivity is important when trying to identify as many cases as possible.

c Sensitivity is the percentage of positive results among individuals who have the disease for which they are being tested.

d Specificity is the percentage of negative test results in patients who actually do not have the disease.

e Specificity is important in trying to include only true cases.

16 All of the following statements regarding functional magnetic resonance imaging (fMRI) are accurate *except*:

a It identifies brain activity while the subject performs a cognitive task.

b The image intensity changes the result from the variable oxygenation levels in the regions of interest.

c Its spatial and temporal resolutions are superior to that of conventional PET and SPECT.

d Its temporal resolution is superior to that of electroencephalography (EEG).

e It is relatively safe in children.

17 All of the following statements regarding diffusion tensor imaging (DTI) are correct *except*:

a It is an application of MRI technology.

b It has a unique strength in providing information about the orientation and integrity of gray matter tracts.

c It measures the net movement of water molecules.

d Initially, it was used to diagnose stroke.

e There are potential uses for studying brain connectivity.

18 All of the following are essential elements of information that should be transmitted to research subjects during the informed consent process *except*:

a Purpose and duration of the research

b Foreseeable risks and benefits

c Confidentiality of records

d Contact information in case of questions

e Specifying loss of benefits because of refusal to participate

19 Which of the following is *most* essential to be obtained from child subjects before they participate in clinical research?

a Assent

b Permission

c Consent

d Authorization

e Acceptance

20 Which of the following EEG waves represents a deeper stage of sleep?

a Alpha

b Beta

c Delta

d Gamma

e Theta

21 Intoxication or withdrawal from which of the following substances appears to have the *least* effect on EEG?

a Alcohol

b Caffeine

c LSD

d Marijuana

e Tobacco

22 Which of the following medications should be definitely avoided during electroconvulsive therapy (ECT)?

a Aripiprazole

b Haloperidol

c Lithium

d Nortriptyline

e Venlafaxine

23 Which of the following tools or devices applies magnetic stimulation to the brain?

a ECT

b Implanted cortical stimulation

c Transcranial direct current stimulation (tDCS)

d Transcranial magnetic stimulation (TMS)

e Vagus nerve stimulation

24 Which type of the following study designs can obtain data regarding incidence rates and incidence rate ratios?

a Case-control study

b Cohort study

c Cross-sectional study

d Ecological study

e None of the above

ANSWERS AND EXPLANATIONS

1 **(c)** Validity does not guarantee reliability, just as reliability cannot ensure validity. Validity may include predictive validity, factorial validity, and construct validity, whereas reliability may include test-retest reliability and interrater reliability. Inter-item consistency is also used to estimate reliability. *(Ref. 3, Ch. 3.1.1, Variables and Their Measurement section)*

2 **(b)** In contrast to the quasi-experimental studies, subjects in randomized studies are assigned randomly to groups (experimental or control), with an advantage of eliminating bias. Single and double blinding further reduces the possibility of bias. This leads to more convincing evidence that the independent variable rather than the dependent or control variable caused the difference. Both experimental designs require an active variable. *(Ref. 3, Ch. 3.1.1, Experimental Designs section)*

3 **(d)** The independent variable can be defined broadly including any predictors, antecedents, or presumed causes or influence under investigation in the study, which can be subtyped into: active independent variables (interventions or therapies that are prescribed to the experimental group, but not to the control group) and attributed to independent variables (gender, age, or ethnic group—cannot be manipulated). *(Ref. 3, Ch. 3.1.1, Variables and Their Measurement section)*

4 **(a)** If the variable is normally distributed, 68% of the youth who participate in the IQ testing will fall within one standard deviation from either side of the mean (100). Ninety-five percent of them will fall within two standard deviations, and 99% will fall within three standard deviations. One standard deviation equals 15. Thus, 68% of the youth will have an IQ between 85 and 115. Only 5% of them will have IQ either lower than 70 or higher than 130. *(Ref. 3, Ch. 3.1.1, Variables and Their Measurement section)*

5 **(c)** Internal structure (not external) is one of five broad types of evidence that can support the validity of a test or measure. They cannot be used alone, and the validation should integrate all the pertinent information gathered from these five types of evidence. *(Ref. 3, Ch. 3.1.1, Variables and Their Measurement section)*

6 **(c)** In applied behavioral sciences, $r \geq 0.3$ represents an acceptable level of support for measurement validation. An $r \geq 0.5$ represents strong support, whereas $r \geq 0.1$ represents weak support even if it is statistically significant. *(Ref. 3, Ch. 3.1.1, Variables and Their Measurement section)*

7 **(b)** The comparative research approach is also called causal-comparative or *ex post facto* (generally a nonexperimental approach). It compares independent variable differences between groups. Among all these approaches, the randomized experimental approach provides the best evidence about cause and effect. The descriptive approach is distinguishable from the other four approaches because only one variable is used and only descriptive statistics are provided, without determination of comparisons or associations. *(Ref. 3, Ch. 3.1.1, Research Approaches, Questions, and Designs section)*

8 **(b)** In associational research designs, the two variables are either independent or dependent. The Pearson product moment correlation is used to estimate the strength of association between the two variables and expresses as coefficient r, ranging from -1 to $+1$, with value > 0.5, indicating a strong positive association. *(Ref. 3, Ch. 3.1.1, Inferential Statistics and their Interpretation section)*

9 **(a)** The p value represents the strength of the correlation between two variables, indicating the probability an outcome could occur if the null hypothesis were true. Statistical significance should not be interpreted as clinical significance or approval of the null hypothesis. The κ value represents the correlation coefficient of reliability. The $x2$ represents the chi-square value. The r family, d family, and the measures of risk potency are proposed measures of sample size. *(Ref. 3, Ch. 3.1.1, Summarizing Statistical Outcomes section)*

10 **(e)** An OR = 1 (not = 0) or odds = 0 indicates a random association. Discriminant analysis requires more assumptions than logistic regression analysis does to make an optimal prediction. The odds are used to express the probability an event will occur in logistic regression, and the odds ratio increases with an increase of a positive association and decreases with a negative association. *(Morgan et al. 2003)*

11 **(b)** MRI is suited to study structural, physiologic, and developmental brain abnormalities in children and to perform repeated measures because it involves no ionizing radiation or radioactive isotopes and has been shown to have an absence of biologic hazards at currently used field strengths. MRS measures concentration and distribution of metabolites and is useful for the assessment of metabolic, mitochondrial, and neurodegenerative disorders. The use of CT exposes the child to x-rays, and PET exposes the child to radiation. Although SPECT provides for functional neuroimaging, it involves small amounts of radioisotopes. *(Ref. 1, Ch. 6, Neuroimaging section)*

12 **(d)** The MRS technique has been used to measure amino acids, neurotransmitters, metabolites related to energy production, and metabolism of lipids and carbohydrates. It has not been used to measure cerebral blood flow that can be measured by fMRI. *(Ref. 1, Ch. 6, Neuroimaging section)*

13 **(b)** The SPECT technique provides a three-dimensional image of brain function. It measures cerebral blood flow and metabolic activity with minimal radiation exposure. PET and SPECT are both useful in identification of focal epileptogenic brain regions. The major disadvantages are the limited clinical experience with it and its inferior spatial resolution compared to that of PET. *(Ref. 1, Ch. 6, Neuroimaging section)*

14 **(c)** A type II error refers to incorrectly deciding no difference exists when there really is a difference (the null hypothesis is not rejected when is false). A type I error refers to deciding a difference exists when there is really no difference (null hypothesis is rejected when it is true). *(Ref. 3, Ch. 3.1.1, Inferential Statistics and Their Interpretation section)*

15 (a) Sensitivity is the proportion of true cases that the test selects. Specificity is the proportion of subjects who do not have the disease in the group that the test identifies as negative. *(Ref. 3, Ch. 3.2.1, Case Identification and Screening section)*

16 (d) Compared to fMRI, EEG has a much better temporal resolution than fMRI. However, fMRI has better resolution than PET and SPECT. fMRI can test subjects undertaking cognitive tasks by identifying changes in oxygenation levels of identified regions of interest. *(Ref. 1, Ch. 6, Neuroimaging section)*

17 (b) DTI specifically focuses on the white matter and evaluates the orientation and integrity of the white matter tracts. DTI images show water diffusion along white matter tracts, providing information regarding neuronal connectivity. Clinically, it was first used to diagnose stroke, and then to show the white matter loss in multiple sclerosis, schizophrenia, dyslexia, and preterm birth. *(Ref. 1, Ch. 6, Neuroimaging section)*

18 (e) According to federal regulations, certain key elements of information must be transmitted to the research subjects during the informed consent process. Participation is on a voluntary basis, and no loss of benefits should result from refusal to participate in research. *(Ref. 3, Ch. 3.1.3, Informed Consent section)*

19 (a) "Assent" is the term that describes children's agreement to participate in a research project. Informed consent is usually given by parents or legal guardians who have ultimate rights to authorize or refuse participation. Permission refers to the collective decision and judgment of the family in deciding to allow the child to participate. *(Ref. 3, Ch. 3.1.3, Assent section)*

20 (c) Delta waves (1–3 Hz) are seen in deeper stages of sleep and in pathological states such as encephalopathy. Alpha activity is seen in awake individuals with their eyes closed, and the high rhythmic waves have a frequency of 8–13 Hz. Faster than alpha waves, beta waves (13–20 Hz) are commonly seen in normal adult awake EEGs, especially over frontal regions. Gamma waves have very high frequency (> 30 Hz) and reflect the mechanism of cortical integration, and are also being investigated in neurobehavioral disorders. Theta waves, with a frequency of 4–7 Hz, are present in awake states in children, but more common in drowsy states. *(Ref. 1, Ch. 6, Electroencephalography section)*

21 (c) Hallucinogens such as LSD and mescaline do not appear to have any major effects on the visualized EEG and do not produce any clinically relevant EEG changes. However, use of or withdrawal from all other listed substances, and others (e.g., barbiturates, cocaine, and inhalants), may produce significant noticeable changes in the EEG. *(Ref. 5, Ch. 1.15, EEG Alterations from Medications and Drugs section)*

22 (c) The combination of lithium and ECT can cause prolonged and/or focal seizures, and can also lead to confusion and serotonin syndrome. Haloperidol and fluphenazine have little effect on seizures induced by ECT, but reserpine should not be combined with ECT. Second-generation antipsychotics are generally considered safe combined with ECT. Antidepressants (except for MAOIs) are commonly used along with ECT. TCAs seem to be safe in patients without significant cardiac comorbidities. Both venlafaxine and nortriptyline are found to increase the response to ECT. *(Ref. 5, Ch. 34.35, Patient Management section)*

23 (d) Among all the listed devices or tools, only transcranial magnetic stimulation (TMS) applies a rapidly changing magnetic field to the superficial layers of the cerebral cortex, and induces small electric currents locally. Normally, it does not induce a seizure, in contrast to ECT. Repetitive transcranial magnetic stimulation (rTMS) may induce a seizure, and that is one of the potential severe side effects of the treatment. All other listed devices or tools use electrical currents. *(Ref. 5, Ch. 34.36, Brain Stimulation Tools section)*

24 (b) The cohort study uses a longitudinal prospective or retrospective design to collect data to compare the group that was or will be exposed to a particular agent(s) or risk factor(s) to the group without such an exposure(s). The incidence rates and incidence rate ratios can be calculated. The cohort study is also called an incidence study. *(Ref. 3, Ch. 3.2.1, General Epidemiology section)*

References

Morgan, G. A., Vaske, J. J., Gliner, J. A., and Harmon, R. J. (2003). Logistic Regression and Discriminant Analysis: Use and Interpretation. *JAACAP*, 42, 994–997.

PART II

CLINICAL CASES

17

CASE HISTORIES, CLINICAL ASSESSMENT, DIFFERENTIAL DIAGNOSIS, FORMULATION, AND TREATMENT PLANNING

DOI: 10.4324/9781003308805-19

QUESTIONS

Case 1

Sam, a 4.5-year-old boy, is brought in by his mother to see a child psychiatrist with concerns about Sam's social difficulties at daycare, where Sam has limited social interactions with other children and only seems to play by himself or to parallel play with other children. His mother reports that Sam does not like to interact with his 6-year-old sister at home; often he lines up his toys and stares at the ceiling fan. He gets frustrated easily, which can lead to body rocking, hand flapping, and at times temper tantrums. His mother reports her first son (current age 14 years) was previously diagnosed with autism spectrum disorder at age 4.

Questions 1–12. Based on the information given in Case 1, answer the following questions.

1   Which of the following differential diagnoses should *not* be considered?

   a   Autism spectrum disorder

   b   Communication disorder

   c   Intellectual disability

   d   Stereotypic movement disorder

   e   None of the above

2   Which of the following is the *most* likely diagnosis based on the case description?

   a   Autism spectrum disorder

   b   Communication disorder

   c   Intellectual disability

   d   Stereotypic movement disorder

   e   Other specified neurodevelopmental disorder

3   Which of the following areas of deficits does *not* need to be present for a formal diagnosis of autism spectrum disorder?

   a   Deficits in social-emotional reciprocity

   b   Deficits in nonverbal communication during social interaction

   c   Deficits in intellectual functioning

   d   Deficits in developing, maintaining, and understanding relationships

   e   Restricted, repetitive patterns of behavior, interests, or activities

4   Which of the following further evaluations or tests is *least* diagnostically and clinically relevant at this point?

   a   Appropriate genetic testing and counseling

   b   Brain MRI

   c   Hearing test

   d   Neurological consultation and evaluation

   e   Speech and language evaluation

5   If a genetic test confirms that Sam has Fragile X syndrome and he also meets the full criteria for autism spectrum disorder, which of the following is the *best* way to document the diagnosis based on DSM-5?

   a   Diagnose him with Fragile X syndrome

   b   Diagnose him with pervasive developmental disorder, NOS (PDD NOS)

   c   Diagnose him with autism spectrum disorder, associated with another neurodevelopmental, mental, or behavioral disorder

   d   Diagnose him with autism spectrum disorder, associated with a known medical or genetic condition or environmental factor

   e   Diagnose him with other specified neurodevelopmental disorder

6   If, during a neurological consultation and evaluation, Sam is found to have café-au-lait spots throughout his body, which of the following conditions does Sam *most* likely have?

   a   Down syndrome

   b   Fragile X syndrome

   c   Landau-Kleffner syndrome

   d   Neurofibromatosis

   e   Tuberos sclerosis

7   Say your history reveals that Sam has a fairly normal early developmental history, he was able to speak normally prior to his age of 4 years, and it was only after his fourth birthday that he gradually lost the language skills he previously acquired, leading to impaired social skills. In addition, his recent EEG indicates severe paroxysmal discharges over both hemispheres, which worsen during his non-REM sleep. Now, which of the following conditions does Sam *most* likely have?

   a   Down syndrome

   b   Fragile X syndrome

   c   Landau-Kleffner syndrome

   d   Neurofibromatosis

   e   Tuberos sclerosis

8   After thorough assessments and evaluation procedures, Sam is confirmed to have a diagnosis of autism spectrum disorder. All of the following statements regarding assessing him for a possible intellectual disability (ID) are correct *except*:

   a   Abilities in reasoning, problem solving, planning, and abstract thinking should be assessed.

   b   Adaptive functioning should be assessed.

   c   Onset of intellectual and adaptive deficits should be clarified.

d Severity should be assessed and determined including mild, moderate, severe, and profound.

e Level of severity depends primarily on IQ scores.

9 Sam is verbal, but he is not interested in carrying on reciprocal conversations with his peers. He presents with low frustration tolerance, irritability, and occasional aggression. He continues to experience high sensitivity to certain sounds and tags on his shirts. He is described by his mother as a picky eater. Which of the following interventions is *least* applicable to him?

a Applied behavior analysis (ABA)

b Speech and language therapy

c Picture Exchange Communication System (PECS)

d Occupational therapy

e Social, Communication, Emotional Regulation, and Transactional Support Treatment (SCERTS)

10 Which of the following medications is FDA approved for treatment of his irritability?

a Aripiprazole

b Clozapine

c Olanzapine

d Quetiapine

e Ziprasidone

11 Which of the following is the *least* important prognostic factor for Sam?

a Cognitive ability

b Functional play skills

c Joint attention

d Neuroimaging findings based on MRI

e Severity of the autistic symptoms

12 Sam's mother brings him back to see the child psychiatrist when he is 6 years old. His mother reports that Sam's teacher has complained that he has not been able to sit still or focus on his schoolwork. He is extremely distracted. He clearly presents with significant symptoms that are consistent with an ADHD, combined presentation. His ADHD symptoms seem to exceed what is typically seen in individuals of comparable mental age. He also continues to demonstrate a spectrum of symptoms of autism spectrum disorder. Which of the following diagnosis/diagnoses should be given to Sam at this time?

a ADHD, combined presentation

b Autism spectrum disorder

c ADHD, combined presentation + autism spectrum disorder

d Other specified ADHD + autism spectrum disorder

e Unspecified ADHD + autism spectrum disorder

Case 2

Eric is a 7-year-old male. He is brought by his foster mother (FM) to your office for evaluation of his behavioral problems both at home and at school. Reportedly, his schoolteacher has noticed that he has been having difficulties with academic performance, getting along with his classmates, and concentrating on his schoolwork. He is reportedly very hyperactive, distracted, unable to follow through with instructions, and very disruptive in class. He is noted to have trouble relating to his peers, and often plays by himself during recess. He was reportedly removed from his biological parents when he was 5 years old because of parental involvement with illegal substances, neglect, and physical abuse.

Questions 13–26. Based on the information given in Case 2, answer the following questions.

13 Which of the following conditions can be excluded from the differential diagnoses?

a ADHD

b Anxiety disorder

c Autism spectrum disorder

d Major depressive disorder

e None of the above

14 During the interview, FM tells you that the information she gathered from the child protective service agency social worker indicates Eric has a fairly normal developmental history. He is a relatively physically healthy child. He is affectionate, caring, very social, and always wants to be the center of attention. He has very good language skills, and he enjoys playing soccer with similar-aged neighbor boys. Which of the following diagnoses is *least* likely?

a ADHD

b Autism spectrum disorder

c Depression

d PTSD

e Specific learning disorder

15 Based on a psychoeducational assessment, over the past whole school year, Eric has had a pattern of mathematic difficulties, specifically in accurate math reasoning. In addition, he has had significant difficulties reading words accurately. Which of the following is *not* an appropriate way to describe his diagnosis?

a Specific learning disorder with impairment in reading and mathematics

b Specific learning disorder with impairment in mathematics and dyslexia, difficulties with word reading accuracy

c Dyslexia, difficulties with word reading accuracy and math reasoning

d Dyscalculia, difficulties with math reasoning and word reading accuracy

e Specific learning disorder

16 Which of the following categories would he *most* likely be qualified in for special education?

a Emotional disturbance (ED)

b Hearing impairment

c Intellectual disability (ID)

d Other health impairment (OHI)

e Specific learning disability (SLD)

17 Which of the following rating scales is *least* useful for assessing him for possible ADHD?

a Behavior Assessment System for Children (BASC-3)

b Child Behavior Checklist (CBCL)

c Children's Global Assessment Scale (CGAS)

d Conners

e Vanderbilt

18 Both FM and Eric report that when he was 5.5 years old, within a few months after he was removed from his biological parents, while staying with his foster family, he often experienced recurrent and intrusive distressing memories of his past physical abuse by his father. He avoided activities, conversations, or places that aroused his recollection of the trauma. He also demonstrated a lot of anger outbursts that often led to physical aggression. FM reports that after receiving counseling and therapies for the past few years, Eric has not experienced any significant occurrence of these symptoms and he has developed good relationships with his current caregivers. Which of the following needs to be added for him to meet the full criteria of PTSD in the past based on DSM-5?

a Diminished interest in activities, such as constriction of play

b Dissociative reactions

c Hypervigilance

d Intense psychological physiological reactions to reminders of the trauma

e Recurrent distressing dreams related to his past trauma

19 At age 6.5 years, Eric was seen by the psychiatrist who had diagnosed him with PTSD, and he prescribed sertraline. Which of the following would be the *least* concern regarding his taking the medication?

a Risk of switching

b Risk of increasing suicidal ideations or behaviors

c Lack of empirical support for benefit

d Risk of cardiovascular complications

e Risk of activation/agitation

20 Which of the following interventions for Eric's PTSD symptoms has the *strongest* supporting published evidence?

a Behavioral therapy

b Cognitive-behavioral therapy (CBT)

c Interpersonal psychotherapy (IPT)

d Psychodynamic psychotherapy

e Trauma-focused cognitive-behavioral therapy (TF-CBT)

21 According to his birth history, Eric was exposed to alcohol during the entire pregnancy. He was previously diagnosed with fetal alcohol syndrome (FAS) and his head size is small. Which of the following is found to be associated with microcephaly?

a Enhanced dopamine receptor

b Inhibited dopamine receptor

c Enhanced NMDA receptor

d Inhibited NMDA receptor

e None of the above

22 All the collateral information and clinical evaluation/observations support an ADHD diagnosis for Eric. As his current child psychiatrist, you consider all of the following as being routinely needed while you consider treating him with stimulant medications *except*:

a Gathering Eric's medical history

b Gathering Eric's family history

c Ensuring that Eric's physical examination indicates no significant medical conditions contraindicating stimulant medications

d Screening EKG

e None of the above

23 Which of the following compounds does lisdexamfetamine dimesylate (Vyvanse) release in a rate-limiting enzymatic hydrolysis process to become the active compound d-amphetamine?

a Cysteine

b Histidine

c Lysine

d Methionine

e Tyrosine

24 Which of the following medications would you *least* likely consider as pharmacologic choices for his ADHD symptoms?

a Aripiprazole

b Atomoxetine

c Guanfacine extended-release

d Clonidine extended-release

e Methylphenidate

25 If one day Eric's teacher calls you and asks you the detailed information about his psychotropic medication treatment, which of the following is your *most* appropriate next step?

a Sharing only names of the medication(s) with the teacher without providing more detailed information

b Refusing to directly communicate with his teacher

c Telling the teacher that you have to write her a formal letter rather than talking to her on the phone

d Obtaining consent for releasing or sharing Eric's medical information first

e Inviting his teacher to come to your office to discuss in person

26 Which of the following should *not* be an aspect of discussion in regard to the informed consent for Eric's psychotropic medication treatment?

a The nature of the condition that requires the treatment

b The nature, benefits, and goals of the proposed treatment

c The risks, side effects, and negative consequence of the proposed treatment

d Alternatives to the proposed treatment

e The way to guarantee a success of the proposed treatment

Case 3

Lisa is a 13-year-old Caucasian girl who is brought to see child psychiatrist Dr. Lee. Lisa presents with weight loss of 19 pounds over an eight-month period from her previous weight of 95 pounds. Her height is 63 inches. Her mother reports that Lisa has been increasingly withdrawn, spending much of her time alone in her room. She has been skipping breakfast and eating little of her school lunch. Her mother describes her daughter as an otherwise perfect child. She is an A student, spends her time studying hard, plays flute, and devotes more than two hours a day to exercise. Her menarche occurred right before her thirteenth birthday, and she has been having irregular menstrual periods since her weight loss. She also has a recent history of engaging in episodic binge eating and self-induced vomiting.

Questions 27–38. Based on the information given in Case 3, answer the following questions.

27 Which of the following conditions is the *least* likely diagnosis for Lisa?

a Anorexia nervosa (AN)

b Avoidant/restrictive food intake disorder

c Binge-eating disorder

d Bulimia nervosa (BN)

e None of the above

28 In Dr. Lee's office, Lisa reveals that she has significant concerns about being "too fat" and not "attractive." Her mother further reports that Lisa likes to measure her waist size many times a day, which often disappoints Lisa because of her perceived large waist size. Which of the following criteria *must* be present to formally diagnose Lisa with AN based on DSM-5?

a Amenorrhea

b Denial of having any problems

c Galactorrhea

d Intense fear of gaining weight

e Using laxatives

29 Based on DSM-5, which of the following should be used to determine whether Lisa has a "significant low body weight" to qualify for the diagnosis of AN?

a Less than minimal normal weight

b BMI-for-age percentile < fifth percentile

c BMI between 16 and 16.99

d BMI between 15 and 15.99

e BMI < 15

30 What is the *minimal* length of time that Lisa must have engaged in recurrent episodes of binge eating or purging behavior to meet criteria for AN, binge-eating/purging type?

a One month

b Three months

c Six months

d Nine months

e Twelve months

31 During the course of Lisa's illness, she continues to lose weight (down to 73 pounds) over time while receiving outpatient psychotherapy. She is hospitalized on a pediatric unit with a plan that a longer hospitalization on a psychiatric unit may be needed. Lisa is *least* likely to show which of the following physical signs?

a Bradycardia

b Emaciation

c Hypertension

d Lanugo

e Peripheral edema

32 Lisa is *least* likely to have which of the following laboratory findings in the hospital?

a Elevated blood urea nitrogen level

b Hypocholesterolemia

c Leukopenia

d Lymphocytosis

e Osteoporosis

33 Lisa's mother asks Dr. Lee what the potential risk of mortality is for Lisa. Which of the following numbers reflecting the crude mortality rate for AN per decade should Dr. Lee use to inform her?

a Approximately 1%

b Approximately 2%

c Approximately 5%

d Approximately 10%

e Approximately 15%

34 During the hospitalization on the pediatric unit, Lisa voices strong suicidal ideation, which results in her being transferred to a psychiatric unit because of safety concerns. Based on the epidemiologic data, what is the reported suicide rate in patients with AN?

a 1/100,000 per year

b 12/100,000 per year

c 23/100,000 per year

d 46/100,000 per year

e 53/100,000 per year

35 Lisa's inpatient treatment for AN will likely include all of the following *except*:

a Calorie prescriptions

b Meal plans

c In-depth psychotherapy exploring disordered thoughts

d Limits on physical activity

e Disruption of compensatory behaviors such as purging

36 During her inpatient treatment, Lisa is monitored for refeeding syndrome. All of the following are signs of refeeding syndrome *except*:

a Hypophosphatemia

b Edema

c Dysrhythmias on EKG

d Hyperkalemia

e Hypomagnesemia

37 Dr. Lee is called by the hospital treatment team, requesting recommendations for treating Lisa with psychotropic medications for her sleeping problems and anxiety around eating. Which of the following medications has case reports/open-label trials data to support its potential usefulness for Lisa?

a Aripiprazole

b Clozapine

c Olanzapine

d Quetiapine

e Ziprasidone

38 After some weight gain and being medically and psychiatrically stabilized, Lisa has no more suicidal ideation and does not meet criteria for inpatient care anymore. She is subsequently discharged back to her home with her family. She is still overall underweight. Per Dr. Lee's recommendation, family-based treatment is initiated. Which of the following is a phase(s) of such treatment?

a Restoration of Lisa's weight

b Handing control over eating back to Lisa

c Discussion of Lisa's developmental issues

d b and c

e All of the above

Case 4

Sophia is a 16-year-old pansexual-identified girl. Her mother took Sophia to the emergency room (ER) after finding her daughter in the bathroom with cuts on her forearms. In the ER, Sophia was found to have multiple superficial lacerations on her left forearm with no need for suturing. Sophia reported to the ER doctor that her girlfriend broke up with her the day before, which made her very angry, and she stated "I just want to feel it" and denied any intent to die.

Questions 39–52. Based on the information given in Case 4, answer the following questions.

39 Which of the following is the *least* appropriate first step that the ER doctor should consider for Sophia?

a Inquiring about previous suicidal ideations and suicide attempts

b Inquiring about the intent of prior suicide acts

c Assessing environmental and family factors

d Asking the availability of transportation for her to go back home with her mother

e Assessing accessibility of suicide methods

40 Which of the following would put Sophia at a lower suicide risk?

a High impulse control

b Low level of hopelessness and helplessness

c Future-orientated mindset

d Communicating openly about her thoughts of suicide

e All of the above

41 In the ER, when interviewed by Dr. Smith (the ER doctor), Sophia revealed that her father has been sexually molesting her repeatedly when she visits him on weekends. Sophia told Dr. Smith she never told this to anyone else. Reportedly, Sophia's parents divorced when she was 14 years old, and she lives with her mother primarily and visits her father on some weekends. The molestation consisted of genital fondling and has not involved penetration. Dr. Smith has a strong suspicion of child sexual abuse. Which of the following actions is *most* appropriate for Dr. Smith to be involved in next?

a Filing a report to appropriate authorities immediately

b Notifying Sophia's father that the suspected child abuse will be reported to authorities

c Instructing the ER social worker to see Sophia and then to decide whether a formal report should be filed

d Allowing Sophia to return home with her father before further evaluation or investigation

e Continuing the ER risk assessment without notifying the authorities because penetration did not occur

42 According to the ER medical records, this was one of many ER visits Sophia had in the past year, which are usually due to self-injurious behaviors (such as cutting, overdosing on drugs, using shoelaces to suffocate herself, etc.). They were usually triggered by depression, child–parent relational conflicts, and breakups with different boyfriends or girlfriends after short-term intimate relationships. Her urine toxicological screen was positive for cannabis, which she admitted was her drug of choice. She also reported recurrent episodes of drinking alcohol excessively and being extremely drunk to the point that she passed out. She further reported recurrent episodes of self-induced vomiting followed by binge-eating episodes. Sophia's mother reported that Sophia has been very moody, and at times her mood changed quickly from intense dysphoria, irritability, and anxiety to being intrusive, giggly, with milder euphoric within a few hours. She was reportedly impulsive and tended to act before thinking. She occasionally maintained sexual relationships with a few teenagers simultaneously. Which of the following personality disorders *most* fits Sophia's presentation and history?

a Antisocial personality disorder

b Avoidant personality disorder

c Borderline personality disorder

d Histrionic personality disorder

e Narcissistic personality disorder

43 Even though Sophia is only 16 years old, her outpatient treating psychiatrist has considered borderline personality disorder as one of the working diagnoses. Based on follow-up studies, in ten years, how likely is it that Sophia will still meet full criteria for borderline personality disorder (BPD)?

a 10%

b 30%

c 50%

d 70%

e 90%

44 Based on epidemiologic studies, all of the following conditions are likely to occur at higher rates in the first-degree relatives of Sophia if her diagnosis of BPD is confirmed *except*:

a Depression

b Other mood disorders

c Substance abuse

d Schizophrenia spectrum disorder

e None of the above

45 Based on structural neuroimaging studies, which of the following is the *least* likely finding from individuals with BPD?

a Increased serotonergic neurotransmission in cortical inhibitory areas

b Bilateral increased activation of the amygdala to affective stimuli

c Increased left amygdala activation to facial emotional expression

d Reduced amygdala size

e Reduced hippocampal size

46 Among all of the following treatment modalities, based on empirical support, which one is *most* useful for not only addressing Sophia's problems related to her repeated suicidal ideation and self-injurious behaviors, but also for helping her depression, anxiety, and social/interpersonal functioning?

a Dialectical-behavioral therapy (DBT)

b Interpersonal psychotherapy

c Mentalization-based treatment (MBT)

d Brief psychodynamic psychotherapy

e None of the above

47 Which of the following is the *least* appropriate antidepressant to be considered for Sophia?

a Bupropion

b Citalopram

c Escitalopram

d Sertraline

e Venlafaxine

48 After thorough evaluation, Sophia was determined to meet the full criteria for major depressive disorder (MDD). Which of the following antidepressants is FDA approved for treating youth (under age 18 years) with MDD?

a Bupropion

b Citalopram

c Escitalopram

d Sertraline

e Venlafaxine

49 During the course of her outpatient treatment (a few months after the discharge from the hospital ER), she suddenly developed symptoms that were consistent with a hypomanic episode when she had not been on any antidepressant and had been sober and clean for approximately two months. Which of the following is the *most* appropriate diagnosis that should be given to her at this time?

a Bipolar I disorder

b Bipolar II disorder

c Cyclothymic disorder

d Disruptive mood dysregulation disorder

e Substance/medication-induced bipolar and related disorder

50 Given the new symptom manifestation by Sophia, which of the following medications should be avoided as a monotherapy agent?

a Fluoxetine

b Lamotrigine

c Lithium

d Seroquel

e Ziprasidone

51 Sophia's outpatient psychiatrist learned that Sophia is a patient of Chinese ancestry. Before considering treating her with carbamazepine, which of the following specific tests should be completed before initiation of the medication?

a TSH

b Kidney functioning test

c Urine analysis

d Test for HLA-B*1502

e CYP 2D6 polymorphism

52 The drug levels of which of the following medications are most likely to be increased if administered together with carbamazepine?

a Aripiprazole

b Lamotrigine

c Lithium

d Valproate

e Oral contraceptives

Case 5

Tommy, a 7-year-old boy, presented with intense eye blinking for the past three weeks. His mother brought him to see his child psychiatrist, Dr. Jackson, for an evaluation and additional intervention because the symptoms were not only noticeable to others, but also interfered with his school functioning. Reportedly, he could not maintain visual attention in the classroom, and peers started making fun of him. His mother recalled that Tommy has experienced recurrent eye-blinking episodes since he was 5 years old, and the symptoms wax and wane in severity. Reportedly, he was seen by a neurologist and the tic symptoms were determined not to be attributable to the physiological effects of any substance or another medical condition. Tommy's mother also noted that he displayed symptoms of inattention and hyperactivity as well as repetitive, intrusive thoughts accompanied by ritualized behaviors.

Questions 53–65. Based on the information given in Case 5, answer the following questions.

53 Based on DSM-5, Tommy meets criteria for which of the following tic disorders?

a Persistent (chronic) motor or vocal tic disorder, with motor tics only

b Persistent (chronic) motor or vocal tic disorder, with vocal tics only

c Provisional tic disorder

d Tourette's disorder

e Transient tic disorder

54 Tommy's mother noted that Tommy's blinking episodes are sometimes followed by shoulder shrugging. Which of the following terms describes his tics accurately?

a Complex motor tics

b Complex vocal tics

c Simple motor tics

d Simple vocal tics

e None of the above

55 Over the next few months, Tommy's tics seemed to become worse. His eye-blinking episodes lasted longer, which, at times, occurred simultaneously with making a throat-clearing noise and repeating his own words. Which of the following terms describes the phenomenon of repeating his own words?

a Coprolalia

b Copropraxia

c Echolalia

d Echopraxia

e Palilalia

56 At this time, Tommy presented to Dr. Jackson's office again. Which of the following tic disorder diagnoses is *most* appropriate for Tommy?

a Persistent (chronic) motor or vocal tic disorder, with motor tics only

b Persistent (chronic) motor or vocal tic disorder, with vocal tics only

c Provisional tic disorder

d Tourette's disorder

e Transient tic disorder

57 Tommy may experience symptoms of other comorbid psychiatric conditions related to his tic disorder. Dr. Jackson is *most* likely to find Tommy experiencing the symptoms associated with which of the following potential comorbid conditions?

a Generalized anxiety disorder (GAD)

b Major depressive disorder (MDD)

c Attention-deficit/hyperactivity disorder (ADHD)

d Obsessive-compulsive disorder (OCD)

e None of the above

58 Tommy's mother asked Dr. Jackson about the genetic risks of Tourette's disorder in regard to her future grandchildren. Based on genetic studies, Dr. Jackson should tell Tommy's mother which of the following numbers *correctly* reflects the approximate chance that Tommy's children will have Tourette's disorder?

a 2–5%

b 5–10%

c 10–15%

d 15–25%

e > 25%

59 Which of the following is the *most* important treatment aspect of Tommy's tic disorder that Dr. Jackson should consider during the initial treatment phase?

a CBT

b DBT

c Psychoeducational interventions

d Neurosurgical intervention

e Pharmacological interventions

60 Dr. Jackson prescribed habit reversal training (HRT) to Tommy for his Tourette's disorder. Dr. Jackson explained to Tommy and his mother that HRT includes two main aspects: (1) awareness training; and (2) competing response practice. The goal of awareness training is to enhance Tommy's awareness of his own tics. Which of the following should *not* be a component of such training?

a Response description

b Response detection

c Early warning procedure

d Situational awareness training

e None of the above

61 Tommy's mother asked Dr. Jackson about the course and prognosis of Tommy's tic disorder. Dr. Jackson should inform her of all of the following *except*:

a Peak severity usually occurs in mid adolescence.

b Tic symptoms may diminish in adulthood.

c Tic symptoms may be persistently severe or even worse in adulthood.

d The tic severity tends to wax and wane.

e When children get older, they are more likely to report premonitory urge.

62 With HRT, Tommy's tics diminished in severity. Teacher and parent reports reflected ongoing impairment from inattention, hyperactivity, and impulsivity. Which of the following medications should Dr. Jackson consider?

a Amphetamine salts

b Methylphenidate

c Guanfacine

d Clonidine

e Any of the above

63 Which of the following medications is FDA approved for the treatment of Tourette's disorder in youth?

a Aripiprazole

b Haloperidol

c Olanzapine

d Quetiapine

e Ziprasidone

64 Dr. Jackson also prescribed an SSRI for Tommy's OCD symptoms. Which of the following is a *better* augmenting agent to enhance the SSRI's anti-OCD effect if OCD symptoms are refractory?

a An antipsychotic

b Another SSRI

c Clonidine

d Lithium

e Valproate acid

65 Many studies have been conducted on the effectiveness of neurosurgical interventions for severe and intractable tics in adults. Which of the following techniques could be a promising alternative to the neurosurgical interventions?

a Deep brain stimulation (DBS)

b Electroconvulsive therapy (ECT)

c Magnetic seizure therapy (MST)

d Transcranial magnetic stimulation (TMS)

e Vagus nerve stimulation (VNS)

Case 6

April was a 9-year-old girl when she was initially brought to see a child psychiatrist (Dr. Schmitt) to evaluate her experience of acute hallucinations and delusions. April's mother reported that April was born full term, and the pregnancy was complicated by a maternal viral illness. The delivery was prolonged, which led to a Cesarean section. Early infancy and childhood development was unremarkable, but the mother of the child (MOC) could not remember clearly the timelines of April's developmental milestones. April's teachers noted she was shy when she was in daycare and subsequently in kindergarten. During her first two years in a public school, she had some difficulty learning and retaining information, and her teachers noted that she had only a limited number of peers with whom she interacted. A few weeks prior to this visit to the child psychiatrist for evaluation, April seemed increasingly withdrawn and was observed talking to herself. In Dr. Schmitt's office, April reported that she had been hearing things (mostly single words) for the past three weeks, but she could not describe them well. She also reported she believed that she would be kidnapped, with a significant fear of being killed. She had not been able to go to school and had locked herself in her bedroom with intense fears for the past ten days.

Questions 66–80. Based on the information given in Case 6, answer the following questions.

66 At this time, which of the following differential diagnoses can Dr. Schmitt rule out?

a Autism spectrum disorder

b Major depressive disorder

c Generalized anxiety disorder or PTSD

d Psychosis, which can potentially lead to childhood-onset schizophrenia (COS)

e None of the above

67 Dr. Schmitt further learned that even though April was shy as a child, she always wanted to play with similar-age children and peers. She had fair relationships with her two older siblings and her parents. There was no history of trauma or any abuse. She never demonstrated any restricted, repetitive patterns of behavior, interests, or activities that were consistent with autism spectrum disorders. According to MOC, April's recent medical evaluations with her pediatrician failed to reveal a specific medical explanation for her presentations. In the office, Dr. Schmitt did not elicit any significant symptoms that were consistent with major mood disorders or anxiety disorders, signs of PTSD, or substance influences. April's anxiety and withdrawn behavior seemed to be the result of her perceptual disturbances. On a mental status examination, April was noticed to have a blunt affect, with loose associations and marked tangential thinking. She also reported seeing monsters and ghost-like images. April appeared to respond to internal stimuli as well. According to MOC, April's father and paternal grandmother were previously diagnosed with schizophrenia. Family psychiatric history was also positive for depression on the maternal side of the family. April's 16-year-old brother was previously psychiatrically hospitalized for psychosis and self-injurious behaviors. Which of the following diagnoses is *most* appropriate based on the new information?

a Brief psychotic disorder

b Delusional disorder

c Schizophreniform disorder

d Separation anxiety disorder

e Schizophrenia (COS)

68 Dr. Schmitt initiated a low dose of risperidone for April. April only had a partial response. Dr. Schmitt also ordered psychological testing. The Rorschach inkblot test for April revealed marked thought problems along with a pattern of odd, bizarre interpretations of the inkblots, which indicated psychotic processes. Her recent brain MRI showed no lesions or tumors. Two months after taking low-dose risperidone, April was psychiatrically hospitalized because of her increasingly disorganized speech and grossly disorganized behaviors along with the ongoing hallucinations. The voices became clearer to her and started making comments about her and instructing her to kill herself. Which of the following diagnoses is *most* appropriate based on the new information?

a Brief psychotic disorder

b Delusional disorder

c Schizophreniform disorder

d Separation anxiety disorder

e Schizophrenia (COS)

69 April's risperidone dose was titrated up during the hospital stay, and her response to the treatment improved during the next six months. However, April continued to experience significant residual hallucinations. She was not able to go back to her regular school. She had to do homeschooling, her academic performance deteriorated over time, and she had significant difficulties catching up. She still believed that she might be kidnapped by someone on the street and was unable to leave her house if not accompanied by her parents. Which of the following diagnoses is *most* appropriate based on the new information?

a Brief psychotic disorder

b Delusional disorder

c Schizophreniform disorder

d Separation anxiety disorder

e Schizophrenia (COS)

70 Which of the following is the *least* likely finding on April's neuropsychological functioning test report?

a Poor performance on tasks involving attention

b Poor performance on tasks involving fine motor coordination

c Poor performance on tasks involving rote language skills and simple perceptual processing

d Poor performance on tasks involving the short-term memory

e Poor performance on tasks involving working memory

71 Based on recent neuroimaging studies, which of the following is *most* likely a finding of follow-up brain MRI scans for April over the next 5–10 years?

a Decreased ventricular volume

b Increased total cortical gray matter

c Increased frontal gray matter

d Increased medial temporal gray matter

e Pattern of back to front gray matter loss

72 Investigating possible genetic causes of April's presentation, which of the following cytogenetic abnormalities is the *most* likely responsible one if her presentation is truly influenced by a genetic syndrome?

a A deletion of a large segment of chromosome 7

b A deletion on 15q11-q13

c A deletion on 22q11

d Mutations on MeCP2 gene

e Numerous CGG repeats in FMR-1 gene

73 April's cytogenetic tests were negative and she continued to take risperidone until she came back to see Dr. Schmitt for one of her follow-up visits at the age of 11 years. According to April and MOC, April had been gaining a lot of weight, and also complained of tenderness, enlargement, and engorgement of her breasts. She also showed signs of hirsutism and galactorrhea. Dr. Schmitt believed April was experiencing significant side effects from risperidone. Which of the follow laboratory tests is *most* likely to clarify the cause of these symptoms?

a Liver function tests

b Lipid profile tests

c Hemoglobin A1C

d Prolactin level

e Complete blood cell counts

74 Which of the following neurotransmission mechanisms can *best* explain April's side effects from the risperidone?

a Alpha adrenergic blockade ($\alpha2$ blockade)

b Dopaminergic blockade (D_2 blockade)

c Histamine blockade (H_1 blockade)

d Muscarinic blockade (M_1 blockade)

e Serotonergic agonist ($5\text{-}HT_{2A}$ agonist)

75 To avoid prolactin-related side effects, which of the following antipsychotics is the *best* alternative to risperidone for treating April's psychosis?

a Aripiprazole

b Haloperidol

c Olanzapine

d Quetiapine

e Ziprasidone

76 Dr. Schmitt continued to see April for the following six years as an outpatient, during which time April was psychiatrically hospitalized twice during major depressive episodes with severe suicidal ideation and intent to die. Different antidepressants were tried in addition to antipsychotic therapy. Based on April's medical records and treatment history, Dr. Schmitt believed that April overall experienced a much longer duration of active depressive symptoms with many recurrent major depressive episodes than psychotic symptoms. April's psychotic symptoms fluctuated over time, and for the most part April seemed able to deal with them well. She was also free of any psychosis during a few major depressive episodes. However, her hallucinations could also continue to be present for more than a few weeks at a time even when her depressive symptoms were minimal. Overall, April had been physically healthy and was not involved with alcohol or any illicit drugs. Which of the following diagnoses is *most* appropriate based on the new information?

a Brief psychotic disorder

b Delusion disorder

c Schizophreniform disorder

d Schizoaffective disorder

e Schizophrenia

77 April's mother was wondering about April's lifetime risk of suicide. Which of the following *accurately* reflects such a rate that Dr. Schmitt should share with MOC?

a 1%

b 5%

c 10%

d 15%

e 20%

78 Discussing with MOC the prevalence, development/course, and risk factors from schizoaffective disorder (SAD), all of the following are accurate for Dr. Schmitt to share with MOC *except*:

a Schizoaffective disorder is only one-third as common as schizophrenia with lifetime prevalence of approximately 0.3%.

b The incidence of SAD is higher in males than in females.

c There is an increased incidence of the depressive type among females.

d People with a family history of schizophrenia, SAD, or bipolar disorder in their first-degree relatives may have an increased risk for SAD.

e African American and Hispanic populations are more likely to be overdiagnosed with schizophrenia compared with SAD.

79 April's mother continued worrying about April's current weight-related issues (at the age of 17 years) after so many years of taking different psychotropic medications. Which of the following is *not* a criterion to define whether she had a metabolic syndrome?

a Adjusted fasting glucose ≥ 100 mg/dL (fasting glucose ≥ 110 mg/dL)

b Blood pressure ≥ 90th percentile for age and sex

c Fasting HDL < 40mg/dL

d Fasting triglyceride ≥ 110 mg/dL

e Waist circumference > 35 inches (88 cm)

80 To qualify for metabolic syndrome, April had to meet how many out of the five criteria?

a 1

b 2

c 3

d 4

e 5

Case 7

Ryan is a 10-year-old male brought in by his divorced parents for challenges with frequent tantrums and irritability. Tantrums tend to occur in the context of limit setting, especially around screen time. They consist of screaming, throwing things, and sometimes hitting. Ryan takes a long time to calm down afterward. His family history is notable for bipolar disorder in his father and ADHD in his older brother.

Questions 81–92. Based on the information given in Case 7, answer the following questions.

81 At this time, which of the following differential diagnoses can be ruled out?

a ADHD

b Disruptive mood dysregulation disorder (DMDD)

c Oppositional defiant disorder (ODD)

d MDD

e None of the above

82 Which of the following does *not* include irritability as part of the diagnostic criteria?

a MDD

b GAD

c ADHD

d ODD

e Bipolar II disorder

83 What question would Ryan's psychiatrist *not* need to ask to make a diagnosis of DMDD?

a What is his mood like between tantrums?

b Does he often make careless mistakes?

c How often does he have tantrums?

d Do these symptoms occur in other settings besides home?

e Has he had discrete episodes of irritability, increased goal-directed activity, and/or decreased need for sleep?

84 Parents describe that Ryan has always been an irritable kid prone to tantrums, but that this has become more problematic as he's gotten older. Smaller tantrums happen daily with large ones at least three times a week. Even small frustrations can trigger them. Between outbursts, he tends to be irritable. Teachers have also reported problems at school with him not following directions, acting impulsively, getting in fights with one of his peers, and getting upset when he doesn't get his way. If Ryan is diagnosed with DMDD, what other diagnosis can he not be given?

a MDD

b GAD

c ADHD

d ODD

e PTSD

85 Which of the following distinguishes DMDD from intermittent explosive disorder (IED)?

a Persistent irritability between outbursts

b Recurrent outbursts

c Presence of ADHD

d Physical aggression

e Impairments in interpersonal functioning

86 Which is an FDA-approved treatment for DMDD?

a Fluoxetine

b Risperidone

c Methylphenidate

d Lamotrigine

e None of the above

87 Ryan's parents are worried that his frequent changes in mood may mean he has bipolar disorder, especially given his family history. Which of the following aspects of Ryan's presentation is most reassuring that he does not currently meet criteria for bipolar disorder?

a He is too young to have bipolar disorder.

b His mood is irritable rather than euphoric.

c His mood changes multiple times per day or week.

d His not following directions and impulsivity suggest ADHD rather than bipolar disorder.

e His not following directions, irritability, and fighting suggest ODD rather than bipolar disorder.

88 To make a diagnosis of ODD, which of the following would need to be true of the symptoms in Ryan's case?

a Symptoms must be present in each of three categories.

b Symptoms must be present in multiple settings.

c Symptoms must be present on most days.

d Symptoms must be present for at least six months.

e Symptoms must be present with at least one individual who is not a parent.

89 If Ryan is diagnosed with ODD, pharmacological treatment of which concurrent disorder, if present, would be most likely to lead to a reduction in oppositional behaviors?

a ADHD

b MDD

c DMDD

d GAD

e ASD

90 Ryan and his family move out of state and return five years later. At age 15, Ryan continues to exhibit many of the same behaviors, and his parents are additionally concerned about more serious aggression and rule violations. He also continues to have impulsive behavior and difficulty staying on task and following directions. To make a diagnosis of conduct disorder, which of the following must be true of Ryan's symptoms?

a Symptoms must be present in each of four categories.

b There must be at least three criteria present in the past 12 months.

c Limited prosocial emotions must be present.

d Criteria must be met by age 15.

e Symptoms must not meet criteria for antisocial personality disorder.

91 Ryan is diagnosed with conduct disorder and ADHD. His parents indicate that the aggressive behavior is the highest priority and ask if the psychiatrist can prescribe medication to treat it. Which of the following statements would most accurately address the inquiry?

a There are FDA-approved medications for aggression occurring in the setting of conduct disorder.

b The only evidence for medication being effective for aggression is for aggression in the setting of autism spectrum disorder.

c The risks outweigh the benefits of using atypical antipsychotics to treat aggressive behavior.

d Stimulant medication may be effective in treating the aggression.

e Stimulant medication should be avoided due to increasing the risk of substance abuse in an adolescent with conduct disorder.

92 Which of the following interventions would be *least* recommended for Ryan's aggressive and antisocial behaviors?

a Pharmacotherapy

b Family therapy

c Individual psychotherapy for Ryan

d Parent training

e Enrollment in a juvenile awareness (deterrence) program

ANSWERS AND EXPLANATIONS

Case 1

1 **(e)** Based on the case description, all of the listed differential diagnoses should be considered because any of them could be the primary diagnosis without knowing additional information. *(Ref. 4, pp. 33–86)*

2 **(a)** Sam does seem to present with a spectrum of symptoms that are commonly seen in children with autism spectrum disorder. However, if Sam does not meet criteria for autism spectrum disorder, other conditions should be considered and evaluated, especially because children with social (pragmatic) communication disorder can present with a similar picture. The lack of abnormal nonverbal communications and the absence of restricted, repetitive patterns of behavior, interests, or activities can help distinguish language disorders or social communication disorder from autism spectrum disorder. *(Ref. 4, pp. 50–59)*

3 **(c)** Intellectual impairment is not required to diagnose autism spectrum disorder based on DSM-5. In DSM-5, autism spectrum disorder can be specified "with or without accompanying intellectual impairment." Additional specifiers can be used to describe the severity level as the following: Level 1—requiring support; Level 2—requiring substantial support; and Level 3—requiring very substantial support. *(Ref. 4, pp. 51–53)*

4 **(b)** A brain MRI is not a current routine diagnostic tool for autism spectrum disorder even though it has been applied in clinical research for neurodevelopmental disorders. However, appropriate medical and neurological consultation and evaluation can help to rule out other medical conditions that can manifest as autism spectrum disorder or are comorbid with autism spectrum disorder, such as tuberos sclerosis, neurofibromatosis, epilepsy (especially because Sam has staring spells—could be an absence seizure). Other listed evaluations or tests are important in the clinical evaluation of Sam. In addition, gathering historical information about early development, medical and family history, assessment of developmental, psychosocial and adaptive functioning, and psychiatric evaluation are applicable to this case. *(Ref. 3, Ch. 5.2.1, Differential Diagnosis section)*

5 **(d)** The correct way to document his diagnosis is with "autism spectrum disorder, associated with a known medical or genetic condition or environmental factor." This is so with the diagnosis of Fragile X syndrome, Down syndrome, or Rett syndrome (mostly applicable for girls), or the patient is confirmed to have a known medical condition, such as epilepsy, or a history of environmental exposure, such as fetal alcohol syndrome, very low birth weight, and valproate, etc. PDD NOS is no longer a diagnosis in DSM-5. *(Ref. 4, pp. 50–53)*

6 **(d)** Neurofibromatosis, an autosomal dominant disease, often presents with café-au-lait spots throughout the body along with neural-derived tumors, and approximately 50% of affected individuals have intellectual disabilities. The associated gene, NF1, has several different mutations and was recently identified. *(Ref. 3, Ch. 3.3.3, Learning section)*

7 **(c)** Landau-Kleffner syndrome is associated with loss of previously acquired language skills, abnormal EEG, and epilepsy. Language regression may affect social skills. The presentation can be confused with autism spectrum disorder. *(Ref. 3, Ch. 7.2.4, Intellectual disability section)*

8 **(e)** Level of severity depends primarily on adaptive functioning, not on IQ score. Both individualized, standardized intellectual testing and clinical assessment are needed to assess deficits in intellectual functions. Adaptive functioning determines the level of support the individual with ID needs, and IQ measures are less valid, especially at the lower end of the IQ ranges. Assessment of ID in individuals with autism spectrum disorder is more of a challenge because of poorer social communication and behavior deficits, which often interfere with understanding or complying with the testing procedures. In addition, IQ scores are less stable, especially in early childhood, for children with autism spectrum disorder. Thus, reassessment over time may be needed. *(Ref. 4, pp. 33–40)*

9 **(c)** Modified from ABA, the Picture Exchange Communication System (PECS) is specifically used for children with an autism spectrum disorder who are nonverbal to help them learn symbolic communication. *(Ref. 1, Ch. 8, Treatment section)*

10 **(a)** Both aripiprazole and risperidone are FDA approved for the treatment of irritability associated with autism spectrum disorder in children (ages: 6–17 years for aripiprazole; 5–17 years for risperidone). *(Ref. 1, Ch. 8, Treatment section)*

11 **(d)** Research studies have shown neurostructural changes associated with autism spectrum disorder, but the significance of these for prognosis is not yet known. Lack of joint attention by age 4 years, lack of functional speech by age 5 years, intellectual disability, seizure, and comorbid medical or psychiatric conditions are all predictors for a poor prognosis. Early intervention, successful inclusion in regular education and community settings, and a higher level of cognitive adaptive functioning predict better outcomes. *(Johnson & Myers 2007)*

12 **(c)** Based on the case description, Sam does meet criteria for both ADHD, combined presentation and autism spectrum disorder. Thus, both diagnoses should be given. In DSM-IV, ADHD and autism spectrum disorder are exclusive to each other. In DSM-5, the two diagnoses are allowed to be given together when ADHD symptoms exceed those typically seen in individuals of comparable age. *(Ref. 4, p. 58)*

Case 2

13 **(e)** The case description does not provide enough specific information to exclude any of the listed conditions as a potential differential diagnosis, which should be broad at this time. *(Ref. 4, pp. 59–66)*

14 **(b)** Based on developmental history and current social and communication skills, autism spectrum disorder is unlikely. However, all other conditions are still possible. *(Ref. 4, pp. 50–51)*

15 **(e)** All answers except (e) capture specific learning disorder with impairment in reading and specific learning disorder with impairment in mathematics, which Eric has. When either the term "dyslexia" or "dyscalculia" is used, DSM-5 requests that the specific difficulties that are present be specified. *(Ref. 4, pp. 66–70)*

16 **(e)** Under IDEA, he will most likely be qualified for special education based on the category of SLD. *(Ref. 3, Ch. 7.3, Special Education section)*

17 **(c)** The Children's Global Assessment Scale (CGAS) is one of the scales used for assessment of functional impairment and adaptive function. *(Ref. 5, Ch. 36.1, Rating Scales section)*

18 **(c)** All the symptoms listed can be supportive of the diagnosis of PTSD. However, based on DSM-5, to diagnose PTSD in children 6 years and younger, there must be two (or more) symptoms existing to support the Criterion D "alternations in arousal and reactivity associated with the traumatic event(s)" including: irritable behavior and anger outbursts, hypervigilance, exaggerated startle response, problems with concentration, and sleep disturbance. *(Ref. 4, pp. 272–273)*

19 **(d)** Among all the listed concerns, cardiac risk is least concerning. There is no strong empirical support for using SSRIs in children with PTSD. Studies also do not demonstrate greater benefit when sertraline is added to trauma-focused CBT. The FDA has a black box warning for suicidal ideation when using antidepressants in youth up to age 24 years. *(Ref. 1, Ch. 16, Treatment section)*

20 **(e)** Among all the listed interventions, trauma-focused cognitive-behavioral therapy (TF-CBT) has the strongest evidence for support from multiple published randomized controlled trials. *(Ref. 1, Ch. 16, Treatment section)*

21 **(d)** Microcephaly associated with FAS is found to be related to the inhibition of NMDA receptor activity, which leads to widespread apoptosis in the immature/developing cortex. *(Ref. 5, Ch. 1.10, Clinical Aspects of Ion Channels section)*

22 **(d)** Routine EKG screening or other specific cardiologic evaluation prior to the initiation of stimulant medications treatment in otherwise healthy youth is not required. However, if the child has a history of a cardiovascular disease or significant cardiac symptoms (e.g., severe palpitation, fainting, and exercise intolerance), a strong family history of sudden death, unexplained chest pain, family history of arrhythmia and syncope, etc., a cardiologic consultation and evaluation is recommended. *(Ref. 1, Ch. 10, Pediatric Evaluation section)*

23 **(c)** D-amphetamine is released from l-lysine via a rate-limiting enzymatic hydrolysis process to become an active stimulant compound. *(Ref. 5, Ch. 45.1, Formulations section)*

24 **(a)** Antipsychotics such as aripiprazole are not indicated in the treatment of ADHD except in severely ill children who are not responding to other choices. They may be needed for youth with ADHD who also have comorbid symptoms such as mood lability and aggression. Stimulants are the first-line drug of choice for ADHD in general. Atomoxetine and alpha-2 agonists such as extended-release guanfacine and clonidine can be considered. *(Ref. 1, Ch. 10, Treatment section)*

25 **(d)** Gathering information from and consulting with other providers, such as primary care physicians, schoolteachers, counselor, speech therapist, and psychologist are important parts of collaboration. However, the Health Insurance Portability and Accountability Act (HIPAA) restricts unauthorized disclosure of medical information to certain parties, such as school, daycare, social welfare departments, and insurance companies. The patient or legal guardian must give consent before such disclosure occurs; otherwise, it can be counted as breach of confidentiality and a HIPAA violation. In Eric's case, because he is living in a foster home, he is likely under state jurisdiction (a dependent of the court). If his parents have lost legal rights to give the consent, only his "legal guardian" or "legal representative" can give such consent. It can be similar to his psychotropic medication informed consent process; his "legal guardian" has such authority to give consent, and he may give assent (as a child). Different states may have different laws or regulations regarding who can be considered a "legal guardian" when parents have lost their legal rights to consent. In certain states, such as in California, it is usually the court that grants the approval for psychotropic medications for children who are court dependent. Minors can consent to treatment on their own behalf in some situations (e.g., to seek treatment for sexually transmitted diseases in all states, and to seek treatment for substance abuse in most states). *(Ref. 3, Ch. 7.4.4, HIPAA section)*

26 **(e)** The way to guarantee success of the proposed treatment is not a part of the discussion. In fact, clinicians are generally not able to guarantee treatment success for a specific treatment proposal. The potential benefits and possible successful rate of the proposed treatment should be included in the discussion. Potential outcomes with and without the proposed treatment should be discussed as well. *(Ref. 3, Ch. 7.4.4, Improper Treatment section)*

Case 3

27 **(c)** Binge-eating disorder is characterized by recurrent eating of unusually large amounts food in discrete periods, with a sense of lack of control over the eating behavior. The binge eating cannot be associated with inappropriate compensatory behaviors such as self-induced vomiting, as seen in AN and BN. It does not usually cause weight loss. Instead, it can lead to weight gain and obesity. *(Ref. 4, pp. 350–351)*

28 **(d)** Based on DSM-5, three criteria have to be present to formally diagnose AN: restricted food intake leading to a significant weight loss (A); intense fear of gaining weight or becoming fat (B); and disturbance in the way one's body weight or shape is experienced (C). Amenorrhea is one of the common physical signs of AN; however, it is no longer a necessary diagnostic criterion for AN in DSM-5. *(Ref. 4, pp. 338–339)*

29 **(b)** Based on DSM-5, "significant low weight" is defined as weight that is less than that minimally expected (not "minimally normal") for children and adolescents. CDC BMI-for-age percentile is often used in youth rather than simple numerical BMI guidelines as used in adults. In general, the CDC-BMI-for-age below the fifth percentile is used to suggest underweight for children and adolescents. However, children with a BMI percentile above this line can be sometimes considered underweight in light of failure to maintain their expected growth trajectory. In DSM-5, the severity of AN in adults is specified by BMI (mild-BMI: ≥ 17; moderate-BMI: 16–16.99; severe-BMI: 15–15.99; extreme-BMI <15). *(Ref. 4, pp. 338–339)*

30 **(b)** Lisa has to engage in recurrent episodes of binge eating or purging behavior during the past three months to meet criteria for AN, binge-eating/purging type. *(Ref. 4, p. 339)*

31 **(c)** Hypotension (not hypertension) is one of the common physical signs of an emaciated patient with AN. Other physical signs may include hypothermia, hypercarotenemia, hypertrophy of the salivary glands, dental enamel erosion, and scars or calluses on the dorsal surface of the hand (some of these signs are due to self-induced vomiting). *(Ref. 4, p. 343)*

32 **(b)** Hypercholesterolemia is one of the common serum chemistry findings in patients with AN. Other serum chemistry changes may include elevated liver enzymes, hypomagnesemia, hypozincemia, hypophosphatemia, and hyperamylasemia. Metabolic alkalosis, hypochloremia, and hypokalemia can be seen because of self-induced vomiting. Mild metabolic acidosis may occur because of laxative abuse. Loss of all cell types (leukopenia) can be seen in the CBC test, but lymphocytosis is also common. *(Ref. 4, pp. 342–343)*

33 **(c)** Even though most patients with AN remit within five years, the crude mortality rate (CMR) is still high, approximately 5%, which is most commonly due to medical complications and/or suicide. *(Ref. 4, p. 342)*

34 **(b)** The estimated suicide risk for patients with AN is 12/100,000 per year. Thus, it is important to assess suicide risk in patients with AN along with common comorbid conditions such as mood disorders, anxiety disorders, OCD, substance use, etc. *(Ref. 4, pp. 343–345)*

35 **(c)** Weight restoration is the primary goal of inpatient treatment for AN. Expectations of regular weight gain in addition to all the strategies listed except (c) are used to help normalize weight. Malnutrition can cause anxiety and depressive symptoms and impair concentration. Thus it is important to focus on weight restoration first, which can be followed by additional therapy addressing disordered thoughts and behaviors and underlying issues; this can often be done at a lower level of care such as day treatment or outpatient. *(Ref. 5, Ch. 22, Treatment section)*

36 **(d)** Hypokalemia is a sign of refeeding syndrome. Refeeding syndrome is a rare but potentially fatal complication of rapidly increasing food intake in malnourished patients characterized by shifts in fluids and electrolytes. *(Ref. 5, Ch. 22, Treatment section)*

37 **(c)** Low-dose use of olanzapine in patients with AN has been studied via several open-label trials and there are some case reports as well that indicate benefits of decreasing anxiety around eating, decreasing rumination about food and body concerns, and improving sleeping, although sedation is a common side effect. *(Ref. 1, Ch. 19, Pharmacotherapy section)*

38 **(e)** Three phases of family-based treatment of AN include: restoration of patient's weight; handing control over eating back to the patient; and discussion of the patient's developmental issues. *(Ref. 1, Ch. 19, Psychotherapy section)*

Case 4

39 **(d)** It is inappropriate to consider discharging the client without an appropriate risk assessment that should involve a comprehensive evaluation, which includes interviewing the adolescent patient and the parent(s) to identify the presence of environmental and family risk factors, current and past suicidal behaviors, intent, methodology, and accessibility to lethal means (such as knives, guns, etc.). Possible patient and parental underlying psychopathologies, substance involvement, cognitive distortions, inadequate coping strategies, and mood/anxiety/possible psychotic symptoms also should be assessed. The most important aspect of the risk assessment is to determine the degree of immediate danger and whether there is a need for psychiatric hospitalization. *(Ref. 3, Ch. 6.3.1, Comprehensive Assessment of Youth in Psychiatric Crisis section)*

40 **(e)** All of the listed factors indicate a lower suicide risk for youth who engage in suicidal behaviors. Other factors include having good judgment and capacity to communicate honestly and openly about their emotions, feelings, worries, etc. A consistent and stable environment, low degree of violence, absence of family psychopathology, and availability of the family to provide sufficient support are positive social factors that may decrease youth suicide risk. *(Ref. 3, Ch. 6.3.1, Comprehensive Assessment of Youth in Psychiatric Crisis section)*

41 **(a)** All physicians are mandatory reporters in all states. Failure to make an appropriate report for suspected child abuse or neglect can be a basis for malpractice. Filing a formal report with appropriate authorities immediately is the most appropriate thing to do next. Because Dr. Smith already has a strong suspicion of child sexual abuse, it is not appropriate to rely on the ER social worker or another staff member to decide whether a formal report is necessary. It will be up to the authorities to determine whether she is safe to go back to her parents upon discharge. *(Ref. 1, Ch. 24, Child and Parent Treatment section)*

42 **(c)** Borderline personality disorder is characterized by a pervasive pattern of instability of interpersonal relationships, self-image, poor impulse control, and poor affect regulation. *(Ref. 4, p. 663)*

43 **(c)** Follow-up studies show that about half of the patients no longer meet full criteria for borderline personality disorder ten years after they were identified through an outpatient mental health clinic. *(Ref. 4, p. 665)*

44 **(d)** Studies did not indicate a higher occurrence of schizophrenia spectrum disorder in the first-degree relatives of patients with BPD. *(Ref. 3, Ch. 5.13, Etiology section)*

45 **(a)** Decreased serotonergic neurotransmission in cortical inhibitory areas is found in patients with BPD. *(Ref. 3, Ch. 5.13, Diagnosis and Clinical Features section)*

46 **(c)** Mentalization-based treatment (MBT) was developed by Bateman and Fonagy. Similar to DBT, it can decrease

hospitalization, medication use, and suicidal ideation and suicidal behaviors. In addition, it can also help reduce anxiety and depression and improve social and interpersonal relationships, aspects where DBT has not been shown to be effective. *(Ref. 3, Ch. 5.13, Treatment section)*

47 **(a)** Bupropion can induce seizures, especially in patients with chronic alcohol abuse and bulimia. Sophia had a history of consuming large amounts of alcohol and engaged in binge-eating/purging episodes, which increases the risk of seizure, especially if she takes bupropion. *(Ref. 1, Ch. 35, Atypical Antidepressants section)*

48 **(c)** Escitalopram is an FDA-approved medication for treating adolescents (ages 12–17) with MDD. The other FDA-approved medication is fluoxetine (ages 8–18). *(Ref. 1, Ch. 35, Selective Serotonin Reuptake Inhibitors section)*

49 **(b)** Bipolar II disorder requires at least one past or current hypomanic episode and at least one past or current major depressive episode, and episodes cannot be attributable to the physiological effects of a substance of abuse, a medication, or other treatment. Intoxication or withdrawal from a substance of abuse or use of a medication has to be within one month preceding the episode to meet criteria for substance/mediation-induced bipolar and related disorder. Bipolar I disorder requires at least one manic episode regardless of whether a major depressive episode has ever been present. A new diagnosis appeared in DSM-5, disruptive mood dysregulation disorder, which is categorized under depressive disorders, but not under bipolar and related disorders. *(Ref. 4, pp. 132–133)*

50 **(a)** Monotherapy with antidepressant for bipolar depression can increase risk of switching. Thus, among the listed medications, fluoxetine is the most appropriate one to avoid. *(Ref. 1, Ch. 14, Treatment section)*

51 **(d)** Tests for HLA-B*1502 should be completed prior to starting carbamazepine for any patients of Chinese ancestry because HLA-B*1502 is associated with the risk of developing Stevens-Johnson syndrome and toxic epidermal necrolysis (TEN). A positive test is considered a contraindication for carbamazepine. *(Ref. 1, Ch. 36, Carbamazepine section)*

52 **(a)** Carbamazepine decreases lithium clearance, increasing the risk of lithium toxicity. Carbamazepine can decrease serum levels of many medications, including atypical antipsychotics, lamotrigine, valproate, and oral contraceptives *(Ref. 1, Ch. 36, Carbamazepine section)*

Case 5

53 **(a)** He has single motor tics that have a waxing and waning pattern for more than one year since the first tic onset. Tourette's disorder must have both multiple motor and one or more vocal tics to be present together at some time during the illness. Provisional tic disorder refers to a single or multiple motor and/or vocal tics that have been present for less than one year since first tic onset. Diagnosis of transient tic disorder was eliminated from DSM-5. *(Ref. 4, p. 81)*

54 **(c)** Tommy's tics are considered as simple motor tics even though he has both eye blinking and shoulder shrugging because they do not occur simultaneously. If occurring simultaneously, they would be considered as complex motor tics. *(Ref. 4, p. 82)*

55 **(e)** Palilalia refers to vocal tics that involve repeating one's own sounds or words. Coprolalia refers to vocal tics that involve uttering socially unacceptable words (e.g., cuss words and/or racial/religious slurs, etc.). Copropraxia refers to motor tics that involve seemingly purposeful sexual or obscene gestures. Echolalia refers to repeating the last-heard words or phrases (not one's own), whereas echopraxia refers to mimicking someone else's movements. *(Ref. 4, p. 82)*

56 **(d)** Tourette's disorder is the most appropriate diagnosis for Tommy at this time because he presented with both motor and vocal tics, and tics have been present for over one year. *(Ref. 4, p. 81)*

57 **(c)** ADHD is the most common coexisting condition with Tourette's disorder, with estimates of upwards of 50% of children with Tourette's disorder having comorbid ADHD *(Ref. 3, Ch. 5.6, Coexisting Conditions section)*

58 **(c)** Approximately 10–15% of the offspring of a patient with Tourette's disorder will also develop Tourette's disorder; 20–29% will develop a tic disorder; and 12–32% will develop OCD. *(Ref. 3, Ch. 5.6, Etiology section)*

59 **(c)** Providing accurate information to patients and parents via psychoeducational activities is the most important aspect of interventions for Tourette's disorder, especially during the initial phase. This helps ensure that patients and parents comprehend the problems, reduce fears, decrease blaming, and enhance cohesiveness in the family. *(Ref. 3, Ch. 5.6, Treatment section)*

60 **(e)** Habit reversal training (HRT) is a behavioral intervention that has shown significant effectiveness in reducing tic symptoms in adults with Tourette's disorder. It also shows similar results in children through unblended studies. Thus, more rigorous studies in youth are needed. All of the listed are the four components of awareness training of HRT. *(Ref. 3, Ch. 5.6, Treatment section)*

61 **(a)** Peak severity usually occurs in pre-pubertal ages (between 10 and 12 years), and the severity tends to decline during adolescence, with a further reduction in adulthood (with occasional exceptions). Premonitory urge refers to a somatic sensation that precedes the tic, which seems more likely to be associated with tics experienced by children when they get older. *(Ref. 4, p. 83)*

62 **(b)** Stimulant medications, including methylphenidate and amphetamine salts, have the highest efficacy of pharmacotherapy options for ADHD symptoms and are not contraindicated in tic disorders despite some controversy around this, with recent studies showing no association between stimulants and increased tics. Alpha-2 agonists, including clonidine and guanfacine, are often used as first-line pharmacotherapy for tic disorders given their relatively favorable side-effect profile, and can also help ADHD symptoms. The choice of treatment should take into consideration individual factors such as the relative severity of each disorder, treatment priorities, side-effect profiles, and willingness or reticence to use multiple medications if needed. *(Ref. 1, Ch. 34, Stimulants section)*

63 (a) Haloperidol, pimozide (Orap), and aripiprazole are approved by the FDA for the treatment of Tourette's disorder in youth. Clinical trials using risperidone, ziprasidone, and olanzapine treating youth with Tourette's have shown some promising data. However, none of them is FDA approved. *(Ref. 1, Ch. 20, Treatment section)*

64 (a) Antipsychotics (either conventional or atypical) can be potentially considered as augmenting agents to SSRIs to reduce commonly difficult-to-treat or refractory OCD symptoms in patients with Tourette's disorder. *(Ref. 3, Ch. 5.6, Treatment section)*

65 (a) Used in patients with other movement disorders, DBS is a relatively reversible, stereotactic technique that can be considered as an alternative to the neurosurgical interventions for intractable and severe tics. However, its usage is still limited to adult patients because youth with tics are likely to get better as they get older. *(Ref. 3, Ch. 5.6, Treatment section)*

Case 6

66 (e) Given limited background or other specific information, the differential diagnoses should be broad. The hallucinations and delusions could also be related to underlying medical conditions and influences from medications or substances. *(Ref. 4, pp. 50–57, 99–105, 161–168, 222–226, 271–280)*

67 (a) April's presentation of core psychotic symptoms occurred within one month. Thus, brief psychotic disorder is the most appropriate diagnosis at this time among all the given options. Delusion disorder requires the presence of one or more delusions for more than one month, and hallucinations, if present, cannot be prominent and should be related to delusional themes. *(Ref. 4, pp. 90–94)*

68 (c) The core symptoms presented are still within the time frame of between one month and six months. Thus, the most appropriate diagnosis at this time is schizophreniform disorder out of all the listed options. *(Ref. 4, pp. 96–97)*

69 (e) Given the updated information, April continued to experience residual psychotic symptoms that are most consistent with schizophrenia. Because of her age, the disorder should be considered as childhood-onset schizophrenia. *(Ref. 3, Ch. 5.3, Background section; Ref. 4, pp. 99–105)*

70 (c) Performance on tasks involving rote language skills and simple perceptual processing is not generally impaired in patients with COS. However, other listed impairments can be seen in COS probands. *(Ref. 3, Ch. 5.3, Phenomenology and Neurobiology of COS section)*

71 (e) Gray matter (GM) loss has been found in adolescents with COS, with a pattern of back to front tissue loss over time during adolescence, which may reflect an exaggeration of normal maturational pruning during a critical period. Over time, the GM loss seems to eventually resemble a pattern similar to that observed in adults with schizophrenia. The GM loss does not seem to be the result of medications, and appears to be a diagnostically specific trait marker. *(Ref. 3, Ch. 5.3, Brain Imaging: Structural, Functional, and Positron Emission Tomography section)*

72 (c) A deletion on 22q11 can lead to velocardio-facial syndrome (VCFS), which can be manifested as psychiatric conditions including psychosis. An increased number of CGG repeats (usually 200 to 1,000) on the FMR-1 gene leads to the phenotype of Fragile X syndrome. Specific deletions of chromosome 15 (15q11-q13) can cause either Prader-Willi syndrome (PWS) or Angelman syndrome. As a contiguous gene syndrome, Williams syndrome is caused by a deletion on chromosome 7. MeCP2 mutations have been found in more than 80% of patients with Rett syndrome. *(Ref. 3, Ch. 5.3, Genetic Studies section)*

73 (d) While other tests may be relevant for individuals who are taking antipsychotics, the prolactin level can confirm prolactinemia, which can explain the side effects that April is experiencing. *(Ref. 1, Ch. 37, Adverse Effects section)*

74 (b) The D_2 blockade of antipsychotics is not only responsible for the antipsychotic efficacy but also responsible for a series of side effects, such as elevated prolactin level, EPS/akathisia, and sexual reproductive system dysfunction. *(Ref. 1, Ch. 37, Pharmacology section)*

75 (a) Being a partial agonist at D_2 receptors, aripiprazole is the best alternative that is least likely to cause prolactinemia. *(Ref. 1, Ch. 37, Adverse Effects section)*

76 (d) Because she is experiencing major depressive symptoms during the majority of the time with her overall active illness, along with hallucinations for more than two weeks in the absence of a major mood episode, April's current diagnosis should be schizoaffective disorder. *(Ref. 4, pp. 105–109)*

77 (b) The lifetime risk of suicide with schizoaffective disorder and schizophrenia is approximately 5%, with a higher risk in North American than in European, South American, and Indian populations. Suicide risk is also associated with the presence of depression. *(Ref. 4, p. 109)*

78 (b) The incidence of SAD is higher in females than in males, which can be due to an increased incidence of the depressive type among females. *(Ref. 4, pp. 107–109)*

79 (e) Waist circumference > 35 inches/88 cm is one of the metabolic syndrome criteria for adult females (for adult males > 40 inches/102 cm). In children and adolescents this criterion is replaced by the waist circumference ≥ 90th percentile, or BMI ≥ 95th percentile for sex and age. All listed other criteria are used for determination of metabolic syndrome in children and adolescents. *(Ref. 1, Ch. 37, Adverse Effect Assessment and Monitoring section)*

80 (c) Three out of five criteria (see question 79) are required to diagnose metabolic syndrome in children and adolescents. *(Ref. 1, Ch. 37, Adverse Effect Assessment and Monitoring section)*

Case 7

81 (e) The case description does not provide enough specific information to exclude any of the listed conditions as a potential differential diagnosis, which should be broad at this time. *(Ref. 4, pp. 59, 156, 160, 462)*

82 (c) Irritability is included in the diagnostic criteria of all the listed diagnoses except ADHD. *(Ref. 4, pp. 59, 132, 160, 222, 462)*

83 (b) The diagnostic criteria for DMDD include having one year or more of severe outbursts occurring three times or more per week with persistently irritable mood between outbursts. These symptoms must be present in at least two settings. The child must never have had a manic or hypomanic episode. Often making careless mistakes is one of the symptoms of ADHD and is not a criterion for DMDD. However, ADHD and DMDD are highly comorbid so patients with DMDD should also be screened for ADHD. *(Ref. 4, p. 156)*

84 **(d)** Rates of comorbidity are very high and most children with DMDD also have other psychiatric disorders such as ADHD, anxiety disorders, and depression. Symptoms of ODD are common in children with DMDD; however, per DSM-5 criteria, if a child meets criteria for both ODD and DMDD, only the diagnosis of DMDD should be given. If the symptoms occur only in the context of a major depressive episode or anxiety-provoking context, DMDD shouldn't be diagnosed. *(Ref. 4, p. 160)*

85 **(a)** Both DMDD and IED entail recurrent outbursts that can be physically aggressive and can impair interpersonal functioning. The presence of persistent irritability between outbursts is a criteria for DMDD, but not IED. DMDD and IED cannot coexist; if criteria are met for both, only a diagnosis of DMDD should be made. Either can be comorbid with ADHD. *(Ref. 4, p. 160)*

86 **(e)** As a relatively new diagnosis, DMDD has limited evidence-based treatment and no FDA-approved treatments. Currently, treatment focuses on targeting symptoms. Since most children with DMDD have comorbid psychiatric disorders, treatment often starts with treatment of these comorbidities such as ADHD, MDD, and anxiety disorders that have more evidence-based treatments. Treatment for DMDD is an active area of research. *(Ref. 6, Ch. 2.11, Treatment section)*

87 **(c)** In order to meet criteria for a manic or hypomanic episode, the change in mood must be present most of the day, nearly every day, and last at least one week for a manic episode or four days for a hypomanic episode. The mood change can be elevated, expansive, or irritable. Bipolar disorder can coexist with ADHD or ODD. Although the typical age of onset is older than Ryan, there is no minimum age to make the diagnosis of bipolar I or bipolar II disorder. *(Ref. 4, p. 123-136)*

88 **(d)** For a diagnosis of oppositional defiant disorder, at least four symptoms must be present across symptom categories (angry/irritable mood, argumentative/defiant behavior, and vindictiveness), but not all categories need to be represented. Symptoms must be present for at least six months and must be present on most days for children younger than five years or weekly for children five years or older (with the exception of vindictiveness, which must be present at least twice within the past six months for children of any age). Symptoms must be present with at least one individual who is not a sibling. The number of settings where the symptoms are present determines the severity level. *(Ref. 4, pp. 462–463)*

89 **(a)** Treatment of comorbid ADHD with stimulants, alpha-2 agonists, and atomoxetine has been shown to lead to reduction in oppositional symptoms. There is no FDA-approved or well-evidenced pharmacological treatment for the core features of DMDD or ASD (and diagnoses of DMDD and ODD cannot be made simultaneously). *(Ref. 1, Ch. 11, Oppositional Defiant Disorder section)*

90 **(b)** For a diagnosis of conduct disorder, at least three criteria must be present in the past 12 months and at least one in the past six months across four categories (aggression to people and animals, destruction of property, deceitfulness or theft, and serious violations of rules), but not all categories need to be represented. Limited prosocial emotions is a specifier, but not a criterion that must be met. There is no age limit by when criteria must have been met. If the individual is over age 18, criteria must not be met for antisocial personality disorder (ASPD), but ASPD is not diagnosed before age 18 *(Ref. 4, pp. 469–471)*

91 **(d)** There are no medications approved by the FDA for aggression in conduct disorder, but there is evidence for several classes of medications for treating aggression, including atypical antipsychotics, mood stabilizers, and alpha-2 agonists. Atypical antipsychotics have a significant side-effect profile, but the risks must be weighed against the potential benefits in deciding whether to prescribe them. Treating the ADHD can reduce aggressive behavior in a patient with comorbid ADHD and conduct disorder. Treating ADHD with a stimulant medication does not increase, and may in fact lower, the risk of substance abuse. *(Ref. 1, Ch. 28, Treatment section)*

92 **(e)** Juvenile awareness programs, also called deterrence programs, such as "Scared Straight," have been found to be ineffective and to lead to increased delinquent behaviors. Individual therapy for an adolescent with a disruptive behavior disorder may not be as effective as interventions involving the family, but individual interventions such as cognitive-behavioral therapy do have evidence to support their role in the treatment of conduct problems. A number of parent- and family-based interventions have evidence of effectiveness. There are a number of pharmacologic options with varying levels of evidence for aggressive behavior. *(Ref. 1, Ch. 11, Conduct Disorder section).*

References

Johnson, C. P. & Myers, S. M. (2007). Identification and Evaluation of Children with Autism Spectrum Disorders. *Pediatrics*, *120*, 1183–1215.

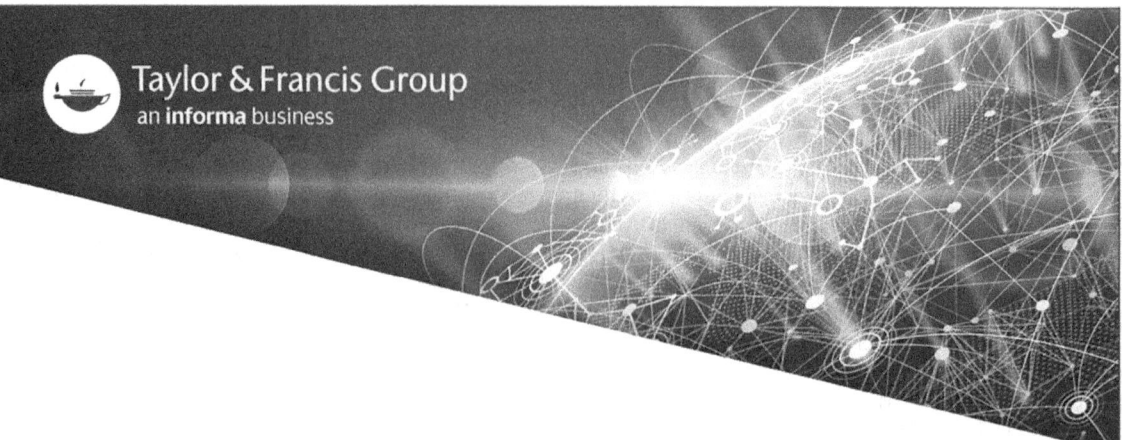
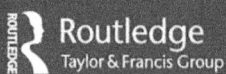
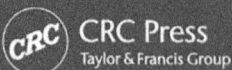